Cognitive-Communication Disorders of MCI and Dementia

Definition, Assessment, and Clinical Management

Third Edition

Cognitive-Communication Disorders of MCI and Dementia

Definition, Assessment, and Clinical Management

Third Edition

Kathryn Bayles, PhD, CCC-SLP
Kimberly McCullough, PhD, CCC-SLP
Cheryl Tomoeda, MS, CCC-SLP

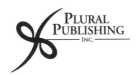

PLURAL PUBLISHING INC.

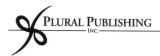

5521 Ruffin Road
San Diego, CA 92123

e-mail: information@pluralpublishing.com
Web site: http://www.pluralpublishing.com

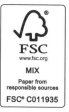

Typeset in 10/12 Palatino by Achorn International
Printed in the United States of America by McNaughton & Gunn, Inc.

Library of Congress Cataloging-in-Publication Data:

Names: Bayles, Kathryn A., 1942- author. | McCullough, Kimberly (Speech-language pathologist), author. | Tomoeda, Cheryl K., author.
Title: Cognitive-communication disorders of MCI and dementia : definition, assessment, and clinical management / Kathryn Bayles, Kimberly McCullough, Cheryl Tomoeda.
Other titles: Cognitive-communication disorders of dementia
Description: Third edition. | San Diego, CA : Plural Publishing, [2020] | Preceded by Cognitive-communication disorders of dementia / Kathryn A. Bayles and Cheryl K. Tomoeda. Second edition. 2014. | Includes bibliographical references and index.
Identifiers: LCCN 2018028636| ISBN 9781635500608 (alk. paper) | ISBN 1635500605 (alk. paper)
Subjects: | MESH: Cognitive Dysfunction—diagnosis | Dementia—diagnosis | Communication Disorders—etiology | Dementia—complications |Communication Disorders—diagnosis | Communication Disorders—therapy
Classification: LCC RC521 | NLM WM 220 | DDC 616.8/3—dc23
LC record available at https://lccn.loc.gov/2018028636

Contents

**Clinical Management Guide: Assessments and Interventions
for Cognitive-Communication Disorders of Dementia**

Preface

Since publication of the second edition of *Cognitive-Communication Disorders of Dementia*, a tsunami of dementia research has been published. More than ever, the focus is MCI, or mild cognitive impairment, typically a harbinger of a dementia producing disease. Historically, however, the term MCI was primarily associated with Alzheimer's disease, though scientists and clinicians recognized that all dementing diseases create subtle early cognitive impairments. This problem was remedied with the publication of the fifth edition of the *Diagnostic and Statistical Manual of Mental Disorders* (2013). The American Psychiatric Association introduced the term "minor neurocognitive disorder" to refer to mild cognitive impairments that are insufficient to be considered frank dementia, and they characterized dementia as a "major neurocognitive disorder." Nonetheless, clinicians and researchers still use the term MCI but with the understanding that it is associated with myriad diseases, and not just Alzheimer's.

Global interest in early identification of individuals with MCI is intense because drug and cognitive stimulation therapies, as well as lifestyle changes, show promise for delaying or preventing development of dementia. *Highly relevant to speech-language pathologists is the well-documented finding that language performance problems are among the earliest signs of MCI.* Moreover, the new recommendations for diagnosing MCI, also known as a "minor neurocognitive disorder," include the evaluation of language. As experts in language and commu-nication science, speech-language pathologists are uniquely qualified to evaluate and treat the cognitive-based communication disorders of MCI and dementia. Thus, in this new edition, greater emphasis is given to the characteristics of MCI, its assessment, and clinical interventions.

The third edition opens with an overview of cognition and communication and why individuals with dementia have serious cognitive-communication disorders. This is followed by a rationale for building cognitive reserve in those with MCI and therapy for individuals with dementia. Chapter 2 provides an overview of cognition, memory, and communication, and how they are interrelated. Thereafter, clinicians and students in training will find up-to-date information about the characteristics of all major dementia-producing diseases and Down syndrome.

The last segment of the book is composed of the new Clinical Guide and is extensive. It begins with a discussion of the process of assessment and a review of reputable tests. Subsequent topics include:

- Cognitive stimulation programming for MCI
- Clinical techniques supported by the principles of neuroplasticity
- Indirect interventions that facilitate communication, quality of life and the safety of individuals with dementia, and caregiver counseling
- Care planning, goal setting, reimbursement, and required documentation

Acknowledgments

Our greatest debt is owed to the many people with dementia and their family members who shared their experiences and generously gave their time to participate in research. They are our heroes. We are also indebted to the teachers, colleagues, and students who shaped our views and supported our endeavors. Since publication of the first edition of *Cognitive-Communication Disorders of Dementia*, voluminous research has been published on dementia-associated diseases, their diagnosis, and treatment. For their cheerful help in locating and organizing the publications relevant to the mission of this book and their care in performing myriad assignments, we thank Maddie Elliot, Kayla Elmore, and Abby Peterson.

1

Speech-Language Pathology, Mild Cognitive Impairment, and Dementia

Introduction

Individuals with mild cognitive impairment (MCI) and dementia are the fastest-growing clinical population, nationally and globally. In fact, every 65 s someone in the United States develops Alzheimer's disease (AD), the leading cause of dementia (Alzheimer's Association, 2018; Ferri, Prince, Brayne, Brodaty, & Fratiglioni, 2005). Currently, 47 million individuals worldwide are believed to be living with dementia; however, by the year 2050, approximately 131.5 million people will have AD or another form of dementia (Alzheimer's Disease International, 2016). More than five million Americans live with AD, and that number may rise to 16 million by 2050. Characterized another way, one in 10 Americans 65 years or older has AD, two-thirds of whom are women. Individuals with dementia need care and an estimated 15 million Americans provide unpaid care. The cost of care in 2018 may exceed $277 billion and a trillion dollars by 2050 (Alzheimer's Association, 2018).

Dementia-associated diseases, such as AD, can begin decades before they are clinically obvious and, once diagnosed, endure for many more years. Most patients are cared for at home by family, typically with serious financial, social, and emotional consequences

for all involved. Those patients and families who have the support of professionals have a higher quality of life (Gaugler, Roth, Haley, & Mittelman, 2008; Mittelman, Roth, Coon, & Haley, 2004) and speech-language pathologists (SLPs) are among the professionals who have an important role in the management of affected individuals. Language performance deficits occur early and worsen as the disease progresses. As experts in language and communication science and the evaluation and treatment of communication disorders, SLPs are uniquely qualified to diagnose and treat the cognitive-communication disorders associated with dementia-producing diseases. Additionally, SLPs provide counseling to professional and personal caregivers about how to best communicate with affected individuals.

The goal of this book is to provide practicing professionals and graduate students the knowledge needed to evaluate and treat individuals who have mild cognitive impairment (MCI), AD, or another type of dementia, as well as counsel professional and personal caregivers. Toward that end, the first order of business is answering the question, why do individuals with dementia have a communication disorder. To answer that question, we need to first define communication.

Communication Defined

Communication is the sharing of information by means of a symbol system. We call communication linguistic when words are used and nonlinguistic when other symbol systems are used, such as mathematical notation. To communicate, either linguistically or nonlinguistically, an individual must have an idea to share and a symbol system through which to express the idea. For example, symphony conductors communicate their ideas about tempo and loudness to orchestra members by moving a baton in prescribed ways. Football coaches communicate plays to players by hand signals. These are examples of nonlinguistic communication, and although nonlinguistic communication can be impaired as a consequence of a dementing disease, the focus of the SLP is impairment in linguistic communication. *Nonetheless, both nonlinguistic and linguistic communications are impaired in AD because both are cognitive processes for sharing and interpreting information and information processing is progressively disrupted.* Another distinction critical to characterizing the effects of dementia on communicative function is the difference between "speech" and "language." For our purposes, the term "speech" refers to the motor production of sounds, and the term "language" refers to the symbol system by which sound is paired with meaning for a particular purpose. As previously noted, "linguistic communication" is the cognitive process of intentionally sharing ideas through language and in *dementia it is the ability to communicate that is typically most affected.*

"Meaningful" communication requires the production and comprehension of ideas. The act of speaking, in and of itself, does not constitute communication because that which is spoken may be structurally and semantically meaningless. Similarly, knowing the grammar of a language does not ensure the ability to communicate. Communication only occurs when words are structured in such a way that the listener comprehends the speaker's idea. Having made this distinction, the question of why communication is affected in dementia can be answered. Communication is affected because the pathophysiologic processes that disrupt multiple cognitive functions and produce dementia also disrupt information processing.

Clients with dementia are said to have a "cognitive-communication" problem because progressive deterioration of cognition interferes with communication. The fact is, *the production and comprehension of language cannot be separated from cognition.* Consider just the simple act of naming an object; for example, a parsnip. First, you must perceive the features of the parsnip. They must be matched to those in long-term memory for recognition to occur. Thereafter, you must form an intention to say the object's name. The linguistic representations of objects are part of long-term lexical memory and must be retrieved and brought to consciousness. Perhaps you are uncertain about how a parsnip looks and therefore are unsure whether you are perceiving a turnip, parsnip, or rutabaga. If so, you have to decide whether to indicate your uncertainty. To articulate uncertainty about the object's name or identity, a motor plan must be formed. Thus, the simple act of object naming requires perception, access to long-term memory, association, recognition, lexical retrieval, decision making, motor planning, and self-monitoring.

Persons with dementia have difficulty *producing* linguistic information because the information-processing capabilities of declarative and working memory systems are compromised, as is the case in AD (Hornberger, Bell, Graham, & Rogers, 2009; Rogers & Friedman, 2008), and in part because of progressive degradation of knowledge (Landin-Romero, Tan, Hodges & Kumfor, 2016), as is the case in semantic dementia. They have difficulty *comprehending* language because of deficits in the cognitive processes of perception, recognition, attention, and memory, as well as degradation of knowledge (Macdonald, Almor, Henderson, Kempler, & Andersen, 2001).

Rationale for Therapy

In the not too distant past, clinicians thought little could be done to improve the functioning of individuals diagnosed with dementia. Early identification of those affected was not the priority it is today; however, as the number of dementia patients skyrocketed, interest in early detection and intervention also skyrocketed. Worldwide, researchers in neuroscience, as well as the behavioral and cognitive sciences, have focused on understanding dementia-associated diseases and their management. Research has revealed that individuals with AD experience subtle cognitive deficits years before the disease impairs their ability to live independently. When these individuals are identified, much can be done to prevent evolution to frank dementia or slow the course of the disease, among them pharmacologic interventions, lifestyle changes, and cognitive stimulation. Consider the following facts that comprise a rationale for intervention:

1. The human brain is plastic and many of the factors that advantage neuroplasticity are known.
2. Humans have multiple systems for learning and information representation that are not equally vulnerable to the pathology of the common dementia-producing diseases and spared systems can be strengthened to compensate for impairments.
3. Individuals with greater cognitive reserve exhibit dementia later than those with less.
4. Cognitive stimulation can produce learning and thus greater cognitive reserve in individuals with MCI.

In sum, SLPs now have evidence-based techniques that stimulate neuroplasticity and the building of cognitive reserve in individuals with MCI to delay conversion to dementia. Furthermore, they have evidence-based techniques for maximizing the functioning of those with clinically apparent dementia.

Neuroplasticity

Neuroplasticity is the lifelong ability of the brain to reorganize as a result of experience (Kleim &

Jones, 2008; Nudo & Bury, 2011). Learning is the byproduct of neuroplasticity. Intuitively, we know this to be true because we add to and refine our knowledge throughout life. Said another way, *neuroplasticity is experience-dependent and behavioral training is key to promoting brain reorganization after brain damage* (Raskin, 2011). Table 1–1 contains a list of empirically demonstrated factors that can be clinically manipulated to support neuroplasticity (Kleim & Jones, 2008; Kolb & Gibb, 2008; Shaffer, 2016). Not listed are hormones and drugs that also affect the capacity for recovery, but are not the province of SLPs.

Of particular significance to clinicians is the fact that the *type* of experience matters (the specificity principle). Learning can be negative or positive. An example of negative learning is the learned nonuse of a paretic limb. An example of positive learning is improvement in a language skill through language therapy.

To trigger neuroplasticity, sufficient stimulation is needed and the *type* of stimulation influences the way in which the brain reorganizes. For example, the presentation of an intensive program to incrementally challenge the auditory processing system can create structural changes in the network of cells that support auditory processing. Visual stimuli influence cell networks that support visual processing. A clinician who knows a client's profile of processing deficits and strengths can design a personalized stimulation program to influence brain response in a positive way. In the case of individuals with a neurodegenerative disease, such as Parkinson's disease or AD, the goal is to strengthen residual knowledge and skills, and if possible, build additional cognitive reserve.

Memory Systems and Their Selective Vulnerability to Disease

In Chapter 2, the various memory systems with their putative neuroanatomical substrates are described. Of significance to clinicians is how the neuropathology of the different dementia-associated diseases affects each disease. For example, as previously noted, the various memory

Table 1–1. Principles of Neuroplasticity

PRINCIPLE	DEFINITION
Attention	Learning requires attention. Attention is a function of stimulus relevance to the individual.
Specificity	Nature of stimulation dictates the nature of brain reorganization. For example, language stimulation produces changes in neuronal networks supporting language.
Use or Lose	Lack of use of knowledge or skills causes both to degrade.
Use and Improve	Use of knowledge and skills strengthens both.
Stimulation	Sensory and/or motor stimulation of sufficient intensity produce changes in brain.
Simultaneity	Concepts, words, actions that occur together become linked in nervous system.
Novelty/Challenge	New, enriching experience stimulates neurogenesis and increases gray matter volume and health of white matter.
Positive Emotion	Enhances mental performance.
Reward	Increases attention and frequency of desired behavior and creates positive emotion.
Constrain	Forced use stimulates the brain to reorganize.
Repetition	Repeated stimulation is essential for creation of long-term memory and skill building.
Intensity	Intense experience is needed for significant brain change.
Duration	The stimulation/experience must be of sufficient duration to create lasting change.
Interference	Brain reorganization in response to one experience can interfere with learning of a similar behavior.
Transference	Brain reorganization in response to one experience can enhance learning of a similar behavior.
Sleep	Regular sleep of 7–8 hours is necessary for consolidation of new information and skills.
Diet	High antioxidant, low fat, low sugar diet nourishes brain cells and reduces damaging free radicals.
Exercise	Exercise increases blood flow to the brain, increases gray matter volume, and energizes motor responses to improve speed of reaction.
Age	Plasticity is greater in childhood.
Time	Different forms of plasticity occur at different times.

Sources: Kleim & Jones (2008); Kolb & Gibb (2008); Shaffer (2016).

systems are not equally vulnerable to the effects of AD, especially early in the disease course. The neural structures that support working and declarative memory, particularly episodic memory, are affected early, whereas those supporting conditioning, motor procedural, and habit memory are relatively spared until advanced dementia (de Vreese, Neri, Fioravanti, Belloi, & Zanetti, 2001; Salmon, Heindel, & Butters, 1992). In Parkinson's disease, the neural structures supporting nondeclarative and

working memory are more vulnerable early, whereas those supporting declarative memory are relatively spared. *Clinicians can use early spared systems to help individuals compensate for disease effects and inform caregivers about how to reduce demands on impaired systems.*

The discovery of the differential vulnerability of the brain's representation systems to AD motivated investigations of the potential of procedural learning treatments and conditioning for improving function and quality of life for AD patients. A considerable literature now exists documenting improved skill learning in AD patients through programs that capitalized on spared procedural memory systems and conditioning (de Werd, Boelen, Rikkert, & Kessels, 2013; Deweer et al., 1994; Deweer, Pillon, Michon, & Dubois, 1993; Dick, Hsieh, Bricker, & Dick-Muehlke, 2003; Dick et al., 1996; Grober, Ausubel, Sliwinski, & Gordon, 1992; Keane, Gabrieli, Fennema, Growdon, & Corkin, 1991; van Halteren-van Tilborg, Scherder, Hulstijn, 2007; Verfaellie, Keane, & Johnson, 2000). For individuals with MCI, who have not evolved to dementia, strengthening their knowledge and skills (cognitive reserve) is the primary goal. Their ability to learn new factual information will be greatly influenced by the degree of their episodic memory impairment. Early on, when episodic memory is minimally affected, new fact learning is easier. As the disease progresses, more emphasis can be placed on using the spared nondeclarative memory/learning systems than on the more impaired declarative systems. Regardless of stage, however, consistent use of retained skills and knowledge helps maintain them.

Cognitive Reserve

The term *"cognitive reserve" refers to the mind's ability to cope with brain damage.* One cannot assume that people with similar amounts of brain damage, by virtue of disease or injury, have similar cognitive abilities. This fact is apparent in individuals with AD. Research has shown that some individuals with extensive brain pathology display few, if any, cognitive deficits in life (Katzman et al., 1988). In fact, approximately 25% of individuals with AD pathology whose brains undergo postmortem examination were symptom free in life (Ince, 2001). Why the discrepancy?

Scientists theorize that some individuals may have had more neurons to begin with; others suggest that some internal or external mechanism prevents the extensive neuronal loss typical of the disease. Yet, others suggest that a richer network of interneuronal connections, as a result of education and life experiences, have had a neuroprotective effect. All of these theories are true.

Katzman and colleagues (1988) found an association between brain size and degree of AD symptomatology. Patients who had few symptoms and extensive pathology had higher brain weights and more neurons. More recently, Perneczky et al. (2012) reported that clinical and epidemiologic studies suggest that AD patients who have larger head sizes have better cognitive performance than those with smaller head circumferences, even though the degree of neuropathology is the same.

One "external mechanism" known to influence susceptibility to the effects of AD is amount of education. Individuals with greater education have a reduced risk of developing AD (Anttila et al., 2002; Evans et al., 1993; Evans et al., 1997; Letenneur, Commenges, Dartigues, & Barberger-Gateau, 1994; Stern et al., 1994; White et al., 1994; Zhang et al., 1990). Furthermore, slower decline in cognitive function has been reported in people with more education (Albert et al., 1995; Butler, Ashford, & Snowdon, 1996; Chodosh, Reuben, Albert, & Seeman, 2002; Christensen et al., 1997; Colsher & Wallace, 1991; Farmer, Kittner, Rae, Bartko, & Regier, 1995; Lyketsos, Chen, & Anthony, 1999; Sando et al., 2008; Snowdon, Ostwald, & Kane, 1989). Similarly, people with more education and cognitively challenging careers have better cognitive reserves that reduce risk of dementia (Cheng, 2016; Katzman, 1993; Stern, 2002; Valenzuela & Sachdev, 2005).

Education provides cognitive stimulation and cognitive stimulation results in synaptogenesis and a richer network of interconnected neurons, or brain reserve. Cognitive reserve is related to brain reserve (physical characteristics of brain, e.g., more neurons). Brain reserve can be characterized in any number of ways including brain size, number of neurons, synapse count, and degree of dendritic branching.

Cognitive Stimulation Therapy Can Build Cognitive Reserve

The brain needs novelty, challenge, and training to maximize its potential for appropriate functional reorganization (Shaffer, 2016). Kleim and Jones (2008) acknowledge that a better understanding is needed of when and how much training should be given for optimal response. Then too, little is understood about how training interacts with aging, brain damage, and self-derived compensatory behaviors. Nonetheless, the fact remains that *novelty, challenge, and training are needed*.

The effects of stimulation on brain reserve are easier studied in animals and, indeed, an extensive literature attests to their positive effects. Animals placed in rich environments have greater neuron density, dendritic branching, increased brain weight, and cortical thickness than those placed in simple environments (Anderson, Eckburg & Relucio, 2002; Briones, Suh, Jozsa, & Woods, 2006; Jones, 2011). Hippocampal neurogenesis in the rat brain is stimulated by exercise (van Praag, Christie, Sejnowski, & Gage 1999; van Praag, Kempermann, & Gage 1999; van Praag, Shubert, Zhao, & Gage, 2005), learning (Gould, Beylin, Tanapat, Reeves, & Shors, 1999), and environmental enrichment (Kempermann, Kuhn, & Gage, 1997; Komitova, Mattsson, Johansson, & Eriksson, 2005). These same factors produce positive results in humans, though they are harder to measure (Vemuri et al., 2014). (For a review of the animal literature see Jones, 2011.)

Researchers worldwide are researching how best to sustain function in individuals with dementia-producing diseases. Later in the book is information on direct interventions like cognitive stimulation programming, transcranial magnetic stimulation (Boggio et al., 2011; Marra et al., 2015), and constraint therapy, as well as indirect interventions such as environmental modifications, use of technology, and caregiver education.

In conclusion, our responsibilities as clinicians are to: (a) assist in the diagnosis of MCI and dementia; (b) provide individuals with MCI the education and stimulation that will produce positive structural and chemical changes in the brain to delay, slow, or prevent the clinical manifestation of dementia; (c) provide those persons with dementia the direct and indirect interventions to maximize their function and quality of life; and (d) counsel personal and professional caregivers about how best to communicate with affected individuals to maximize their ability to function. This book contains chapters on MCI, the common dementia-producing diseases, assessment, and a special section on treatment.

Summary of Important Points

- Individuals with MCI and dementia are the profession's fastest-growing clinical population, nationally and globally.
- Communication disorders are an inherent part of the dementia syndrome because the production and comprehension of language cannot be separated from cognition and cognitive functions progressively deteriorate.
- The neuropathological processes that disrupt multiple cognitive functions sufficient to warrant the diagnosis of dementia disrupt information generation and processing.
- Neuroplasticity is the lifelong ability of the brain to reorganize as a result of experience.
- Neuroscientists have identified key factors that advantage neuroplasticity and learning: attention, novelty/challenge, stimulation, reward, use or lose, use and improve, specificity, simultaneity, repetition, intensity, sufficient duration, constraint or forced use, interference, transference, exercise, sleep, diet, time, and age.
- Neuroplasticity is informing clinical interventions to advantage rehabilitation.
- Dementia-producing diseases affect the various memory systems of the brain differently and each disease produces a typical profile of deficits and residual abilities.
- By understanding the brain systems that process information, their neural architecture, and the relation of communication to

cognition, clinicians can reasonably predict the types of cognitive-communication disorders associated with damage to different brain areas.

- Building cognitive reserve through new learning in individuals with MCI may delay conversion to frank dementia.
- Clinicians can use spared memory/learning systems to compensate for those impaired to create new learning, maintain function, and improve quality of life.

References

Albert, M. S., Jones, K., Savage, C. R., Berkman, L., Seeman, T., Blazer, D., & Rowe, J. W. (1995). Predictors of cognitive change in older persons: MacArthur studies of successful aging. *Psychology and Aging, 10,* 578–589.

Alzheimer's Association. (2018). Alzheimer's disease facts and figures. *Alzheimer's and Dementia, 14,* 367–429.

Alzheimer's Disease International. (2016). *World Alzheimer's Report 2016: Improving healthcare for people living with dementia.* London, UK: Author.

Anderson, B. J., Eckburg, P. B., & Relucio, K. I. (2002). Alterations in the thickness of motor cortical subregions after motor-skill learning and exercise. *Learning and Memory, 9,* 1–9.

Anttila, T., Helkala, E. L., Kivipelto, M., Hallikainen, M., Alhainen, K., Heinonen, H., . . . Nissinen, A. (2002). Midlife income, occupation, APOE status, and dementia: A population-based study. *Neurology, 59,* 887–893.

Boggio, P. S., Valasek, C. A., Campanha, C., Giglio, A. C., Baptistia, N. I., Lapenta, O. M., & Fregni, F. (2011). Non-invasive brain stimulation to assess and modulate neuroplasticity in Alzheimer's disease. *Neuropsychological Rehabilitation, 5,* 703–716.

Briones, T. L., Suh, E., Jozsa, L., & Woods, J. (2006). Behaviorally induced synaptogenesis and dendritic growth in the hippocampal region following transient global cerebral ischemia are accompanied by improvements in spatial learning. *Experimental Neurology, 198,* 530–538.

Butler, S. M., Ashford, J. W., & Snowdon, D. A. (1996). Age, education, and changes in the Mini-Mental State Exam scores of older women: Findings from the nun study. *Journal of the American Geriatrics Society, 44,* 675–681.

Cheng, S-T. (2016). Cognitive reserve and the prevention of dementia: The role of physical and cognitive activities. *Current Psychiatry Reports, 18,* 85.

Chodosh, J., Reuben, D. B., Albert, M. S., & Seeman, T. E. (2002). Predicting cognitive impairment in high-functioning community-dwelling older persons: MacArthur Studies of Successful Aging. *Journal of the American Geriatrics Society, 50,* 1051–1060.

Christensen, H., Korten, A. E., Jorm, A. F., Henderson, A. S., Jacomb, P. A., Rodgers, B., & Mackinnon, A. J. (1997). Education and decline in cognitive performance: Compensatory but not protective. *International Journal of Geriatric Psychiatry, 12,* 323–330.

Colsher, P. L., & Wallace, R. B. (1991). Longitudinal application of cognitive-function measures in a defined population of community-dwelling elders. *Annals of Epidemiology, 1,* 215–230.

de Vreese, L. P., Neri, M., Fioravanti, M., Belloi, L., & Zanetti, O. (2001). Memory rehabilitation in Alzheimer's disease. *International Journal of Geriatric Psychiatry, 16,* 794–809.

de Werd, M. M., Boelen, D., Rikkert, M., & Kessels, R. (2013). Errorless learning of everyday tasks in people with dementia. *Clinical Interventions in Aging, 8,* 1177–1190.

Deweer, B., Ergis, A. M., Fossati, P., Pillon, B., Boller, F., Agid, Y., & Dubois, B. (1994). Explicit memory, procedural learning and lexical priming in Alzheimer's disease. *Cortex, 30,* 113–126.

Deweer, B., Pillon, B., Michon, A., & Dubois, F. (1993). Mirror reading in Alzheimer's disease: Normal skill learning and acquisition of item specific information. *Journal of Clinical and Experimental Neuropsychology, 15,* 789–804.

Dick, M. B., Hsieh, S., Bricker, J., & Dick-Muehlke, C. (2003). Facilitating acquisition and transfer of a continuous motor task in healthy older adults and patients with Alzheimer's disease. *Brain and Cognition, 29,* 294–306.

Dick, M. B., Shankel, R. W., Beth, R. E., Dick-Muehlke, C., Cotman, C. W., & Kean, M. L. (1996). Acquisition and long-term retention of a fine motor skill in Alzheimer's disease. *Brain and Cognition, 29,* 294–306.

Evans, D. A., Beckett, L. A., Albert, M. S., Hebert, L. E., Scherr, P. A., Funkenstein, H. H., & Taylor, J. O. (1993). Level of education and change in cognitive function in a community population of older persons. *Annals of Epidemiology, 3,* 71–77.

Evans, D. A., Hebert, L. E., Beckett, L. A., Scherr, P. A., Albert, M. S., Chown, M. J., . . . Taylor, J. O. (1997). Education and other measures of socioeconomic status and risk of incident Alzheimer disease in a defined population of older persons. *Archives of Neurology, 54,* 1399–1405.

Farmer, M. E., Kittner, S. J., Rae, D. S., Bartko, J. J., & Regier, D. A. (1995). Education and change in cognitive function: The epidemiologic catchment Area Study. *Annals of Epidemiology, 5,* 1–7.

Ferri, C. P., Prince, M., Brayne, C., Brodaty, H., & Fratiglioni, L. (2005). Global prevalence of dementia: A Delphi consensus study. *Lancet, 366,* 2112–2117.

Gaugler, J. E., Roth, D. L., Haley, W. E., & Mittelman, M. S. (2008). Can counseling and support reduce

Alzheimer's caregivers' burden and depressive symptoms during the transition to institutionalization? Results from the NYU caregiver intervention study. *Journal of the American Geriatrics Society, 56,* 421–428.

Gould, E., Beylin, A., Tanapat, P., Reeves, A., & Shors, T. J. (1999). Learning enhances adult neurogenesis in the hippocampal formation. *Nature Neuroscience, 2,* 260–265.

Grober, E., Ausubel, R., Sliwinski, M., & Gordon, B. (1992). Skill learning and repetition priming in Alzheimer's disease. *Neuropsychologia, 30,* 849–858.

Hornberger, M., Bell, B., Graham, K. S., & Rogers, T. T. (2009). Are judgments of semantics relatedness systematically impaired in Alzheimer's disease? *Neuropsychologia, 47,* 3084–3094.

Ince, P. (2001). Pathological correlates of late-onset dementia in a multicenter community-based population in England and Wales. *Lancet, 357,* 169–175.

Jones, T. A. (2011). Experience-dependent changes in non-humans. In S. Raskin (Ed.), *Neuroplasticity and rehabilitation* (pp. 103–116). New York, NY: Guilford Press.

Katzman, R. (1993). Education and the prevalence of dementia and Alzheimer's disease. *Neurology, 43,* 13–20.

Katzman, R., Terry, R., DeTeresa, R., Brown, T., Davies, P., Fuld, P., . . . Peck, A. (1988). Clinical, pathological, and neurochemical changes in dementia: A subgroup with preserved mental status and numerous neocortical plaques. *Annals of Neurology, 23,* 138–144.

Keane, M. M., Gabrieli, J. D. E., Fennema, A. C., Growdon, J. H., & Corkin, S. (1991). Evidence for a dissociation between perceptual and conceptual priming in Alzheimer's disease. *Behavioral Neuroscience, 105,* 326–342.

Kempermann, G., Kuhn, H. G., & Gage, G. H. (1997). More hippocampal neurons in adult mice living in an enriched environment. *Nature, 386,* 493–495.

Kleim, J. A., & Jones, T. A. (2008). Principles of experience-dependent neural plasticity: Implications for rehabilitation after brain damage. *Journal of Speech, Language, and Hearing Research, 51,* 225–239.

Kolb, B., & Gibb, R. (2008). Principles of neuroplasticity and behavior. In D. Stuss, G. Winocur, & I. Robertson (Eds.), *Cognitive neurorehabilitation* (pp. 6–21). Cambridge, UK: Cambridge University Press.

Komitova, M., Mattsson, B., Johansson, B. B., & Eriksson, P. S. (2005). Enriched environment increases neural stem/progenitor cell proliferation and neurogenesis in the subventricular zone of stroke-lesioned adult rats. *Stroke, 36,* 1278–1282.

Landin-Romero, R., Tan, R., Hodges, J., & Kumfor, F. (2016). An update on semantic dementia: Genetics, imaging and pathology. *Alzheimer's Research and Therapy, 8,* 52.

Letenneur, L., Commenges, D., Dartigues, J. F., & Barberger-Gateau, P. (1994). Incidence of dementia and Alzheimer's disease in elderly community residents of southwestern France. *International Journal of Epidemiology, 23,* 1256–1261.

Lyketsos, C. G., Chen, L., & Anthony, J. C. (1999). Cognitive decline in adulthood: An 11.5-year follow-up of the Baltimore epidemiologic catchment area study. *American Journal of Psychiatry, 156,* 58–65.

Macdonald, M. C., Almor, A., Henderson, V. W., Kempler, D., & Andersen, E. S. (2001). Assessing working memory and language comprehension in Alzheimer's disease. *Brain and Language, 78,* 17–42.

Marra, H. L. D., Myczkowski, M. L., Memoria, C. M., Arnaut, D., Ribeiro, P. L., Mansur, C. G. S., . . . Marcolin, M. A. (2015). Transcortical Magnetic Stimulation to address mild cognitive impairment in the elderly: A randomized controlled study. *Behavioural Neurology,* Article ID 287843, 1–13.

Mittelman, M. S., Roth, D. L., Coon, D. W., & Haley, W. E. (2004). Sustained benefit of supportive intervention for depressive symptoms in Alzheimer's caregivers. *American Journal of Psychiatry, 161,* 850–856.

Nudo, R. J., & Bury, S. (2011). Motor and sensory reorganization in primates. In S. Raskin (Ed.), *Neuroplasticity and rehabilitation* (pp. 65–88). New York, NY: Guilford Press.

Perneczky, R. S., Lunetta, K. L., Cupples, L. A., Green, R. C., Decarli, C., Farrer, L. A., . . . MIRAGE Study Group. (2012). Group head circumference, atrophy and cognition: Implications for brain reserve in Alzheimer disease. *Neurology, 75,* 137–142.

Raskin, S. A. (Ed.). (2011). *Neuroplasticity and rehabilitation.* New York, NY: Guilford Press.

Rogers, S. L., & Friedman, R. B. (2008). The underlying mechanisms of semantic memory loss in Alzheimer's disease and semantic dementia. *Neuropsychologia, 46,* 12–21.

Salmon, D. P., Heindel, W. C., & Butters, N. (1992). Semantic memory, priming and skill learning in Alzheimer's disease. *Advances in Psychology, 89,* 99–118.

Sando, S. B., Melquist, S., Cannon, A., Hutton, M., Sletvold, O., Saltvedt, I., . . . Aasly, J. (2008). Risk-reducing effect of education in Alzheimer's disease. *International Journal of Geriatric Psychiatry, 11,* 1156–1162.

Shaffer, J. (2016). Neuroplasticity and clinical practice: Building brain power for health. *Frontiers in Psychology, 7,* 1118.

Snowdon, D. A., Ostwald, S. K., & Kane, R. L. (1989). Education, survival and independence in elderly Catholic sisters, 1936–1988. *American Journal of Epidemiology, 130,* 999–1012.

Stern, Y. (2002). What is cognitive reserve? Theory and research application of the reserve concept. *Journal of the International Neuropsychological Society, 8,* 448–460.

Stern, Y., Gurland, B., Tatemichi, T. K., Tang, M. X., Wilder, D., & Mayeux, R. (1994). Influence of education and occupation on the incidence of Alzheimer's disease. *Journal of the American Medical Association, 271,* 1004–1010.

Valenzuela, M. J., & Sachdev, P. (2005). Brain reserve and dementia: A systematic review. *Psychological Medicine, 35,* 1–14.

van Halteren-van Tilborg, I., Scherder, E., & Hulstijn, W. (2007). Motor-skill learning in Alzheimer's disease: A review with an eye to the clinical practice. *Neuropsychology Review, 17,* 203–212.

van Praag, H., Christie, B. R., Sejnowski, T. J., & Gage, F. H. (1999). Running enhances neurogenesis, learning, and long-term potentiation in mice. *Proceedings of the National Academy of Sciences of the United States of America, 96,* 13427–13431.

van Praag, H., Kempermann, G., & Gage, F. H. (1999). Running increases cell proliferation and neurogenesis in the adult mouse dentate gyrus. *Nature Neuroscience, 2,* 266–270.

van Praag, H., Shubert, T., Zhao, C., & Gage, F. H. (2005). Exercises enhances learning and hippocampal neurogenesis in aged mice. *Journal of Neuroscience, 25,* 8680–8685.

Vemuri, P., Lesnick, T. G., Przybelski, S. A., Machulda, M., Knopman, D. S., Mielke, M. M., . . . Jack, C. R. (2014). Association of lifetime intellectual enrichment with cognitive decline in the older population. *JAMA Neurology, 71,* 1017–1024.

Verfaellie, M., Keane, M. M., & Johnson, G. (2000). Preserved priming in auditory perceptual identification in Alzheimer's disease. *Neuropsychologia, 38,* 1581–1792.

White, L., Katzman, R., Losonczy, K., Salive, M., Wallace, R., Berkman, L., . . . Havlik, R. (1994). Association of education with incidence of cognitive impairment in three established populations for epidemiologic studies of the elderly. *Journal of Clinical Epidemiology, 47,* 363–374.

Zhang, X., Katzman, R., Salmon, D., Jin, H., Cai, G., Wang, Z., . . . Liu, W. T. (1990). The prevalence of dementia and Alzheimer's disease in Shanghai, China: Impact of age, gender, and education. *Annals of Neurology, 27,* 428–437.

2

Cognition, Memory, and Communication

Cognition and Memory

"Cognition" is a general term that refers to our information processing systems and stored knowledge. Basically, the human brain is a pattern recognition system, and memories are stored patterns. The processes that enable us to perceive and interpret patterns enable us to modify our behavior to ensure survival as well achieve more modest objectives.

The "Company of Cognition"

A helpful analogy for conceptualizing cognition is to think of it as a large company whose mission is to analyze sensation, detect and remember regularities in incoming sensory information, and use experience to guide behavior. The "company of cognition" has numerous departments (lobes of the brain) whose personnel perform unique functions but, nonetheless, work in parallel with personnel in other departments. Each department is responsible for analyzing a certain kind of sensory input (auditory, visual, tactile, gustatory, and olfactory). For example, there is a department for processing auditory sensations, a department for processing visual stimuli, and so on. Ultimately, all departments report to an executive division that analyzes information, makes

decisions, and plans action. Each department in the "company of cognition" has unique neural architecture. The department that processes auditory sensations is the province of the temporal lobes. Processing visual sensations is the province of the occipital lobes, and somatic sensations are processed by the parietal lobes. The frontal lobes make decisions and carry out executive functions. All departments share information by virtue of fiber tracts connecting them and all send their output via fiber tracts to the frontal lobes. In similar fashion, the lobes of the brain are connected to the limbic system, which is responsible for linking emotion with sensation. The limbic system, in turn, is linked to the frontal executive system.

Thinking of cognition as a company, with many departments working together to process information, is similar to how Alexander Luria (1973), the late renowned Soviet psychologist, described cognitive functioning. In Luria's three-unit model, one neural unit governs arousal and tone, another unit processes sensory information, and a third unit makes decisions and initiates action. The integrity of all three units is essential to normal cognitive functioning. If the level of arousal is poor, then information processing by other units is compromised. If a sensory processing system is damaged, individuals can develop agnosias and/or other processing deficits. When the executive unit is dysfunctional, judgment, attention, and decision making are compromised.

Memory Defined

Memory is not a unitary phenomenon (Eichenbaum, 2012; Schacter, Wagner, & Buckner, 2000; Squire, Stark, & Clark, 2004), *nor does it serve a single psychological function*. Consider that you have memory for facts, faces, sensations, various procedures, music, symbol systems, words, and contexts. As Karpicke and Lehman (2013) write, "Memory can manifest itself in various ways." In fact, many memory systems exist (Cohen & Squire, 1980; Eichenbaum, 2012; Gaffan, 1974; Hirsh, 1974; Nadel & O'Keefe, 1974; Schacter, 1985). A popular and clinically useful schema (after Squire, 2004) for characterizing the types of memory is shown in Figure 2–1. These different memory systems rely on distinct neurologic substrates, process different kinds of information, and have different rules of operation. *Of great importance to clinicians is that these systems can be separately impaired by neurologic disease and injury*. Thus, clinicians need an understanding of the different memory systems, their operational principles, and neural architecture to understand why an individual with a particular type and distribution of neuropathology has certain symptomatology.

Sensory Memory

The earliest stage of information processing is the registration of sensation. Sensations are received by our peripheral receptor organs (e.g., eyes, ears, chemical receptors) and interpreted in sensory cortices. A helpful way to think about sensory memory is as a playback system in which incoming sensory information is sustained long enough that it can be reviewed for further processing (Emery, 2003). The auditory playback system is known as *echoic memory*. The visual playback system is called *iconic memory*.

Sensory Memory: A Preattentive System

The term "sensory memory" applies to sensations that occur at the level of the peripheral receptor organs and create "change-specific cortical activation in visual, auditory, and somatosensory systems" (Downar, Crawley, Mikulis, & Davis, 2000; Ogmen & Herzog, 2016; Tanaka, Inui, Kida, & Kakigi, 2009; Tanaka, Kida, Inui, & Kakigi, 2009) before they are consciously realized. Higher order attentional processes bring some sensations to consciousness, although not all. As you might suspect, information in sensory memory rapidly decays to make way for the representation of new incoming sensations. The duration of sensory memory is estimated to range from .33 s

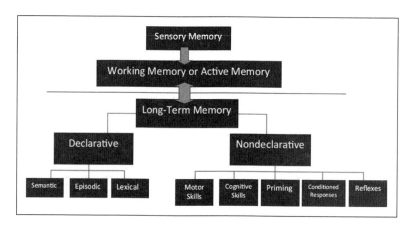

Figure 2–1. A model of memory. (After Bayles & Tomoeda, 1997; Squire, 2004)

to as long as 2 s (Dick, 1974; Harrell, Parente, Bellingrath, & Lisicia, 1992).

When an individual has a deficit in a peripheral receptor organ, sensation is altered and the quality of information coming from the environment is degraded. To facilitate sensory memory, clinicians must ensure that clients with sensory impairments, such as impaired vision or hearing, wear their glasses and hearing aids.

Working Memory

When sensations are consciously realized, they are in what is widely known as *"working memory."* Alan Baddeley (1986) introduced the term *to refer to information in conscious awareness and the processes active in the conscious, awake person.* The term is popular because it implies that much work is going on in consciousness and, indeed, there is. One activity is the focusing of attention that enables individuals to bring certain sensations to consciousness. But attention is only one of the many processes referred to by the term "working memory." Consider that when sensation is brought to consciousness it must be interpreted. Multiple working memory subsystems enable us to review newly received information; two that are of particular relevance to speech-language pathologists (SLPs) are the *articulatory/phonologic loop* and the *visuospatial sketchpad.* The articulatory/phonologic loop makes possible the subvocal rehearsal of what we have just heard, and the visuospatial sketchpad enables us to recirculate, in our "mind's eye," what we have just seen.

To interpret new information, we rely on previous experience; thus, working memory must activate past experience and bring that knowledge to consciousness. Generally, decisions must be made about the new information the organism is receiving. Baddeley called the decision-making component of working memory the *central executive.* The central executive system focuses attention, encodes information, retrieves information from long-term stores, plans action, and solves problems.

When information in working memory is encoded in long-term memory, it is linked with other similar memories. For example, new concepts are linked with those previously learned, new procedures are linked with other procedures, and new words with other words. The two-way arrows in Figure 2–1 signify that information is transferred from working memory to long-term memory and is retrieved from long-term memory when needed. Encoding and retrieval are carried out by the working memory system.

Active Memory

A synonym for working memory is active memory. It is whatever is on your mind. Said another way, it is what you are thinking. Working memory can be conceptualized as containing buffers that store incoming sensory information, but the buffers have a limited capacity. In a classic experiment in 1956, Miller demonstrated that the buffer span capacity of working memory is, on average, seven plus or minus two units of unrelated information. When the amount of information exceeds buffer capacity, some falls from consciousness. The terms used to refer to the buffer span capacity of an individual's working memory are *"short-term memory," "primary memory,"* or *"memory span."* Encoded information that has fallen from consciousness, regardless of whether it was a few seconds or years ago, is long-term memory (James, 1890). Many people mistakenly refer to information that fell from consciousness a short time ago as short-term memory; however, short-term memory only refers to the amount of information that can be *held* in consciousness. Long-term memory refers to information that has fallen from consciousness even if it was a short time ago.

Neural Substrates of Working Memory

As you may have surmised, the frontal lobes are essential to working memory, particularly prefrontal regions, which are extensively connected with the sensory processing systems of the brain and the structures that underlie emotion. Eichenbaum (2012) notes that prefrontal cortex (PFC) has the capacity to hold items in consciousness for manipulation and encoding stimuli and events. Its subdivisions are "highly connected with one another and with posterior areas of the cortex to operate as a complex and widespread network for conscious control over memory and other intellectual functions" (p. 336). The dorsolateral prefrontal cortex bilaterally comprises the CEO of the "company of cognition" (Smith & Jonides, 1999).

The articulatory/phonologic loop is subserved by Broca's area and the surrounding cortex as well as inferior parietal and inferior temporal cortices. The visuospatial sketchpad is supported by the occipitoparietal cortex, which mediates the visual and spatial components, respectively (Baddeley, 2003). Individuals with dementia typically have damage to the frontal lobes and structures that input to the frontal lobes. As a consequence, the functioning of working memory is compromised in dementia.

Long-Term Memory

Long-term memory is commonly dichotomized as *declarative* knowledge and *nondeclarative* knowledge (Squire, 2004). Declarative knowledge is factual information that can be declared. A synonym for declarative memory is explicit memory because fact knowledge can be made explicit. Nondeclarative memory is a broader term referring to movement or motor memory, certain cognitive skills, priming, conditioned responses, and reflexes.

Declarative Memory

Declarative knowledge, or fact memory, can be subdivided into three related systems: semantic memory (SM), episodic memory (EM), and lexical memory (LM).

Semantic Memory

Concept: Elemental Unit. Semantic memory (SM) is that domain in the nervous system in which conceptual knowledge is represented. The term SM was introduced by Quillian (1966) who proposed a theory of information processing that included a long-term store of conceptual knowledge (Cohen, 1983; Tulving, 1972; Wickelgren, 1979). Concepts are constructs we form about the world based on our experiences. As Smith and Medin (1981) wrote in their book about categories and concepts, "Without concepts, mental life would be chaotic. If we perceived each entity as unique, we would be overwhelmed by the sheer diversity of what we experience and unable to remember more than a minute fraction of what we encounter" (p. 1).

The word "semantic" in the term "semantic memory" may make some readers think that the contents of SM are words; however, *the elemental unit of SM is theorized to be the concept*, not the word. If you find the previous sentence hard to accept, consider that humans can conceptualize things for which they have no words. For example, you can conceptualize the following for which no word exists: an amorphous mass of gelatinous material about the size of a basketball seeming to have a self-contained propulsion system that enables it to continually change shape.

Other evidence that the units of SM are not in one-to-one correspondence with words is that many concepts can be referred to by a single word, for example "net." "Net" is associated with a worldwide system for sharing information, a tennis court barrier, a fisherman's tool, what is left after expenses, and a material used to make prom formals, just to name a few of its referents. Conversely, one concept can be associated with many words. For example, the concept "religion" is associated with Taoism, Protestantism, Catholicism, Judaism, Buddhism, Islam, and so forth.

Concepts can be activated by words, but conceptual activation can also result from nonlinguistic stimuli; for example, from objects and pictures. A picture of a parallelogram may activate the spatial concepts of parallel lines and opposing lines of equal length, but not the word parallelogram. Every day, individuals obtain new information by nonlinguistic means and, unless the need arises, much of this knowledge is never given linguistic representation. Consider that individuals who are profoundly deaf develop concepts without forming a linguistic representation for them. When a deaf child touches a hot stove, the concept of hot is encoded; however, without language training, the child will never develop the word "hot." Also, consider that an individual can lose the word for a concept without losing the concept; namely, individuals with anomic aphasia.

Words certainly help us conceptualize and, indeed, are so helpful that much thinking is done in words. However, when information is stored, the words that conveyed the information are generally forgotten; instead, we remember the concepts expressed by the words.

Learning can be thought of as the formation of new concepts (Cowan, 2015) that develop when existing concepts are joined together. SM is a hierarchically organized network of associations in which related concepts are linked; thus, when a concept such as "storm" is activated, the related concepts of "wind," "rain," and "lightning" are also activated. Although the concept is the elemental structural unit of SM, it is not the only unit. Propositions and schemata, which are combinations of concepts, also have representation.

Proposition. *A proposition can be defined as a relational expression.* It is grammatically analogous to a clause and contains a relational term, such as a verb, and one or more nouns or noun phrases that function as subjects and objects of the relation. For example, the following statements are propositions:

Children like to play dress up.

Solar power is clean energy.

Kale is a nutritious vegetable.

These propositions have been given linguistic representation, though not all propositions are translated into words.

Considerable evidence exists for the psychological reality of propositions. For example, regardless of the grammatical form of a sentence, it is reducible to the same constituent propositions, that is, it makes no difference whether the propositions are couched in a complex syntactic frame, a compound construction, or a simple construction (Franks & Bransford, 1974; Wang, 1977). People can recognize when two sentences or clauses are equivalent paraphrases because they perceive the relational expression, or proposition, contained in them. The following two sentences, which are equivalent paraphrases, illustrate this fact:

1. He desires to purchase an acre of land with a panoramic view of Tucson.
2. He really wants to buy an acre-sized lot with a valley-wide view of the "old Pueblo."

Sachs (1967) demonstrated that people remember propositions (or conceptual meaning) and ultimately forget the grammatical form in which they were expressed. Some investigators have demonstrated that it is the number of propositions, rather than the number of words, that affects the memorability of the meaning of a sentence (Kintsch & Glass, 1974; Rochon, Waters, & Caplan, 1994).

Schemata. *A schema is an attentional set formed by the simultaneous activation of a group of related concepts* (Figure 2–2). Schemata are another structural unit of SM. People have schemata for a multitude of activities; for example, packing a carry-on bag for an airplane, being a member of a wedding party, using a cell phone, making an appointment with a doctor, and so forth.

The process of building new schemata involves learning the associations between a particular set of concepts and propositions. For example, individuals exposed to the game of golf learn a host of propositions: that certain clothes and shoes are worn when playing golf, the angle of the club face influences the trajectory of the golf ball, different clubs are used for different kinds of shots, the person who had the fewest strokes on the previous hole

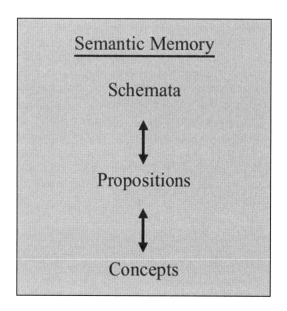

Figure 2–2. Semantic memory: a hierarchically organized representational system.

hits first on the new hole, and it is rude to talk when someone is hitting the ball. By playing golf, the schema is strengthened until the conventions of golf become second nature. Schemata help us know what to expect and guide our behavior.

Episodic Memory. *Episodic memory (EM) is the system that "receives and stores information about temporally dated episodes or events, and temporal-spatial relations among them"* (Tulving, 1984, p. 223). One way to think about episodic memory is that it is semantic memory plus a context. Consider that "golf" is a concept represented in SM. Now, let us assume that you played golf last Sunday morning. That was an event, an episode. If you can remember the event of having played golf last Sunday morning, that is EM. Notice that a context, "last Sunday morning," was added to the conceptual base of golf as a game in the EM example. SM is what you *know*, you know golf is a game. EM is an event you can *remember*; namely, playing golf last Sunday. Likely you do not remember the context in which you learned that golf is a game, it is just something you know, like knowing that

an apple is a fruit. However, being able to remember the last time you played golf or ate an apple is EM.

A synonym for EM is chronologic memory. EM enables us to travel back in time to recall past events. It is more fragile than SM. In fact, we forget most of the events of our lives. Likely you cannot remember what you ate for dinner on the 25th of last month, or the color of the car parked next to yours in the parking lot last Friday, or how the napkins were arranged at the last dinner party you attended. Insignificant events are forgotten.

Lexical Memory. *Lexical memory (LM) refers to our knowledge of words, their form, and meaning.* Certainly, concepts and their linguistic representations are intimately connected; however, people can have concepts for which they have no lexical representation and lexical information can be impaired without impairment of conceptual knowledge. Individuals with aphasia typically have preserved conceptual knowledge but struggle with lexical representations. Word knowledge also includes knowledge of the rules for composing syntactically correct and grammatical sentences. It is theorized that these operations rely on the neural systems that support procedural memory.

Neural Substrates of Declarative Memory. The declarative memory system is supported by three primary components: the cortex, parahippocampal region, and the hippocampus. Together, these brain regions enable us to acquire factual knowledge and remember events. Recall that the cortex is the endpoint for incoming sensory information. Within each sensory modality (or lobe), sensations are analyzed by a hierarchy of cells that perform increasingly complex analyses. The results of the analyses are sent to association areas of the cortex that have the capacity to form multimodal representations of information. These multimodal association areas have extensive inputs to the medial temporal lobes and parahippocampal regions. The parahippocampal region is able to sustain this input for short periods of time thereby enabling the hippocampus to "process comparisons among the various current stimuli and events and between current stimuli and representations of previous stimuli and events" (Eichenbaum, 2002, p. 235). It is the hippocampus that makes possible the addition of new cortical representations of information or the restructuring of existing cortical representations (Nadel & Hardt, 2011). Cells in the hippocampi have the capacity for long-term potentiation, meaning they can stay active for extended periods of time enabling them to replay information recently received. The replay of information during sleep provides the cortex the opportunity to repeatedly strengthen the link between new, recently experienced sensations and previously existing representations of knowledge. Because the hippocampi function like an index to link new, incoming information with previously learned information, individuals with hippocampal damage have difficulty remembering recent events and therefore making new semantic memory.

Just anterior to the hippocampi lie the amygdalae, which are important in the processing of emotion (Cahill, Babinsky, Markowitsch, & McGaugh, 1995; Hyman, 1998; Iversen, Kupfermann, & Kandel, 2000). There is strong evidence that the amygdalae modulate declarative memory on the basis of emotion (Cahill et al., 1995; Cahill et al., 1996). Emery (2003) theorizes that autobiographical memory developed phylogenetically from emotional memory, a theory that has considerable appeal because the emotional significance of an event greatly influences its memorability.

Factual knowledge is said to be "distributed" throughout the cortex; that is, it is not stored in a single area. Take, for example, your fact knowledge of your maternal grandmother. You have knowledge of what she looks like, how her voice sounds, what she smells like, how she feels when you hug her, as well as event knowledge about times you have spent with her. This diverse knowledge is not represented in one cell or cell assembly. Rather, it is believed that your knowledge of how grandmother looks has representation in the visual

association cortex, how her voice sounds in the auditory association cortex, and so on. The multimodal association cortex, where information from the various sensory processing systems converges, contains a more complex representation of grandmother. This explanation is very simplistic but makes the point that conceptual knowledge is distributed across cortical sensory association areas. For a more in-depth account of the brain system that supports declarative memory, the reader is referred to *The Cognitive Neuroscience of Memory* by Eichenbaum (2012).

Word knowledge is fact knowledge and as such is supported by the neural systems that underlie declarative memory (Ullman, 2008). Although lexical knowledge is represented throughout both cerebral hemispheres (Huth, de Heer, Griffiths, Theunissen, & Gallant, 2016), the left temporal lobe is key in the processing of word forms and meanings in both expressive and receptive language tasks (Damasio, 1992; Dronkers, Redfern, & Knight, 2000; Farah & Grossman, 1997; Ullman, 2004). By studying the naming errors of people with brain damage and brain activation patterns of neurologically normal adults during picture naming, Damasio, Grabowski, Tranel, Hichwa, and Damasio (1996) identified three brain regions of particular importance to word knowledge: the anterior inferior temporal pole, the middle part of the inferior temporal gyrus, and the posterior region of the temporal lobe. However, not all lexical operations rely on the same temporal lobe structures. Phonologic processing relies on the middle and posterior regions of the superior temporal cortex, whereas conceptual-semantic knowledge appears reliant on areas in front of and below these areas (Indefrey & Cutler, 2004; Martin & Chao, 2001). Numerous brain areas have been shown to be sensitive to both lexical and syntactic information, but inferior frontal and posterior temporal regions may have a more fine-grained representation (Fedorenko, Nieto-Castanon, & Kanwisher, 2011). Other brain structures also support lexical processing, among them subcortical and cerebellar structures. Word knowledge also includes knowledge of the rules for composing syntactically correct and grammatical sentences. These operations are theorized to rely on the neural systems that support procedural memory (see Ullman, 2007, for an overview).

Nondeclarative Memory

As previously mentioned, *nondeclarative memory is a general term referring to several kinds of memory and processes: motor skills, cognitive skills, priming, conditioned responses, and reflexes (nonassociative learning)*. A characteristic of these different types of nondeclarative memory is that they are strengthened by repetition and practice.

Motor Skill Memory. Motor skill memory refers to motor procedures that are learned and the processes that support them. Examples of motor skill memory are riding a bicycle, driving a car, typing, and articulating (Figure 2–3). Unlike declarative memory, which comprises factual knowledge that can be stated, motor procedural memory refers to the *performance* of an action. One can think about the mechanics of driving a car, but that is not procedural memory. Motor procedural memory is exhibited in the act of actually driving the car. One has knowledge about how to ski or play tennis, but motor procedural memory is evident only when one actually skis or hits the tennis ball.

Neural Substrate of Motor Skill Memory. Motor skill memory (also known as motor procedural memory) is supported by the corticostriatal system including premotor and motor cortex, basal ganglia, and cerebellum (Mishkin, Malamut, & Bachevalier, 1984; Mishkin, Siegler, Saunders, & Malamut, 1982; Zola-Morgan, Squire, & Mishkin, 1982).

Cognitive Skill Memory. The term "cognitive skill memory" is an umbrella term for various cognitive procedures that occur without conscious awareness. Examples are mirror-reversed reading and recognizing holographic images nested in pictures. The neural substrates for various cognitive skills differ, making it impossible to specify a single neural architecture.

Priming. *Priming is the facilitation of performance as a consequence of previous experience with a stimulus* and is typically measured in terms of accuracy of judgment or latency of response. Priming can

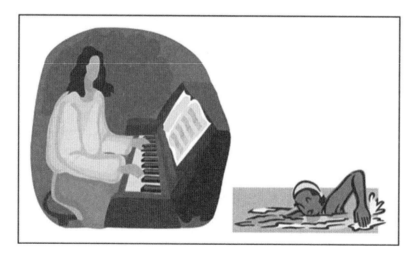

Figure 2–3. Examples of motor skill memory include playing a piano and swimming.

be conceptual or perceptual. Conceptual priming is the spreading of activation between related concepts. An example of conceptual priming is the activation of the concepts "cold," "hard," and "water" when we hear the word "ice."

In perceptual priming, the prior exposure to perceptual features of the stimulus facilitates the response. For example, the word "cake" may be activated by having previously seen the word "cake" or a word similar in appearance such as "make."

Neural Substrates of Priming. Priming occurs in the neocortex, but certain subcortical structures may facilitate priming, notably the basal ganglia. The areas of the cortex involved depend on the nature of the stimulus, that is, whether it is a concept or a set of perceptual features. When the stimulus is visual, areas of the occipital lobe and/or inferior temporal lobe are involved. When the stimulus is auditory, both the left and right auditory cortices are involved. The left auditory cortex processes cues related to phonologic information; the right auditory cortex processes cues related to the speaker's voice.

Habits and Conditioned Behaviors. *Habits are chains of behavioral events.* The events in the chain are associated with each other such that the execution of one behavior triggers the next behavior. Most of us have a chain of behaviors we follow upon awakening and before we go to bed. We can carry out this routine while thinking about something else. Humans can develop habits because of the brain's capacity to form associations between repeated events. In fact, Eichenbaum (2012) defines habit as "an acquired and well-practiced response to a particular stimulus."

Conditioned behaviors are behaviors that are automatically produced in response to a particular stimulus or set of stimuli. The behavior is associated with the stimulus and reinforced by the events subsequent to the behavior or the eradication of an unpleasant antecedent event. An example is feeling afraid when approached by a growling dog.

Neural Substrates of Habit Memory and Conditioned Behaviors. The corticostriatal system, in particular the striatum, underlies the formation of habits (Knowlton, Mangels, & Squire, 1996). Eichenbaum (2012) explains that the striatum receives cortical sensory input and has direct motor outputs that make possible the association of stimuli with behavioral outputs. The striatum also has pathways for reward signals that enhance the association of stimuli and responses. Individuals with damage to the striatum are impaired in developing stimulus-response sequences.

The cerebellum is important in motor conditioning (Squire, 2004). Its circuitry enables it to make a topographic representation of the entire body surface because it receives vestibular, visual, and auditory inputs, and has complex connections with the brain stem (Eichenbaum, 2012). Individuals with damage to the cerebellum are impaired in the acquisition of classically conditioned responses.

Relation of Cognition and Memory to Communication

Production of Linguistic Information

Ideation begins the process of producing meaningful linguistic output. The ideas that people communicate can be reduced to concepts represented in their SM. Once an idea or idea sequence has been formulated, it must be translated into a symbol system for linguistic communication to occur. A point to be underscored is that a translation process occurs, that is, ideation and thinking may be done in a different language than what is seen on the written page or heard in a lecture. The brain appears to have a language of its own—a machine language—or as Fodor (1975) described, a language of thought, the output of which is translatable into human natural language. To utter or write an idea, we rely on complex motor skills (articulation or writing) that are forms of nondeclarative procedural memory. To ensure that what we say is what we intended to say, we monitor our utterances and make judgments about them; thus, the production of linguistically expressed information uses semantic memory, lexical memory, working memory, motor procedural memory, and the central executive system. Although this is an oversimplification of what occurs in producing language, it makes the point that our *cognitive-memorial systems underlie communication.*

Comprehension of Linguistic Information

Linguistic comprehension ultimately involves deriving the right concepts and propositions. Said another way, it involves activation of the intended concepts in lexical and semantic memory. Like linguistic production, linguistic comprehension is the product of sequential and parallel processes involving many parts of the nervous system. For example, the perception of a spoken concept (word) or proposition (sentence) can be traced from its detection by the auditory system in which feature, segmental, and word analyses occur to the level of semantic memory and consciousness. Through their nervous system journey, linguistic stimuli undergo lexical, structural, and logical analyses, the output of which is awareness of the intended concept or proposition. Additionally, the context in which a communicative exchange occurs influences the interpretation of information exchanged. Context refers to the physical setting, emotional climate, social organization between participants, and the purpose of the communicative exchange. Tracking these variables is a complex constructive process and participants in a communicative exchange must attend to phonetic and paraverbal features such as pitch, intonation, gestures, and facial expressions, as well as the physical setting.

Now the question of why communication is affected in Alzheimer's disease can be answered. Communication is affected because the pathophysiologic processes of Alzheimer's disease disrupt information generation and

processing. Patients are said to have a "cognitive-communication" problem because progressive deterioration of cognition interferes with communication. The fact is, the production and comprehension of language cannot be separated from cognition.

Summary of Important Points

- Communication is the sharing of information by means of a symbol system and is a manifestation of cognition.
- Persons with dementia have trouble with intentional communication because by definition they have multiple cognitive deficits.
- Cognition is stored knowledge and the processes for making and manipulating knowledge.
- Cognition can be likened to a large company whose mission is to analyze sensation, detect and remember regularities in incoming sensory information, and use experience to guide behavior.
- Memory is stored knowledge and the processes for making and manipulating it.
- Humans have many memory systems each with distinct neural architecture that can be separately impaired by trauma or disease.
- Sensory memory is the brief registration of sensation at the level of the peripheral receptor organ. It is preattentive and sensations rapidly fade making way for new sensations.
- Working memory is information in conscious awareness and the processes active in the reception, encoding, and retrieving of information.
- Considerable work goes on in working memory that is directed by a central executive that enables us to make decisions and plan action.
- Long-term memory can be dichotomized as declarative knowledge and nondeclarative knowledge.
- Declarative memory is fact memory and can be subdivided into semantic, episodic, and lexical memory.

- Semantic memory comprises our conceptual knowledge; it is what we know. The elemental unit is the concept.
- Episodic memory enables us to remember the events of our life. It is our autobiographical memory and the most fragile of the memory systems.
- Lexical memory is our memory for words, their referents and meaning, spelling, and pronunciation.
- Nondeclarative memory is a general term that refers to several kinds of memory: skills (motor and cognitive), habits, priming, conditioned responses, and reflexes.
- Motor skill memory is often referred to as procedural memory. It is realized in the doing of a skill such as driving a car or hitting a tennis ball.
- Cognitive skill memory refers to myriad cognitive operations that occur without conscious awareness, one of which is mirror-reversed reading.
- Priming is the facilitation of performance as a consequence of previous experience with a stimulus or its associates. Priming can be conceptual or perceptual.
- Habits are chains of behavioral events in which the execution of one behavior triggers the next behavior.
- The production and comprehension of linguistic information cannot be separated from cognition but rather reflect cognition.
- Persons with dementia have difficulty producing linguistic information because they have trouble thinking, generating, and ordering ideas. They have difficulty comprehending language because of deficits in the cognitive processes and degradation and loss of knowledge.
- With an understanding of the types of memory and their neural substrates, clinicians can reasonably predict the cognitive-communication disorders associated with damage to different brain areas.
- Aging affects the functioning of working memory, particularly executive functions.
- Of the declarative memory systems, episodic memory is most affected by age. From midlife on, individuals experience gradual deterioration in their ability to recall names, faces, and events.
- Motor procedural memory holds well with age, although individuals may be slower in performing motor skills.
- In normal aging, individuals slow down physically and psychologically. Aging affects the processing and retrieval of information more than the fund of knowledge.
- Great variability exists in the psychological and physical status of individuals over age 65.
- Knowledge of vocabulary and grammar are preserved in aging and reported effects of aging on language are primarily the consequence of decrements in sensory processing and psychomotor slowing, rather than loss of linguistic knowledge.

References

Baddeley, A. D. (1986). *Working memory*. Oxford, UK: Clarendon Press.

Baddeley, A. D. (2003). Working memory: Looking back and looking forward. *Nature Reviews Neuroscience, 4*, 829–839.

Cahill, L., Babinsky, R., Markowitsch, H. J., & McGaugh, J. L. (1995). The amygdala and emotional memory. *Nature, 377*, 295–296.

Cahill, L., Haier, R. J., Fallon, J., Alkire, M. T., Tang, C., Keator, D., . . . McGaugh, J. L. (1996). Amygdala activity at encoding correlated with long-term, free recall of emotional information. *Proceedings of the National Academy of Science USA, 93*, 8016–8021.

Cohen, G. (1983). *The psychology of cognition*. New York, NY: Academic Press.

Cohen, J. N., & Squire, L. (1980). Preserved learning and retention of pattern-analyzing skill in amnesia: Dissociation of "knowing how" and "knowing that." *Science, 210*, 207–209.

Cowan, N. (2015). Working memory underpins cognitive development, learning, and education. *Educational Psychology Review, 26*(2), 197–223.

Damasio, A. R. (1992). Aphasia. *New England Journal of Medicine, 326*, 531–539.

Damasio, H., Grabowski, T. J., Tranel, D., Hichwa, R. D., & Damasio, A. R. (1996). A neural basis for lexical retrieval. *Nature, 380*, 499–505.

Dick, A. O. (1974). Iconic memory and its relation to perceptual processes and other memory mechanisms. *Perception and Psychophysics, 16*, 575–596.

Downar, J., Crawley, A. P., Mikulis, D. J., & Davis, K. D. (2000). A multimodal cortical network for the detection of changes in the sensory environment. *Nature Neuroscience, 3,* 277–283.

Dronkers, N. F., Redfern, B. B., & Knight, R. T. (2000). The neural architecture of language disorders. In M. S. Gazzaniga (Ed.), *The new cognitive neurosciences* (pp. 949–958). Cambridge, MA: MIT Press.

Eichenbaum, H. (2002). *The cognitive neuroscience of memory.* Cambridge, UK: Oxford University Press.

Eichenbaum, H. (2012). *The cognitive neuroscience of memory* (2nd ed.). New York, NY: Oxford University Press.

Emery, V. O. B. (2003). "Retrophylogenesis" of memory in dementia of the Alzheimer type. In V. O. B. Emery & T. E. Oxman (Eds.), *Dementia: Presentation, differential diagnosis, and nosology* (pp. 177–236). Baltimore, MD: Johns Hopkins University Press.

Farah, M. J., & Grossman, M. (1997). Semantic memory impairments. In T. E. Feinberg & M. J. Farah (Eds.), *Behavioral neurology and neuropsychology* (pp. 473–477). New York, NY: McGraw-Hill.

Fedorenko, E., Nieto-Castanon, A., & Kanwisher, N. (2011). Lexical and syntactic representations in the brain: An fMRI investigation with multivoxel pattern analyses. *Neuropsychologia, 50,* 499–513.

Fodor, J. (1975). *The language of thought hypothesis.* New York, NY: Crowell Press.

Franks, J. J., & Bransford, J. D. (1974). Memory for syntactic form as a function of semantic context. *Journal of Experimental Psychology, 103,* 1037–1039.

Gaffan, D. (1974). Recognition impaired and association intact in the memory of monkeys after transection of the fornix. *Journal of Comparative and Physiological Psychology, 86,* 1100–1109.

Harrell, M., Parente, F., Bellingrath, E. G., & Lisicia, K. A. (1992). *Cognitive rehabilitation of memory: A practical guide.* Gaithersburg, MD: Aspen.

Hirsh, R. (1974). The hippocampus and contextual retrieval from memory: A theory. *Behavioral Biology, 12,* 421–444.

Huth, A. G., de Heer, W. A., Griffiths, T. L., Theunissen, F. E., & Gallant, J. L. (2016). Natural speech reveals the semantic maps that tile human cerebral cortex. *Nature, 532,* 453–459.

Hyman, S. E. (1998). A new image of fear and emotion. *Nature, 393,* 417–418.

Indefry, P., & Cutler, A. (2004). Prelexical and lexical processing in listening. In M. S. Gazzaniga (Ed.), *The cognitive neurosciences* (pp. 759–774). Cambridge, MA: MIT Press.

Iversen, S., Kupfermann, I., & Kandel, E. R. (2000). Emotional states and feelings. In E. R. Kandel, J. Schwartz, & T. M. Jessell (Eds.), *Principles of neural science* (pp. 982–997). New York, NY: McGraw-Hill.

James, W. (1890). *The principles of psychology.* New York, NY: H. Holt & Company.

Karpicke, J. D., & Lehman, M. (2013). Human memory. In D. S. Dunn (Ed.), *Oxford bibliographies online: Psychology.* New York, NY: Oxford University Press.

Kintsch, W., & Glass, G. (1974). Effects of propositional structure upon sentence recall. In W. Kintsch (Ed.), *The representation of meaning in memory* (pp. 140–151). Hillsdale, NJ: Lawrence Erlbaum Associates.

Knowlton, B. J., Mangels, J. A., & Squire, L. R. (1996). A neostriatal habit learning system in humans. *Science, 273,* 1399–1402.

Luria, A. (1973). *The working brain.* New York, NY: Basic Books.

Martin, A., & Chao, L. L. (2001). Semantic memory and the brain: Structure and processes. *Current Opinion in Neurobiology, 11,* 194–201.

Miller, G. A. (1956). The magical number seven, plus or minus two: Some limits on our capacity for processing information. *Psychological Review, 63,* 81–97.

Mishkin, M., Malamut, B., & Bachevalier, J. (1984). Memories and habits: Two neural systems. In G. Lynch, J. McGaugh, & N. Weinberger (Eds.), *Neurobiology of learning and memory* (pp. 65–77). New York, NY: Guilford Press.

Mishkin, M., Siegler, B., Saunders, R. C., & Malamut, B. J. (1982). An animal model of global amnesia. In S. Corkin, K. L. Davis, J. H. Growdon, E. Usdin, & R. J. Wurtman (Eds.), *Toward a treatment of Alzheimer's disease* (pp. 235–247). New York, NY: Raven Press.

Nadel, L., & Hardt, O. (2011). Update on memory systems and processes. *Neuropsychopharmacology, 36,* 251–273.

Nadel, L., & O'Keefe, J. (1974). The hippocampus in pieces and patches: An essay on modes of explanation in physiological psychology. In R. Bellairs & E. G. Gray (Eds.), *Essays on the nervous system. A festschrift for JZ Young.* Oxford, UK: Clarendon Press.

Ogmen, H., & Herzog, M. H. (2016). A new conceptualization of human visual sensory memory. *Frontiers in Psychology, 7,* 830.

Quillian, M. R. (1966). *Semantic memory* (Unpublished doctoral dissertation). Carnegie Institute of Technology, Pittsburg, PA. Reprinted in part in M. Minsky (Ed.). (1968). *Semantic information processing.* Cambridge, MA: MIT Press.

Rochon, E., Waters, G. S., & Caplan, D. (1994). Sentence comprehension in patients with Alzheimer's disease. *Brain and Language, 46,* 329–349.

Sachs, J. S. (1967). Recognition memory for syntactic and semantic aspects of connected discourse. *Perception and Psychophysics, 2,* 437–444.

Schacter, D. L. (1985). Multiple forms of memory in humans and animals. In N. Weingerger, J. McGaugh, & G. Lynch (Eds.), *Memory systems of the brain: Animal and human cognitive processes* (pp. 351–379). New York, NY: Guilford Press.

Schacter, D. L., Wagner, A. D., & Buckner, R. L. (2000). Memory systems of 1999. In E. Tulving & F. I. M. Craik (Eds.), *Oxford handbook of memory* (pp. 627–643). New York, NY: Oxford University Press.

Smith, E. E., & Jonides, J. (1999). Storage and executive processes in the frontal lobes. *Science, 283,* 1657–1661.

Smith, E. E., & Medin, D. L. (1981). *Categories and concepts*. Cambridge, MA: Harvard University Press.

Squire, L. R. (2004). Memory systems of the brain: A brief history and current perspective. *Neurobiology of Learning and Memory, 82,* 171–177.

Squire, L. R., Stark, C. E. L., & Clark, R. E. (2004). The medial temporal lobe. *Annual Review of Neuroscience, 27,* 279–306.

Tanaka, E., Inui, K., Kida, T., & Kakigi, R. (2009). Common cortical responses evoked by appearance, disappearance, and change of the human face. *BMC Neuroscience, 10,* 38.

Tanaka, E., Kida, T., Inui, K., & Kakigi, R. (2009). Change-driven cortical activation in multisensory environments: An MEG study. *NeuroImage, 24,* 464–474.

Tulving, E. (1972). Episodic and semantic memory. In E. Tulving & W. Donaldson (Eds.), *Organization of memory* (pp. 381–403). New York, NY: Academic Press.

Tulving, E. (1984). Elements of episodic memory (precis). *Behavioral and Brain Sciences, 7,* 223–268.

Ullman, M. T. (2004). Contributions of memory circuits to language: The declarative/procedural model. *Cognition, 92,* 231–270.

Ullman, M. T. (2007). The biocognition of the mental lexicon. In M. G. Gaskell (Ed.), *The Oxford handbook of psycholinguistics* (pp. 268–286). Oxford, UK: Oxford University Press.

Ullman, M. T. (2008). The role of memory systems in disorders of language. In B. Stemmer & H. A. Whitaker (Eds.), *Handbook of the neuroscience of language* (pp. 189–198). Oxford, UK: Academic Press.

Wang, M. D. (1977). Frequency effects in the abstraction of linguistic ideas. *Bulletin of the Psychonomic Society, 9,* 303–306.

Wickelgren, W. A. (1979). *Cognitive psychology.* Englewood Cliffs, NJ: Prentice-Hall.

Zola-Morgan, S., Squire, L., & Mishkin, M. (1982). The neuroanatomy of amnesia: Amygdala-hippocampus versus temporal stem. *Science, 218,* 1337–1339.

3

MCI: Mild Cognitive Impairment a.k.a. Mild Neurocognitive Disorder

Introduction

The two terms mentioned in the title of this chapter are used to refer to the same condition. Historically, the term mild cognitive impairment (MCI) was used to refer to the prodromal stage of Alzheimer's disease (AD). However, diseases other than AD have an early stage in which the affected individual has modest cognitive impairment. To avoid the problem of MCI being associated with a particular etiology, criteria were developed in the fifth edition of the *Diagnostic and Statistical Manual of Mental Disorders* for "mild neurocognitive disorder" (a.k.a., mild cognitive impairment) and "major neurocognitive disorder" (American Psychiatric Association, 2013). The criteria for diagnosing mild neurocognitive disorder are essentially the same as those that have been designated for diagnosing MCI (McKhann et al., 2011). The DSM-V criteria for "major neurocognitive disorder" incorporate the syndrome of dementia.

In this chapter, the term MCI will be used with the understanding that it does not connote etiology. Nonetheless, the most common cause of MCI is AD. Regardless of etiology, MCI has the attention of clinicians and researchers worldwide because of its association with dementia-producing diseases. Intense interest exists in early detection to enable affected individuals to seek intervention while they retain the capacity to benefit from cognitive stimulation (Sachdev et al., 2013), pharmacologic interventions, and lifestyle changes. Moreover, public health care costs and caregiver burden would be significantly reduced. An intervention that delays the onset of dementia by just 5 years would result in a 57% reduction in the number of people with dementia and save approximately $283 billion annually in Medicare costs (Sperling et al., 2011).

Prevalence of MCI

Prevalence of MCI is estimated to be 10% to 20% of individuals 65 years old and older (Hanninen, Hallikainen, Tuomainen, Vanhanen, & Soininen, 2002; Lopez et al., 2003; Petersen et al., 2010) and it increases with age (Plassman et al., 2008). Prevalence estimates vary considerably because of methodologic differences in the age of study subjects (higher prevalence in older individuals), the measures used to evaluate cognitive function, and the stringency of the criteria used for diagnosing MCI. Results of a large community-based study of 2,000 randomly recruited individuals, between the ages of 70 and 89 years of age, indicated that the prevalence in this older group approximates 16% to 20% (Petersen et al., 2010).

MCI can take many forms and individuals with amnestic MCI are 2 to 3 times more common than those with nonamnestic. Prevalence is higher in men, people who never marry, and those who carry one or two copies of the APOE e4 allele. It is less common in those with more years of education.

Diagnostic Criteria for MCI

In 2011, the National Institute on Aging and the Alzheimer's Association Task Force recommended biomarker and neurobehavioral criteria for diagnosing MCI (McKhann et al., 2011). *Biomarkers* are physiological, biochemical, and anatomical parameters that reflect the effects of disease-related pathophysiologic processes (Jack et al., 2011). Some markers indicate molecular neuropathology such as the presence of signature proteins that accumulate in the brain and spinal fluid during disease evolution. Others include structural and functional changes such as loss of hippocampal volume, reduction of glucose metabolism or perfusion in temporoparietal cortex that are apparent with positron emission tomography or single photo emission computed tomographic scanning (Jack et al., 2011). Yet, other biomarkers indicate biochemical events such as inflammation (Albert et al., 2011; Jack et al., 2011). Petersen and colleagues (2010) report that the majority of individuals with MCI have biomarker evidence of amyloid deposits or neurodegeneration or both.

Neurobehavioral diagnostic criteria for MCI include:

1. *Concern regarding change in cognition compared to prior level.* Concern can be expressed by the patient, an informant, or a clinician.
2. *Impairment in one or more cognitive domains.* A performance in one or more cognitive areas (memory, executive function, attention, language, and visuospatial skills) that is lower than expected for the patient's age and educational background. Most commonly seen is impairment in episodic memory. If repeated assessments are available, decline should be apparent.
3. *Preservation of independence in functional abilities.* Although individuals in the preclinical stage retain the ability to manage their daily affairs, they are less efficient doing so, make more errors, and require more time to task completion.
4. *Not demented.* The cognitive and behavioral changes are sufficiently mild, failing to significantly interfere with social or occupational functioning.

Neuropsychological testing to detect MCI is more common than biomarker screening, which is expensive and infrequently used. However, evidence of neurobehavioral changes plus biomarkers increase clinician confidence in making the diagnosis of MCI and help in predicting time-to-dementia conversion.

Risk and Protective Factors

The most significant risk factor for MCI is age (Keyimu, Zhou, Miao, & Zou, 2015). As previously noted, prevalence is greater in older individuals. Another risk is apolipoprotein APOE (ApoE) carrier status. APOE transports cholesterol and other types of fat in the bloodstream. The APOE gene is found on chromosome 19 and has three major variants: e2, e3, and e4. Individuals inherit a variant from each parent, most commonly APOE e3, which is carried by more than half the population. Those individuals who carry the less common APOE e4 variant have a significantly greater risk of developing MCI that will evolve to AD, especially if they have two copies (Aggarwal, Wilson, Beck, Bienias, & Bennett, 2005; Tierney et al., 1996). Older individuals who have APOE e4 status are at greater risk of MCI than younger carriers (Qian et al., 2017). Nonetheless, almost half the individuals with AD do *not* have the APOE e4 genotype and the presence of an e4 variant accounts for a relatively small percentage of cases (Evans et al., 1997; Myers et al., 1996; Qian et al., 2017).

Other significant risk factors for MCI include diabetes, hyperlipidemia, current smoking, depression, high blood pressure, increased cholesterol, lack of exercise, high alcohol consumption, infrequent social participation (Etgen, Sander, Bickel, & Förstl, 2011), and certain genes whose significance is being studied. APOE carrier status has also been associated with deficits in episodic memory and executive function (Albert, Moss, Blacker, Tanzi, & McArdle, 2007).

Causes and Clinical Presentations of MCI

MCI has many causes—neurodegenerative, vascular, metabolic, psychiatric, and traumatic. As previously noted, the most common cause is AD that has three recognized stages (Albert et al., 2011): a *preclinical phase* associated with measurable changes in biomarkers before memory loss, *MCI* characterized by measurable changes in cognitive function with sparing of basic activities of daily living, and frank *dementia*.

The most common symptom of MCI is episodic memory impairment, an unsurprising fact given that AD is the most common cause and episodic memory impairment is a signature AD characteristic. However, clinicians should be aware that AD sometimes presents in atypical ways in which memory impairment is not an early symptom (Albert et al., 2007). For example, neither the syndromes of posterior cortical atrophy (PCA) (Alladi et al., 2007) or primary progressive aphasia (PPA) necessarily present with memory impairment (Rabinovici et al., 2008). PCA typically presents with visual processing deficits, such as difficulty reading or recognizing faces, that reflect pathology in the back of the brain.

Then too, these symptoms typically appear when individuals are in their 50s or early 60s. In PPA, language impairment is the presenting symptom and can persist for up to 2 years before memory and other cognitive impairment(s) become apparent (Mesulam & Weintruab, 2008).

A challenge to clinicians is differentiating the cognitive changes associated with healthy aging from those associated with pathology. In healthy aging, changes occur in frontal-striatal circuitry that affects processing speed, attention, source memory, and temporal ordering of events (Hedden & Gabrieli, 2004). Healthy elders typically process more slowly, are less efficient in a divided attention tasks, often have difficulty remembering from whom they learned a fact, and the order in which two or more events occurred; however, *they do not have an episodic memory deficit*. Episodic memory deficit develops when pathologic changes develop in entorhinal cortex and the hippocampal area. It is these changes that distinguish individuals with AD related MCI from healthy elders (Braak & Braak, 1991; Sabbagh et al., 2010).

Neuropsychological Deficits Associated with MCI

The most widely reported deficits in MCI are in working and episodic memory (Kirova, Bays, & Lagalwar, 2015), executive function, and language (Albert et al., 2011). Of clinical significance is the fact that language deficits reflect impairments in working and episodic memory and executive function. Individuals with MCI typically do not suffer loss of linguistic knowledge (though there are rare exceptions), but rather exhibit language *performance* problems because of deficits in the previously noted cognitive functions. For this reason, it is appropriate to make a distinction between a "language deficit," which implies loss of linguistic knowledge, and a "language *performance* deficit," which more appropriately describes the behaviors seen in individuals with MCI.

Table 3–1. Four Widely Recognized Subtypes of Mild Cognitive Impairment *(MCI)*

Subtype	Characteristics
Amnestic MCI Single Domain	Subjective or proxy cognitive complaint Objective memory impairment Relatively intact functional ability Not demented
Amnestic MCI Multiple Domain	Subjective or proxy cognitive complaint Objective impairment in memory and at least one other cognitive domain Relatively intact functional ability Not demented
Nonamnestic MCI Single Domain	Subjective or proxy cognitive complaint Objective impairment in one nonmemory domain Relatively intact functional ability Not demented
Nonamnestic MCI Multiple Domain	Subjective or proxy cognitive complaint Objective impairment in two or more nonmemory domains Relatively intact functional ability Not demented

Consider that language comprehension and production are subserved by myriad cognitive processes—memory, perception, speed of processing, attention, and various executive functions (Brandt et al., 2009; Kirova et al., 2015; Saunders & Summers, 2010; Storandt, 2008; Storandt, Grant, Miller, & Morris, 2006; Taler & Phillips, 2008; Twamley, Ropacki, & Bondi, 2006; Visser, 2003)—and *a strong correlation exists between scores on language measures and scores on measures of the cognitive functions needed to complete language tasks* (Cottingham & Hawkins, 2010). The type and number of neuropsychological deficits have been used to create four types of MCI: amnestic single domain (one cognitive function is impaired), amnestic multidomain (more than one cognitive function is impaired), nonamnestic single domain, and nonamnestic multidomain (Table 3–1). The most common type is amnestic multidomain.

Language Performance Deficits

Language performance deficits came on the radar of clinicians as an early marker of dementia with the publication of the now-famous nun study (Riley, Snowdon, Desrosiers, & Markesbery, 2005; Snowdon, Grenier, & Markesbery, 2000; Snowdon et al., 1996). Investigators had access to the written autobiographies of almost 200 American Roman Catholic sisters between the ages of 75 and 103 who were members of the School Sisters of Notre Dame. All wrote autobiographies decades earlier as novices. Linguistic analyses of their autobiographies revealed differences in the idea density and grammatical complexity of those written by sisters who developed AD later in life. Their texts had fewer ideas and less grammatical complexity. These findings were particularly compelling because the nuns were in the same order, lived under similar conditions, and the majority worked as teachers (85%). Since the report of Snowdon and colleagues, other investigators have reported a relation between cognitive performance early in life and vulnerability to late-life dementia (Dekhtyar et al., 2015; McGurn, Deary, & Starr, 2008; Whalley et al., 2000).

Although few researchers have been so fortunate as to be able to compare the language performance of their older subjects to their subjects' performance as young adults, many have included language testing as part of a neuropsychological evaluation of individuals with MCI and reported language performance impairment (Taler & Phillips, 2008). Oulahaj, Wilcock, Smith, and De Jager (2009) followed a cohort of 241 normal healthy individuals for up to 20 years for the purpose of identifying early markers of MCI and dementia. Subjects were periodically administered the Cambridge Cognitive Examination (CAMCOG), a widely used comprehensive neuropsychological battery comprising subtests of orientation, comprehension, expression, recent memory, remote memory, learning, abstract thinking, perception, praxis, attention, and calculation, as well as a derived Mini-Mental State Examination (MMSE) score. Only the subscores for language expression and learning/memory were predictors of time to conversion to MCI. The CAMCOG expression subtest includes verbal fluency, spoken language descriptions, definitions, and comprehension. For each point lower on the CAMCOG expression score, the time to conversion was 17% shorter; for each point lower on the learning score, the time to conversion was 15% shorter; and for every 5 years of age, time to conversion was 14% shorter. The investigators emphasized that although memory impairment is the signature criterion of amnestic MCI and the recommended type of measure for assessing pre-dementia AD, "expression" or language ability was a stronger predictor of duration to conversion than either "learning" or memory.

Since the nun study, various language performance deficits have been reported in individuals with MCI. Typically, the more dependent the language performance task is on memory and executive functions, the more likely it is that impairment will be present. The literature contains reports of impairment in naming and word retrieval, verbal fluency, language comprehension, discourse processing and production, picture description, the ability to define words, and repetition (Cuetos, Arango-Lasprilla, Uribe, Valencia, & Lopera, 2007; McCullough & Bayles, 2017; Twamley et al., 2006).

Naming and Word Retrieval

Many investigators have examined the confrontation naming skills of individuals with MCI, mild AD, and healthy older adults and reported significant differences in the performance of those with MCI compared to both healthy elders (Dwolatzky et al., 2003; Grundman et al., 2004; Katsumata et al., 2015; Petersen et al., 1999) and those with mild AD (Goldman et al., 2001; Petersen et al., 1999). However, it is also the case that some investigators failed to observe a significant difference in confrontation naming ability of individuals with MCI and healthy elders (Albert, Moss, Tanzi, & Jones, 2001; Chen et al., 2001; Devanand, Folz, Gorlyn, Moeller, & Stern, 1997; Ritchie, Artero, & Touchon, 2001; Schmidtke & Hermeneit, 2008). Results differ because the diagnostic criteria differed in the various investigations as did the type and length of the naming tests used. Perhaps the most important reason for differences is that only a segment of the MCI population has confrontation naming problems.

Saunders and Summers (2010) compared individuals with subjective memory impairment ($n = 32$) to those with confirmed amnestic MCI ($n = 60$), mild AD ($n = 14$), and healthy individuals of a similar age ($n = 25$). All were given the Cambridge Automated Neuropsychological Assessment Battery (CANTAB), which is known to be sensitive to progressive declines in cognitive function over the course of AD. They were also given numerous other neuropsychological tests: WTAR, Dementia Rating Scale, Boston Naming Test, Rey Auditory Verbal Learning Test, and Paired Associates Learning. Study results revealed that individuals with subjective memory impairment and those with confirmed amnestic MCI displayed impairment in language retrieval and other cognitive functions, though language retrieval deficits were larger for the amnestic MCI group. Furthermore, all subjects with subjective memory complaint and 83% of those with amnestic MCI displayed impaired performance on at least one measure of attention or working memory despite the fact that the Dementia Rating Scale-2 (DRS-2; Mattis, 2001) did not detect impairment in these areas. These data suggest that MCI classification criteria based exclusively on the presence of attention, initiation, construction and conceptualization, and memory (components of the DRS-2) will exclude many aging adults who, in fact, have significant decline in other cognitive domains, among them language use. Furthermore, 35% of the subjects who had informant-corroborated memory decline did not display episodic memory impairment but did display impaired attention or working memory deficits.

Verbal Fluency

Verbal fluency, also known as generative or category naming, has been widely studied with semantic and letter category naming tests. Verbal fluency tasks require examinees to generate exemplars of items in a category—such as animals or vegetables—or words beginning with a certain letter in a specified period of time, typically 1 min. Examinees must remember the category while searching lexical and semantic memory. Extensive literature documents deficits in individuals with MCI in both semantic and letter category naming, though semantic category naming is widely reported as more impaired (Amieva et al., 2005; Auriacombe et al., 2006; Blackwell et al., 2004; Chen et al., 2001; Cottingham & Hawkins, 2010; Fabrigoule et al., 1998; Grober et al., 2008; Guarch, Marcos, Salamero, Blesa, 2004; Hanninen et al., 1995; Hodges, Erzinçlioglu, & Patterson, 2006; Howieson et al., 2008; Jorm, Masaki, Petrovitch, Ross, & White, 2005).

Cottingham and Hawkins (2010) hypothesized a relation between verbal fluency and memory test performance in individuals with MCI. Both letter and semantic category tasks were given to 92 individuals referred for neuropsychological assessment by geriatricians because of cognitive complaints. Study results indicated that increasing levels of memory impairment, as measured by performance on the

Wechsler Memory Scale III, were accompanied by increasingly poorer performance in generating category items. Moreover, the verbal fluency scores of subjects were weaker than their reading scores, indicating the greater sensitivity of verbal fluency tests to cognitive decline. Based on results of a meta-analysis of 153 studies of category naming (Henry, Crawford, & Phillips, 2004), not only is semantic category naming more sensitive to early AD, it is more strongly correlated with verbal intelligence.

Demetriou and Holtzer (2017) reported that individuals with MCI generated fewer words compared to controls during the first 20 s and in succeeding intervals in both phonemic and category verbal fluency tests. They reported a group by time interaction and concluded that MCI is characterized by deficits in "early automatic retrieval processes."

Discourse Processing and Production

A substantive literature now exists about changes in the ability of individuals with MCI to process and produce discourse. One early report came from Chapman and colleagues (2002) who had 69 individuals (20 with MCI, 24 with mild AD, and 25 cognitively normal elders) listen to a 578-word narrative and give an account of what they heard including the story's gist. Subjects had a copy of the story to follow while it was read to them and 5 min to study it before recounting it and answering questions about story details. Both the MCI and AD subjects were impaired on all measures of "gist-level" processing and answering questions about story details.

In 2005, the effects of early AD on the characteristics of the writings of a well-known author were published. Garrard, Maloney, Hodges, and Patterson (2005) analyzed the text of three of Iris Murdoch's novels, one written early in her career in her 30s, a second written during her 50's, and her final novel written a few years before her death from AD at age 76. Comparisons of the degree of lexical diversity in the three works were made. In Murdoch's last and least highly regarded work, vocabulary was more restricted and there were fewer unique word types relative to overall word count.

In 2008, Harris, Kiran, Marquardt, and Fleming reported subtle changes in the discourse of 10 adults with MCI compared with 30 neurologically healthy young adults and 22 neurologically healthy older adults. Subjects were instructed to describe, in detail, activities associated with preparing for and taking a trip to New York City. They were advised to think about trip preparation, packing, and activities while there. A variety of discourse analyses were conducted: calculation of mean length of utterance (MLU), proportion of definite nouns, indefinite nouns, verbs and modifiers, pronouns, and "mazed" words (repetitions, false starts, reformulations, and self-corrections). Count was also made of the number of core concepts related to the story theme. Data analyses revealed that individuals with MCI provided less thematic information, more irrelevant comments, and were more verbose than normal subjects. Significantly, performance on the discourse task was associated with performance on cognitive measures including the MMSE.

In a related study, Fleming and Harris (2008) sought to determine whether performance on the trip to New York discourse task differentiated normal elders from eight physician-diagnosed individuals with MCI in terms of discourse length, complexity, and quality using SALT analysis (Miller & Inglesias, 2006). Other analyses included counting the number of words and core elements plus calculating the average number of morphemes per t-units. MCI subjects produced significantly fewer words and core elements than control subjects, though the groups did not differ in average length of t-unit.

In a 2015 study of the narrative production ability of individuals with amnestic MCI, carefully screened participants were asked to narrate a story based on visually presented scenes of a car accident (Drummond et al., 2015). The narratives were videotaped, transcribed, and evaluated in terms of total time required to perform the task, total number of words, cohesion, and overall coherence. The investigators also calculated an "index of discourse effectiveness" by dividing the total number of words produced by the number of relevant macropropositions produced. This index was the only parameter that differentiated the control, amnestic MCI, and AD groups. The amnestic MCI group's performance was worse than that of the normal control subjects' but better than that of the AD subjects'.

In their 2015 review of the literature on language performance deficits in MCI and early AD, Szatloczki, Hoffman, Vincze, Kalman, and Pakaski concluded that *language performance deficits are apparent in the MCI stage of AD and should play a major role in early detection of the disease*. They also suggest that an analysis of the temporal parameters of speech may be a promising method for early detection, specifically articulation rate, speech tempo, hesitation ratio, and grammatical error ratio. Individuals with AD have been reported to have longer hesitations than healthy elders as well as a slower speech rate, more pauses, and an artic rate that is significantly different (Hoffman et al., 2010; López-de-Ipiña et al., 2013).

In a 2016 study, Mueller and colleagues had 39 individuals with psychometric evidence of amnestic MCI and 39 cognitively healthy adults describe the Cookie Theft picture from the Boston Diagnostic Aphasia Examination. Their language was analyzed in terms of content, syntactic complexity, and speech fluency. The individuals with MCI produced significantly fewer semantic units, unique words, and had less idea density. They also performed worse on both phonemic and semantic category naming tasks.

Fraser, Meltzer, and Rudzicz (2015) used an exploratory factor analysis to identify the dimensions of speech most indicative of early dementia in the narratives of 167 individuals diagnosed with possible or probable AD and 97 control subjects. Four factors were identified: *semantic impairment*—use of overly simple words; *acoustic impairment*—slower speech; *syntactic impairment*—use of less complex grammar; and *information impairment*—failure to clearly identify the main aspects of a picture. Although the analyses were based on the narratives of individuals presumed to have AD, the results reflect what researchers are reporting about individuals with MCI and can serve as a guide for how to analyze the language of individuals at risk for AD.

Ability to Define Words

The ability of individuals with amnestic and nonamnestic MCI to define concrete and abstract nouns was examined by Kim, Kim, Baek, and Kim (2015) who had subjects define five concrete and five abstract nouns. The amnestic MCI group scored significantly poorer than normal controls in the abstract word condition. McCullough and Bayles (2017) administered the Concept Definition Subtest of the Arizona Battery for Cognitive Communication Disorders of Dementia to 83 individuals at risk for MCI by virtue of age and self-report of concern about cognitive function and found that 35.5% performed at least one standard deviation or more below the mean of healthy older adults on this test.

Ability to Repeat

The ability to repeat, especially phrases that are nonsensical, is particularly sensitive to MCI. McCullough and Bayles (2017) administered a repetition task that had two levels of difficulty: six and nine syllable nonmeaningful phrases. Fifty-four percent of the 83 individuals who were at risk for MCI because of age and their concern about cognitive status scored one standard deviation or more below the mean of healthy older adults on this test.

Conversion to Dementia

The percentage of individuals with MCI who convert to dementia (Summers & Saunders, 2012) is of great interest. Unfortunately, it is difficult to definitively specify a rate as different investigators have used different criteria for defining MCI. Moreover, the subjects have varied considerably in age. Those investigators who used more stringent diagnostic criteria (1.5 standard deviation below the mean performance of healthy age-matched individuals on neuropsychological tests) had higher rates of conversion over shorter periods of time. Mitchell and Shiri-Feshki (2009) analyzed the results of 41 high-quality studies, some conducted on community populations and others on participants involved in clinical trials, and derived an annual conversion rate of approximately 5% to 10%. However, after 10 years, *more than half* the individuals originally diagnosed with MCI had not progressed to AD or any other dementia. On the other hand, elders with MCI in the Mayo Alzheimer's Research Center study converted at a rate of 12% per year, and after 6 years, 80% had converted (Petersen & Morris, 2003). According to Bruscoli and Lovestone (2004), individuals with amnestic MCI are more likely to progress to dementia than those with nonamnestic MCI. Using a clinical index based on gender and behavioral characteristics—evidence of resisting help, becoming upset when separated from caregiver, difficulty shopping alone, forgetting appointments, word recall, clock drawing, and orientation—Lee, Ritchie, Yaffe, Stijacic Cenzer, and Barnes (2014) found that 43% of a group of 382 MCI diagnosed individuals progressed to probable AD. Of those deemed at high risk, by virtue of performance on the clinical index, 91% converted within 3 years.

Simply stated, the greater the number of cognitive deficits, the greater the probability of conversion to dementia (Bozoki, Giordani, Heidebrink, Berent, & Foster, 2001). Hodges and colleagues (2006) conducted a longitudinal study of 10 individuals with MCI who were given extensive neuropsychological testing annually. All ultimately developed dementia (defined as <24 on the MMSE) and/or a significant problem with activities of daily living. However, the onset of dementia ranged from 1 to 8 years. Those who presented with multiple cognitive deficits early, including language, converted faster and were more likely to develop AD (Alexopoulos, Grimer, Perneczky, Domes, & Kurz, 2006; Sacuiu, Sjögren, Johansson, Gustafson, & Skoog, 2005).

Rates of *reversion to normal* also vary. Ritchie and colleagues (2001) reported a rate of 15%, whereas Busse, Hensel, Gühne, Angermeyer, and Riedel-Heller (2006) reported a rate of 18% to 22%. Improved cognition was most common in those with nonamnestic MCI. Also worth noting is that 4% to 13% of individuals diagnosed with MCI in the Busse et al. (2006) study had a different diagnosis at follow-up evaluation.

Conclusion

MCI is the state of having one or more cognitive impairments that are *insufficient* to significantly affect basic ADLs. Although MCI has many causes, the most common is AD and, in fact, MCI is now a recognized stage of AD. Because cognitive stimulation, pharmacologic intervention, and lifestyle changes may prevent or delay evolution to frank dementia, early detection is critical. Language performance impairments occur early and are typically present in individuals with MCI. Thus, clinicians should incorporate measures of language performance in clinical evaluations.

Summary of Important Points

- Mild cognitive impairment is a psychogeriatric syndrome with many causes that frequently evolves to dementia, thus early detection is critical.
- Another name for MCI is "mild neurocognitive disorder." This term is used in the fifth edition of the *Diagnostic and Statistical Manual of Mental Disorders*.
- The prevalence of MCI in community-based individuals between the ages of 70 and 89 years approximates 16%.
- Alzheimer's disease is the most common cause of MCI; other causes include vascular

disease, depression, Lewy body disease, and Parkinson's disease.
- The four neurobehavioral criteria that define MCI are concern regarding change in cognition compared to prior level, demonstrated impairment in one or more cognitive domains, preservation of independence in functional abilities, and not demented.
- The recognized subtypes of MCI include *amnestic* single and multiple domain and *nonamnestic* single and multiple domain.
- Amnestic multiple domain, in which memory and other cognitive functions are impaired, is the most common, and single nonamnestic domain is the least common.
- The greatest risk factor for MCI is age; the older the individual, the greater the risk.
- The more cognitive deficits an individual has, the greater the probability of conversion to dementia.
- Individuals with MCI have cognitive deficits and deficits in language functions because language use is a manifestation of cognition.
- Since the famous nun study, reported by Snowden and colleagues, other investigators have reported a relation between cognitive-linguistic performance early in life and vulnerability to late-life dementia.
- Individuals with MCI have been reported to have language performance deficits on myriad language tasks, among them naming and word retrieval, verbal fluency, discourse comprehension and production, defining words, and repetition.

References

Aggarwal, N. T., Wilson, R. S., Beck, T. L., Bienias, J. L., & Bennett, D. A. (2005). Mild cognitive impairment in different functional domains and incident Alzheimer's disease. *Journal of Neurology, Neurosurgery and Psychiatry, 76,* 1479–1484.

Albert, M., DeKosky, S., Dickson, D., Dubois, B., Feldman, H., Fox, N., ... Snyder, P. (2011). The diagnosis of mild cognitive impairment due to Alzheimer's disease: Recommendations from the national institute on Aging–Alzheimer's Association workgroups on diagnostic guidelines for Alzheimer's disease. *Alzheimer's and Dementia, 7*, 270–279.

Albert, M., Moss, M. B., Blacker, D., Tanzi, R., & McArdle, J. J. (2007). Longitudinal change in cognitive performance among individuals with mild cognitive impairment. *Neuropsychology, 21*, 158–169.

Albert, M. S., Moss, M. B., Tanzi, R., & Jones, K. (2001). Preclinical prediction of AD using neuropsychological tests. *Journal of the International Neuropsychological Society, 7*, 631–639.

Alexopoulos, P., Grimer, T., Perneczky, R., Domes, G., & Kurz, A. (2006). Progression to dementia in clinical subtypes of mild cognitive impairment. *Dementia and Geriatric Cognitive Disorders, 22*, 27–34.

Alladi, S., Xuereb, J., Bak, T., Nestor, P., Knibb, J., Patterson, K., & Hodges, J. (2007). Focal cortical presentations of Alzheimer's disease. *Brain, 130*, 2636–2645.

American Psychiatric Association. (2013). *Diagnostic and statistical manual of mental disorders* (5th ed.). Arlington, VA: American Psychiatric Publishing.

Amieva, H., Jacqmin-Gadda, H., Orgogozo, J. M., Le Carret, N., Helmer, C., Letenneur, L., . . . Dartigues, J. F. (2005). The 9-year cognitive decline before dementia of the Alzheimer type: A prospective population-based study. *Brain, 128*, 1093–1101.

Auriacombe, S., Lechevallier, N., Amieva, H., Harston, S., Raoux, N., & Dartigues, J. F. (2006). A longitudinal study of quantitative and qualitative features of category verbal fluency in incident Alzheimer's disease subjects: Results from the PAQUID study. *Dementia and Geriatric Cognitive Disorders, 21*, 260–266.

Blackwell, A. D., Sahakian, B. J., Vesey, R., Semple, J. M., Robbins, T. W., & Hodges, J. R. (2004). Detecting dementia: Novel neuropsychological markers of preclinical Alzheimer's disease. *Dementia and Geriatric Cognitive Disorders, 17*, 42–48.

Bozoki, A., Giordani, B., Heidebrink, J. L., Berent, S., & Foster, N. L. (2001). Mild cognitive impairments predict dementia in nondemented elderly patients with memory loss. *Archives of Neurology, 58*, 411–416.

Braak, H., & Braak, E. (1991). Neuropathological staging of Alzheimer disease-associated neurofibrillary pathology using paraffin sections and immunocytochemistry. *Acta Neuropathologica, 112*, 389–404.

Brandt, J., Aretouli, E., Neijstrom, E., Samek, J., Manning, K., Bandeen-Roche, K., & Albert, M. S. (2009). Selectivity of executive function deficits in mild cognitive impairment. *Neuropsychology, 23*, 607–618.

Bruscoli, M., & Lovestone, S. (2004). Is MCI really just early dementia? A systematic review of conversion studies. *International Psychogeriatrics, 16*, 129–140.

Busse, A., Hensel, A., Gühne, U., Angermeyer, M. C., & Riedel-Heller, S. G. (2006). Mild cognitive impairment: Long-term course of four clinical subtypes. *Neurology, 67*, 2176–2185.

Chapman, S. B., Zientz, J., Weiner, M., Rosenberg, R., Frawley, W., & Burns, M. (2002). Discourse changes in early Alzheimer disease, mild cognitive impairment, and normal aging. *Alzheimer Disease and Associated Disorders, 16*, 177–186.

Chen, P., Ratcliff, G., Belle, S. H., Cauley, J. A., DeKosky, S. T., & Ganguli, M. (2001). Patterns of cognitive decline in presymptomatic Alzheimer disease: A prospective community study. *Archives of General Psychiatry, 58*, 853–858.

Cottingham, M. E., & Hawkins, K. A. (2010). Verbal fluency deficits co-occur with memory deficits in geriatric patients at risk for dementia: Implications for the concept of mild cognitive impairment. *Behavioural Neurology, 22*, 73–79.

Cuetos, F., Arango-Lasprilla, J. C., Uribe, C., Valencia, C., & Lopera, F. (2007). Linguistic changes in verbal expression: A preclinical marker of Alzheimer's disease. *Journal of the International Neuropsychological Society, 13*, 433–439.

Dekhtyar, S., Wang, H-X., Scott, K., Goodman, A., Koupil, I., & Herlitz, A. (2015). A life-course study of cognitive reserve in dementia—From childhood to old age. *American Journal of Geriatric Psychiatry, 23*, 885–896.

Demetriou, E., & Holtzer, R. (2017). Mild cognitive impairments moderate the effect of time on verbal fluency performance. *Journal of the International Neuropsychological Society, 23*, 44–55.

Devanand, D. R., Folz, M., Gorlyn, M., Moeller, J. R., & Stern, Y. (1997). Questionable dementia: Clinical course and predictors of outcome. *Journal of the American Geriatrics Society, 45*, 321–328.

Drummond, C., Coutinho, G., Fonseca, R., Assuncao, N., Teldeschi, A., de Oliverira-Souza, R., . . . Mattos, P. (2015). Deficits in narrative discourse elicited by visual stimuli are already present in patients with mild cognitive impairment. *Frontiers in Aging Neuroscience, 7*, 96.

Dwolatzky, R., Whitehead, V., Doniger, G. M., Simon, E. S., Schweiger, A., Jaffe, D., & Chertkow, H. (2003). Validity of a novel computerized cognitive battery for mild cognitive impairment. *BMC Geriatrics, 3*, 4.

Etgen, T., Sander, D., Bickel, H., & Förstl, H. (2011). Mild cognitive impairment and dementia: The importance of modifiable risk factors. *Deutsches Ärzteblatt International, 108*, 743–750.

Evans, D. A., Beckett, L. A., Field, T. S., Feng, L., Albert, M. S., Bennett, D. A., ... Mayeux, R. (1997). Apolipoprotein episilon4 and incidence of Alzheimer disease in a community population of older persons. *Journal of the American Medical Association, 277*, 822–824.

Fabrigoule, D., Rouch, I., Taberly, A., Letenneur, L., Commenges, D., Mazaux, J. M., ... Dartigues, J. F. (1998). Cognitive processes in preclinical phase of dementia. *Brain, 121*, 135–141.

Fleming, V. B., & Harris, J. L. (2008). Complex discourse production in mild cognitive impairment: Detecting subtle changes. *Aphasiology, 22*, 729–740.

Fraser, K., Meltzer, J., & Rudzicz, F. (2015). Linguistic features identify Alzheimer's disease in narrative speech. *Journal of Alzheimer's Disease, 49*, 407–422.

Garrard, P., Maloney, L. M., Hodges, J. R., & Patterson, K. (2005). The effects of very early Alzheimer's disease on the characteristics of writing by a renowned author. *Brain, 128*, 250–260.

Goldman, W. P., Price, J. O., Storandt, M., Grant, E. A., McKeel, D. W., Rubin, E. H., & Morris J. C. (2001). Absence of cognitive impairment or decline in preclinical Alzheimer's disease. *Neurology, 56*, 361–367.

Grober, E., Hall, C. B., Lipton, R. B., Zonderman, A. B., Resnick, S. M., & Kawas, C. (2008). Memory impairment, executive dysfunction, and intellectual decline in preclinical Alzheimer's disease. *Journal of the International Neuropsychological Society, 14*, 266–278.

Grundman, M., Petersen, R. C., Ferris, S. H., Thomas, R. G., Aisen, P. S., Bennett, D. A., ... Thal, L. J. (2004). Mild cognitive impairment can be distinguished from Alzheimer disease and normal aging for clinical trials. *Archives of Neurology, 61*, 59–66.

Guarch, J., Marcos, T., Salamero, M., & Blesa, R. (2004). Neuropsychological markers of dementia in patients with memory complaints. *International Journal of Geriatric Psychiatry, 19*, 352–358.

Hanninen, T., Hallikainen, M., Koivisto, K., Helkala, E. L., Reinikainen, K. J., Soininen, H., ... Riekkinen Sr., P. J. (1995). A follow-up study of age-associated memory impairment: Neuropsychological predictors of dementia. *Journal of the American Geriatrics Society, 43*, 1212–1222.

Hanninen, T., Hallikainen, M., Tuomainen, S., Vanhanen, M., & Soininen, H. (2002). Prevalence of mild cognitive impairment: A population based study in elderly subjects. *Acta Neurologica Scandinavica, 106*, 148–154.

Harris, J. L., Kiran, S., Marquardt, T., & Fleming, V. B. (2008). Communication Wellness Check-Up: Age-related changes in communicative abilities. *Aphasiology, 22*, 813–825.

Hedden, T., & Gabrieli, J. D. E. (2004). Insights into the ageing mind: A view from cognitive neuroscience. *Nature Reviews Neuroscience, 5*, 87–96.

Henry, J. D., Crawford, J. R., & Phillips, L. H. (2004). Verbal fluency performance in dementia of the Alzheimer's type: A meta-analysis. *Neuropsychologia, 42*, 1212–1222.

Hodges, J. R., Erzinçlioglu, S., & Patterson, K. (2006). Evolution of cognitive deficits and conversion to dementia in patients with mild cognitive impairment: A very long-term follow-up study. *Dementia and Geriatric Cognitive Disorders, 21*, 380–391.

Hoffmann, I., Németh, D., Dye, C., Pákáski, M., Irinyi, T., & Kálmán, J. (2010). Temporal features of spontaneous speech in Alzheimer's disease. *International Journal of Speech Language-Pathology, 12*, 29–34.

Howieson, D. B., Carlson, N. E., Moore, M. M., Wasserman, D., Abendroth, C. D., Payne-Murphy, J., & Kaye, J. A. (2008). Trajectory of mild cognitive impairment onset. *Journal of the International Neuropsychological Society, 14*, 192–198.

Jack, C., Jr., Albert, M., Knopman, D., McKhann, G., Sperling, R., Carillo, M., ... Phelps, C. (2011). Introduction to the recommendations from the National Institute on Aging and the Alzheimer's Association workgroup on diagnostic guidelines for Alzheimer's disease. *Alzheimer's and Dementia, 7*, 257–262.

Jorm, A. F., Masaki, K. H., Petrovitch, H., Ross, G. W., & White, L. R. (2005). Cognitive deficits 3 to 6 years before dementia onset in a population sample: The Honolulu-Asia aging study. *Journal of the American Geriatric Society, 53*, 452–455.

Katsumata, Y., Mathews, M., Abner, E., Jicha, G., Caban-Holt, A., Smith, C. . . . Fardo, D. (2015). Assessing the discriminant ability, reliability, and comparability of multiple short forms of the Boston Naming Test in an Alzheimer's disease center cohort. *Dementia and Geriatric Cognitive Disorders, 39*, 215–227.

Keyimu, K., Zhou, X-H., Miao, H-J., & Zou, T. (2015). Mild cognitive impairment risk factor survey of the Xinjiang Uyghur and Han elderly. *International Journal of Clinical and Experimental Medicine, 8*, 13891–13900.

Kim, S. R., Kim, S. Y., Baek, M. J., & Kim, H. (2015). Abstract word definition in patients with amnestic mild cognitive impairment. *Behavioural Neurology, Article ID 580246*, 1–8.

Kirova, A. M., Bays, R. B., & Lagalwar, S. (2015). Working memory and executive function decline across normal aging, mild cognitive impairment, and Alzheimer's disease. *BioMed Research International, 2015*, 1–9.

Lee, S. J., Ritchie, C. S., Yaffe, K., Stijacic Cenzer, I., & Barnes, D. E. (2014). A clinical index to predict progression from mild cognitive impairment to dementia due to Alzheimer's disease. *PLOS ONE. 9*, 1–15.

Lopez, O., Jagust, W., DeKosky, S., Becker, J. T., Fitzpatrick, A., Dulberg, C. . . . Kuller, L. (2003). Prevalence and classification of mild cognitive impairment in the cardiovascular health study cognition study: Part 1. *Archives of Neurology, 60*, 1385–1389.

López-de-Ipiña, K., Alonso, J. B., Travieso, C. M., Solé-Casals, J., Egiraun, H., Faundez-Zanuy, M., . . . Martinez de Lizardui, U. (2013). On the selection of non-invasive methods based on speech analysis oriented to automatic Alzheimer disease diagnosis. *Sensors, 13*, 6730–6745.

Mattis, S. 2001. *Dementia Rating Scale–2 (DRS–2)*. Odessa, FL: Psychological Assessment Resources.

McCullough, K., & Bayles, K. (2017, November). *Why SLPs have an important role in early identification of MCI*. Session presented at the American Speech-Language Hearing Association annual convention, Los Angeles, CA.

McGurn, B., Deary, I. J., & Starr, J. M. (2008). Childhood cognitive ability and risk of late-onset Alzheimer and vascular dementia. *Neurology, 71*, 1051–1056.

McKhann, G., Knopman, D., Chertkow, H., Hyman, B. T., Jr., Jack, C. R., Jr., Kawas, C. H., ... Phelps, C. H. (2011). The diagnosis of dementia due to Alzheimer's disease: Recommendations from the National Institute on Aging–Alzheimer's Association workgroups on diagnostic guidelines for Alzheimer's disease. *Alzheimer's and Dementia, 7,* 263–269.

Mesulam, M., & Weintraub, S. (2008). Primary progressive aphasia and kindred disorders. *Handbook of Clinical Neurology, 89,* 573–587.

Miller, J., & Inglesias, A. (2006). *Systematic Analysis of Language Transcripts (SALT),* English and Spanish (Version 9) [Computer software]. Madison, WI: Language Analysis Lab, University of Wisconsin.

Mitchell, A. J., & Shiri-Feshki, M. (2009). Rate of progression of mild cognitive impairment to dementia: Meta-analysis of 41 robust inception cohort studies. *Acta Psychiatrica Scandinavica, 119,* 252–265.

Mueller, K. D., Koscik, R. L., LaRue, A., Clark, L. R., Hermann, B., Sager, M. A., . . . Riedeman, S. K. (2016). Connected language in late middle-aged adults at risk for Alzheimer's disease. *Journal of Alzheimers Disease, 54,* 1539–1550.

Myers, R. H., Schaefer, E. J., Wilson, P. W. F., D'Agostino, R., Ordovas, J. M., Espino, A., ... Wolf, P. A. (1996). Apoliprotein E epsilon 4 association with dementia in a population-based study: The Framingham study. *Neurology, 46,* 673–677.

Oulahaj, A., Wilcock, G., Smith, A. D., & De Jager, C. A. (2009). Predicting the time of conversion to MCI in the elderly: Role of verbal expression and learning. *Neurology, 73,* 1436–1442.

Petersen, R. C., & Morris, J. C. (2003). Clinical features. In R. C. Petersen (Ed.), *Mild cognitive impairment: Aging to Alzheimer's disease* (pp. 15–40). New York, NY: Oxford University Press.

Petersen, R. C., Roberts, R. O., Knopman, D. S., Geda, Y. E., Cha, R. H., Pankratz, V. S., . . . Rocca, W. A. (2010). Prevalence of mild cognitive impairment is higher in men: The Mayo Clinic Study of Aging. *Neurology, 75,* 889–897.

Petersen, R. C., Smith, G. E., Waring, S. C., Ivnik, R. J., Tangalos, E. G., & Kokmen, E. (1999). Mild cognitive impairment: Clinical characterization and outcome. *Archives of Neurology, 56,* 303–308.

Plassman, B. L., Langa, K. M., Fisher, G. G., Heeringa, S. G., Weir, D. R., Ofstedal, M. B., . . . & Wallace, R. B. (2008). Prevalence of cognitive impairment without dementia in the United States. *Annals of Internal Medicine, 148,* 427–434.

Qian, J., Wolters, F. J., Beiser, Al., Haan, M., Ikrma, M. A., Karlawish, J., . . . Blacker, D. (2017). APOE-related risk of mild cognitive impairment and dementia for prevention trials: An analysis of four cohorts. *PLOS Med, 14,* e1002254.

Rabinovici G. D., Jagust W. J., Furst, A. J., Ogar, J. M., Racine, C. A., Mormino, E. C., ... Gornotempini, M. L. (2008). A beta amyloid and glucose metabolism in three variants of primary progressive aphasia. *Annals of Neurology, 64,* 388–401.

Riley, K. P., Snowdon, D. A., Desrosiers, M. F., & Markesbery, W. R. (2005). Early life linguistic ability, late life cognitive function, and neuropathology: Findings from the nun study. *Neurobiology of Aging, 26,* 341–347.

Ritchie, K., Artero, S., & Touchon, J. (2001). Classification criteria for mild cognitive impairment: A population-based validation study. *Neurology, 56,* 37–42.

Sabbagh, M. N., Cooper, K., DeLange, J., Stoehr, J. D., Thind, K., . . . Beach, T. G. (2010). Functional, global and cognitive decline correlates to accumulation of Alzheimer's pathology in MCI and AD. *Current Alzheimer Research, 7,* 280–286.

Sachdev, P. S., Lipnicki, D. M., Crawford, J. Reppermund, S., Kochan, N. A., Trollor, J. N. . . . . The Sydney Memory, and Ageing Study Team. (2013). Factors predicting reversion from mild cognitive impairment to normal cognitive functioning: A population-based study. *PLOS ONE. 8,* e59649.

Sacuiu, S., Sjögren, M., Johansson, B., Gustafson, D., & Skoog, I. (2005). Prodromal cognitive signs of dementia in 85-year-olds using four sources of information. *Neurology, 65,* 1894–1900.

Saunders, N. L. J., & Summers, M. J. (2010). Attention and working memory deficits in mild cognitive impairment. *Journal of Clinical and Experimental Neuropsychology, 32,* 350–357.

Schmidtke, K., & Hermeneit, S. (2008). High rate of conversion to Alzheimer's disease in a cohort of amnestic MCI patients. *International Psychogeriatric, 20,* 96–108.

Snowdon, D. A., Greiner, L. H., & Markesbery, W. R. (2000). Linguistic ability in early life and the neuropathology of Alzheimer's disease and cerebrovascular disease: Findings from the nun study. *Annals of the New York Academy of Sciences, 903,* 34–38.

Snowdon, D. A., Kemper, S. J., Mortimer, J. A., Greiner, L. H., Wekstein, D. R., & Markesbery W. R. (1996). Linguistic ability in early life and cognitive function and Alzheimer's disease in late life: Findings from the nun study. *Journal of the American Medical Association, 275,* 528–532.

Sperling, R. A., Aisen, P. S., Beckett, L. A., Bennett, D. A., Craft, S., Fagan, A. M., . . . Phelps, C. H. (2011). Toward defining the preclinical stages of Alzheimer's disease: Recommendations from the National Institute on Aging–Alzheimer's Association workgroups on diagnostic guidelines for Alzheimer's disease. *Alzheimer's and Dementia, 7,* 280–292.

Storandt, M. (2008). Cognitive deficits in the early stages of Alzheimer's disease. *Current Directions in Psychological Sciences, 17,* 198–202.

Storandt, M., Grant, E. A., Miller, J. P., & Morris, J. C. (2006). Longitudinal course and neuropathologic outcomes in original vs. revised MCI and pre-MCI. *Neurology, 67,* 467–473.

Summers, M. J., & Saunders, N. L. J. (2012). Neuropsychological measures predict decline to Alzheimer's dementia from mild cognitive impairment. *Neuropsychology, 26,* 498–508.

Szatloczki, G., Hoffmann, I., Vincze, V., Kalman, J., & Pakaski, M. (2015). Speaking in Alzheimer's disease, is that an early sign? Importance of changes in language abilities in Alzheimer's disease. *Frontiers in Aging Neuroscience, 7*, 195.

Taler, V., & Philips, N. A. (2008). Language performance in Alzheimer's disease and mild cognitive impairment: A comparative review. *Journal of Clinical and Experimental Neuropsychology, 30*, 501–556.

Tierney, M. C., Szalai, J. P., Snow, W. G., Fisher, R.G., Tsuda, T., Chi, H., . . . St. George-Hyslop, P. H. (1996). A prospective study of the clinical utility of APOE genotype in the prediction of outcome in patients with memory impairment. *Neurology, 46*, 149–154.

Twamley, E. W., Ropacki, S. A. L., & Bondi, M. A. (2006). Neuropsychological and neuroimaging changes in preclinical Alzheimer's disease. *Journal of the International Neuropsychological Society, 12*, 707–735.

Visser, P. J. (2003). Diagnosis of predementia AD in a clinical setting. In R. W. Richter & B. Zoeller-Richter (Eds.), *Alzheimer's disease. A physician's guide to practical management* (pp. 157–164). New York, NY: Humana Press.

Whalley, L. J., Starr, J. M., Athawes, R., Hunter, D., Pattie, A., & Deary, I. J. (2000). Childhood mental ability and dementia. *Neurology, 55*, 1455–1459.

4

Alzheimer's Dementia

Alzheimer's Disease (AD) Introduction

Alzheimer's disease (AD) is the most common cause of dementia and the number of affected individuals in the world population is near epidemic proportions (World Health Organization, 2017) with more than 50 million people affected. This number is predicted to increase, reaching 82 million in 2030 and 152 million in 2050! Someone in the world develops dementia every 3 s. In the United States, 5.7 million people are living with AD and it has become the sixth leading cause of death (Alzheimer's Association, 2018). Since the turn of the century, deaths from AD have increased by 123% (Alzheimer's Association, 2018).

The cost of AD is staggering, reaching approximately $277 billion in the United States, a figure that includes direct costs for medical care plus the cost of informal care provided by family and others (Alzheimer's Association, 2018; Alzheimer's Disease International, 2016). More than 15 million Americans provide unpaid care to individuals with dementia. The estimated lifetime cost of care for an individual living with dementia is $341,840 (Alzheimer's Association, 2018).

Diagnosing AD is challenging and is typically made by excluding other conditions associated with cognitive changes. Computer tomography (CT) and magnetic resonance imaging (MRI) are used to rule out tumors, cerebrovascular disease, and normal pressure hydrocephalus, and to detect disease-associated atrophy in the medial temporal lobe and amygdalohippocampal system (Knopman et al., 2001). Increasingly, physicians are using biomarker data from scans, results of blood tests, and analysis of cerebrospinal fluid to make the diagnosis, and, when paired with behavioral data, accuracy is high.

Diagnostic Criteria for AD

Three stages of AD are recognized (Albert et al., 2011): a *preclinical phase* associated with demonstrable changes in biomarkers that occur before memory loss; *mild cognitive impairment (MCI)* that is characterized by measurable changes in cognitive function in which the basic activities of daily living are spared; and *frank dementia*. Because dementia is a syndrome associated with myriad etiologies, core diagnostic criteria exist for *all-cause* dementia that include: (1) cognitive and behavioral symptoms that interfere with the ability to function at work or at usual activities; (2) behavior that represents a decline from previous levels of functioning and is not explained by delirium or major psychiatric disease; and (3) cognitive or behavioral impairment involving at least two of the following: (a) ability to acquire and remember new information, (b) impaired reasoning and handling of complex tasks, (c) poor judgment, (d) impaired visuospatial abilities, and (e) impaired language functions (e.g.,

Probable AD

Meets core criteria for all-cause dementia

Gradual onset over months/years

Demonstrable impairment in at least two cognitive domains (memory, language, visuospatial, executive, or mood or behavioral symptoms)

Amnestic presentation, the most common, is characterized by deficits in the recall of new information

Evidence of progressive worsening of memory and other cognitive functions

Insidious onset and clear history of worsening

Absence of cerebrovascular disease or other neurologic disorders that could affect cognition

Symptoms cannot be explained by delirium or other major psychiatric disorder

Biomarker evidence from MRI, positron emission tomography (PET), and cerebrospinal fluid increases certainty of disease as does evidence of a causative gene

Possible AD

Meets the core clinical criteria for AD, but there is evidence of other systemic or neurologic disorder that could affect cognition

speaking, reading, writing) (Lopez, Mcdade, Riverol, & Becker, 2011; McKhann et al., 2011).

Specific additional clinical features distinguish AD from other disorders and the textbox contains an overview of the criteria for diagnosing *probable* and *possible* Alzheimer's dementia.

Alzheimer's disease affects the processes that sustain neuronal health and ultimately destroys interneuronal communication. Historically, it was thought to begin in the cortex; however, recent evidence indicates that its genesis may be in the locus coeruleus (Braak & Del Tredici, 2011), a nucleus in the pons near the base of the brainstem that is involved with homeostatic mechanisms. In a retrospective study, Braak and Del Tredici observed "pretangle material" in the locus coeruleus in individuals under the age of 30 years. Over time, the disease proliferates in the perirhinal cortex (Figure 4–1), the hippocampal complex in the temporal lobes, and the basal forebrain—areas important to episodic memory (Braak, Braak, & Bohl, 1993; Van Hoesen, 1997). Eventually, struc-

tural changes occur in the frontal, temporal, and parietal lobes. The brain areas most spared are the motor and visual cortices (Farkas et al., 1982; Haxby et al., 1986; Haxby et al., 1990), a fact that accounts for the sparing of speech.

Motor symptoms can develop late in the disease, among them change in muscle tone, cogwheel phenomenon, postural instability, and difficulty walking. Collectively, these motor changes are referred to as "extrapyramidal signs" (Wilson et al., 2000) and their presence is associated with greater dementia severity (Mayeux, Stern, & Spanton, 1985; Soininen, Laulumaa, Helkala, Hartikainen, & Riekkinen, 1992; Stern, Albert, et al., 1994; Stern, Mayeux, Sano, & Hauser, 1987).

When tissue from the brain of an AD patient is examined microscopically, changes are apparent in the form of neuritic plaques, neurofibrillary tangles, atrophy, and areas of granulovacuolar degeneration. Deposits of amyloid within blood vessels may also be seen.

Neuritic plaques (Figure 4–2), called senile plaques in the older literature, are bits and

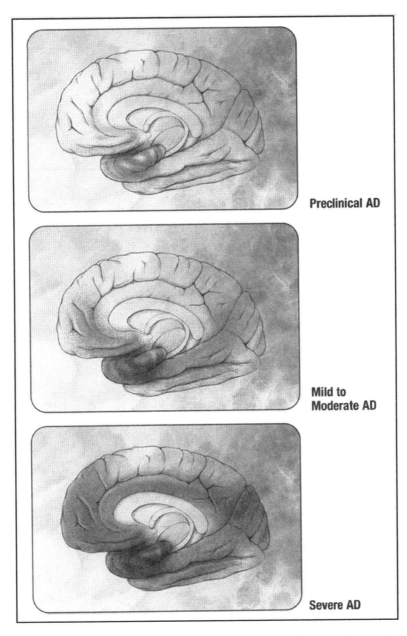

Preclinical AD

Mild to
Moderate AD

Severe AD

Figure 4–1. Brain areas affected by AD over the course of the condition. *Darker shades* indicate areas affected at the various stages of AD. From the National Institute on Aging/National Institutes of Health (2008).

pieces of degenerating neurons that clump together and have an amyloid core. Amyloid-beta is a protein fragment that has been separated from a larger protein called amyloid precursor protein. The disjoined amyloid-beta fragments aggregate and mix with other molecules, neurons, and nonnerve cells. Neuritic plaques are most prevalent in the outer half of the cortex where the number of neuronal connections is largest.

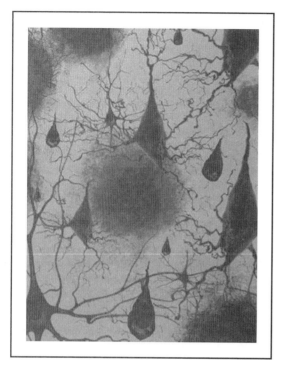

Figure 4–2. Neuritic plaques (*center clump*) and neurofibrillary tangles (*tadpole-shaped bodies*). From the National Institute on Aging/National Institutes of Health (2008).

Neurofibrillary tangles (see Figure 4–2) are disintegrating microtubules (microtubules are part of the internal support structure of healthy neurons). Microtubules disintegrate because of changes in tau protein which binds them and gives them support in healthy brains. Tau is overphosphorylated in AD by enzymes that cause its detachment from the microtubules. As they disintegrate, they become tangled and are a signature morphologic change that confirms the presence of AD.

Atrophy, or the shrinking of tissue, is common in AD (Figures 4–3, 4–4, and 4–5), though it may not be visible on CT scan if the patient is in the early stage of the disease. Positron emission tomography (PET) scans show prominent changes in the temporal and parietal lobes and inconsistent changes in frontal lobes. Magnetic resonance imaging (MRI) shows substantial atrophy in the entorhinal cortex (Krasuski et al.,

1998; Pearlson et al., 1992) and the hippocampal complex (Jack, Petersen, O'Brien, & Tangalos, 1992; Johnson, Saykin, Flashman, & Riordan, 1998).

Granulovacuolar degeneration refers to fluid-filled spaces within cells that contain granular debris. Together these changes (neuritic plaques, neurofibrillary tangles, and granulovacuolar degeneration) in brain cells interrupt intercellular communication and thus information processing.

Risk Factors for AD

The following factors place an individual at increased risk for developing AD:

- Age
- Family history of the disease
- Less education
- Head trauma
- Loneliness
- Gender
- Age of mother at individual's birth
- Having two copies of the type 4 allele of apolipoprotein E
- Lack of consistent and sufficient sleep
- MCI

Age

The greatest risk factor for AD is age, the older you are, the greater the risk (Khachaturian & Radebaugh, 1998). Most individuals with AD are 65 years or older. According to the Alzheimer's Association (2018), the likelihood of developing the disease doubles every five years after age 65.

Family History of AD

People with a first-order relative with AD are four times more likely to develop it; however, the majority of cases are sporadic with

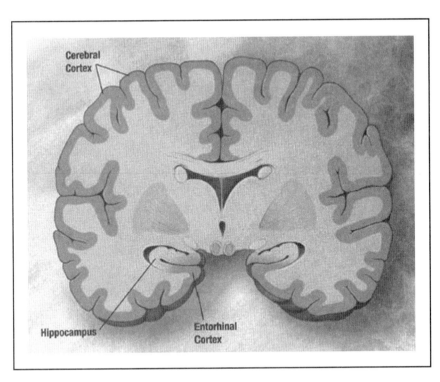

Figure 4–3. Brain regions affected in the preclinical stage of AD. From the National Institute on Aging/ National Institutes of Health (2008).

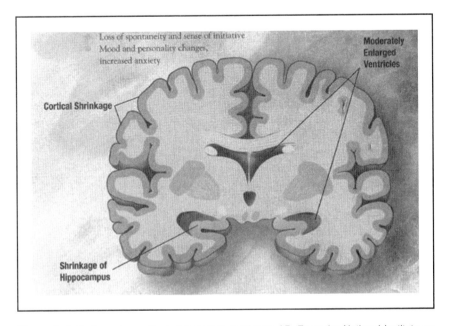

Figure 4–4. Brain regions affected in mild to moderate AD. From the National Institute on Aging/National Institutes of Health (2008).

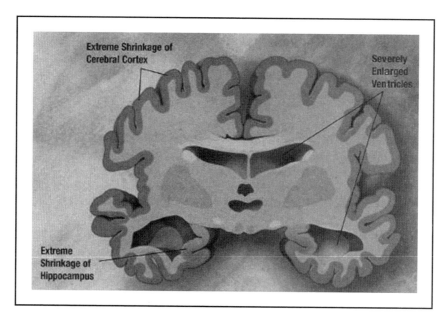

Figure 4–5. Brain regions affected in severe AD. From the National Institute on Aging/National Institutes of Health (2008).

only 5% having familial/autosomal dominant inheritance. Familial AD often develops when individuals are in their 40s and is associated with a more fulminating course (Jacobs, Sano, Marder, & Bell, 1994; Lovestone, 1999; Selkoe, 2000). Results of twin studies indicate that heritability for AD is high. In the 2006 study by Gatz et al., heritability ranged between 58% and 79% depending on the statistical model used, and genes were more influential than environment in accounting for the disease. These percentages are higher than those reported in an earlier study by Breitner and colleagues (1993) who observed that both twins were affected in only 35% to 50% of cases.

Three genes are linked to early-onset AD: the amyloid precursor protein gene on chromosome 21, the presenilin gene 1 on chromosome 14, and the presenilin gene 2 on chromosome 1. Note that the amyloid precursor protein gene is located on the same chromosome that is affected in Down syndrome, chromosome 21. The presenilin gene 1 on chromosome 14 is suspected of being responsible for the majority of early-onset AD cases.

> ## Definitions
>
> *Familial:* Something that occurs in more members of a family than would be expected by chance.
> *Autosomal:* The gene is located on a chromosome other than the sex chromosome, so the disease is not sex linked. Males and females are equally likely to be affected.
> *Dominant:* The defective gene dominates its normal partner gene from the unaffected parent.

Education

Traditionally, having more education was thought to lower your risk of AD (Katzman, 1993; Kawas & Katzman, 1999; Plassman et al., 1995; Sando et al., 2008). The explanation for this view is that educated individuals have a richer network of interneuronal connections and therefore greater cognitive reserve. However, results of a 2011 review of the relation of education to dementia revealed that in 42% of the studies no relation was found (Sharp & Gatz, 2011). Sharp and Gatz describe the education–dementia relationship as strongly tied to the demands of an individual's environment, personality, and life events, such as the nature of their work.

History of Head Trauma

Individuals with prior head injury may be at higher risk for AD (Kawas & Katzman, 1999). Although the specific mechanism underlying the association of AD and head injury is not well understood, scientists theorize that head injury can alter the brain's protective system. Many investigators have addressed the question of the relation of head injury to the development of dementia, but the literature is conflicted. Researchers found head injury to be a risk factor only for those individuals with the APOE e4 allele (Mayeux et al., 1995). However, in a systematic review of case-control studies, Fleminger, Oliver, Lovestone, Rabe-Hesketh, and Giora (2003) reported that head injury was a risk factor for AD but only in males. In a 2012 study by Shively, Scher, Perl, and Diaz-Arrastia, traumatic brain injury was found to be associated with a 2 to 4 fold increased risk of dementia in late life compared with the general population. More recently, results of a review of data from 32 studies representing over 2 million individuals indicated that head injury is associated with increased risk of dementia and AD (Li et al., 2017).

Loneliness

Loneliness is associated with greater risk of AD (Wilson et al., 2007). In a 4-year longitudinal study of the relation of loneliness and social isolation to the presence of dementia, Wilson and colleagues found that cognitive decline more than doubled in lonely persons compared with nonlonely individuals. Wilson and colleagues suggested that the neural systems that support social behavior might be less elaborate in lonely individuals making them less able to compensate for other neural systems being compromised by age and disease-related neuropathology. In fact, forced social isolation is well known to have a deleterious effect on the brains of animals.

Results of a large study in the Netherlands by Tjalling et al. (2014) indicate that feelings of loneliness, rather than social isolation, are associated with dementia onset. They followed 2,173 nondemented, community-dwelling individuals for 3 years who were evaluated for dementia. Feeling lonely, rather than being alone, was associated with an increased risk of dementia.

Gender

Women have higher age-specific prevalence (Hebert et al., 1995; Schoenberg, Anderson, & Haeren, 1985) and incidence (Kokmen, Chandra, & Schoenberg, 1988; McGonigal et al., 1993) of AD than men. In fact, two-thirds of affected individuals are women (Alzheimer's Association, 2018; Hebert, Weuve, Scherr, & Evans, 2013). The gender effect has been attributed to the greater longevity of women (Jagger, Clarke, & Stone, 1995), but research has also shown that the rates of development of atrophy and other biomarkers of AD are earlier in women and cognitive decline occurs faster in women. More research is needed to fully understand why women are more susceptible to AD (Lin & Doraiswamy, 2015).

Maternal Age

The mother's age at the time of one's birth may influence one's risk of developing AD. Both advanced (Cohen, Eisdorfer, & Leverenz, 1982) and early (Van Duijn, Hoffman, & Kay, 1991) maternal age have been reported as influential. The pathogenetic mechanism underlying the association of advanced or early maternal age and AD remains open for speculation.

Apolipoprotein E4 Allele

A type of cholesterol-carrying protein is a known risk factor for late-onset AD, namely, the type 4 allele of apolipoprotein APOE. APOE in the body varies in composition across individuals. The specific composition of APOE is influenced by the presence or absence of three major variants of the gene called e2, e3, and e4. An individual inherits one gene that codes for the APOE protein from each parent. The most common type is APOE e3 and most people inherit one or two copies. People who develop AD more commonly have the APOE e4 allele, and those with two copies of the APOE e4 gene have an **8 times greater risk of developing late-onset** AD than individuals with no copies (Corder et al., 1993). However, almost half the individuals with AD do not have the APOE e4, and the presence of an e4 allele accounts for a relatively small percentage of the cases of AD (Evans et al., 1997; Myers et al., 1996).

Chronic Lack of Sleep

Poor sleep has been linked to higher levels of two Alzheimer's-associated proteins (Pase et al., 2017). Scientists have discovered that during sleep the brain has a waste removal system that removes proteins and other neural waste, such as amyloid-beta that can aggregate and form neuritic plaques (Solan, 2017). Researchers have examined cerebrospinal fluid in individuals who had disturbed sleep and those who had uninterrupted sleep. Both amyloid-beta and tau levels rose with several nights of bad sleep. Moreover, memory consolidation is poorer in individuals with poor sleep (Mander et al., 2015). These findings have raised concern for individuals who have chronic sleep deprivation.

Mild Cognitive Impairment

Although MCI can have many causes and the cognitive status of a significant percentage of affected individuals does not worsen, MCI is recognized as a predementia stage of AD. People with amnestic MCI are more likely to evolve to clinically apparent AD than those with the nonamnestic type.

Predictors of Disease Progression

The **average duration of AD is 8 years**, though many victims suffer for 12 or more years. More rapid decline in AD is linked to:

- Early age at onset
- Presence of delusions or hallucinations
- Presence of extrapyramidal signs

Protective Factors

Besides having a higher level of education, having a socially and cognitively active lifestyle later in life reduces the risk of AD (Weuve et al., 2004). Regular physical exercise also appears to have a neuroprotective effect (Ahlskog, Geda, Graff-Radford, & Petersen, 2011; Etgen et al., 2010; Paillard, Rolland, de Souto Barreto, 2015; Singh-Manoux, Hillsdon, Brunner & Marmot, 2005). A meta-analysis of 15 prospective studies of 33,816 individuals without dementia revealed that moderate and intense exercise reduced the risk of developing MCI by 35% (Pappolla et al., 2003).

Effects of AD on Cognitive and Communicative Functions

As stated in Chapter 3, the onset of AD is insidious and occurs many years before a clinical diagnosis is typically made (Braak, Thal,

Ghebremedhin, & del Tredici, 2011; Collie & Maruff, 2000; Grober, Lipton, Hall, & Crystal, 2000; Hodges, 1998). Early neuropsychological deficits have been demonstrated by investigators using a variety of neuropsychological measures: psychomotor speed (Masur, Sliwinski, Lipton, Blau, & Crystal, 1994), perceptual speed (Rainville, Fabrigoule, Amieva, & Dartigues, 1998), abstract reasoning (Fabrigoule, Lafont, Letenneur, Rouch, & Dartigues, 1996), visuospatial performance (Howieson et al., 1997), verbal ability (Ferris, & Farlow, 2013; Jacobs, Sano, Dooneief, & Marder, 1995; Szatloczki, Hoffmann, Vincze, Kalman, & Pakaski, 2015), and episodic memory (Collie & Maruff, 2000; Grober et al., 2000; Hodges, 1998). Elias and colleagues (2000) reported that lower scores on measures of memory and abstract reasoning are particularly strong predictors of probable AD. Szatloczki and colleagues (2015) emphasize the need for language-based screening as a diagnostic tool for early AD.

The ever-present features of AD are impairment of episodic and working memory, especially executive functions. Other symptoms are more variable and reflect differences in the distribution of neuropathology (Galton, Patterson, Xuereb, & Hodges, 2000; Perry & Hodges, 2000). Some patients have greater visuospatial deficits than language deficits; for others, the reverse is true (Fisher, Rourke, Bieliauskas, & Giordani, 1996; Martin et al., 1986). Those individuals with early-onset AD typically have less hippocampal involvement and greater atrophy in occipital and parietal cortices that results in poorer performance on visuospatial tests than memory tests (Frisoni et al., 2007; Fujimori et al., 1998).

Results of longitudinal studies, using the Mini-Mental Status Examination (MMSE), indicate that the average amount of cognitive decline per year is two to four points (Ballard et al., 2001). On the Alzheimer's Disease Assessment Scale–Cognitive (ADAS-COG; see Clinical Guide Section 1 for description), the average decline is eight points per year (Stern, Mohs, et al., 1994).

Early Stage

As previously stated, the pathophysiologic changes associated with AD begin years before behavioral and cognitive deficits are apparent; thus, specifying the duration of the early stage is problematic. What is known, however, is the median age of survival after medical diagnosis of individuals in their 80s or 90s. Investigators in England followed more than 13,000 men and women aged 65 years and older for 14 years (Xie, Brayne, & Matthews, 2008). In that period, 438 people were diagnosed with dementia, most of whom died. Study results revealed that men did not live as long as women: 4.1 years for men, 4.6 years for women; and frail individuals died earlier than those more physically fit. The investigators concluded that once an individual is medically diagnosed, life expectancy is approximately half that of a healthy individual of the same age.

When caregivers were asked to specify behavioral changes they observed before the diagnosis of AD was made (Bayles, 1991), they reported:

1. difficulty handling finances;
2. memory problems;
3. concentration problems;
4. difficulty with complex tasks;
5. forgetting the location of objects; and
6. decreased awareness of recent events.

Mental Status

In early-stage AD, the affected individual is disoriented for time but not place or person. Table 4–1 shows the average score, or range of scores, of early-stage AD patients on commonly used mental status tests.

Motor Function

Motor function is good and the patient is ambulatory.

Table 4–1. Early Stage AD Scores

ABCD Mental Status Test	7.3–12.5
Mini-Mental State Examination	16–24
Clinical Dementia Rating Scale	1
Global Deterioration Scale	3

Memory Function

The typical first symptom of AD is a problem with episodic memory; for example, forgetting where the car is parked, getting lost, being repetitious, or not remembering having taken medication. Working memory is also affected early and is manifested by decreased efficiency of encoding and retrieval of information. Individuals have difficulty sustaining attention (Bäckman, Small, & Fratiglioni, 2001; Grady et al., 1988; Morris, 1996; Perry, Watson, & Hodges, 2000) and memory span is modestly attenuated in some individuals, though not all.

Activities of Daily Living

Individuals in early-stage AD are generally able to carry out the basic activities of daily living (ADLs), such as bathing, dressing and feeding themselves, and going to the bathroom independently. However, they have difficulty with the instrumental activities of daily living, such as managing their finances.

Linguistic Communication of Individuals with Alzheimer's Dementia

The linguistic communication skills of individuals with mild, moderate and severe Alzheimer's dementia have been well documented. Those whose dementia is mild generally have longer hesitations and a slower speech rate in spontaneous speech (Hoffman et al., 2010; Jarrold et al., 2014; Satt, Hoory, Konig, Aalten, & Robert, 2014). Nonetheless, speech is fluent with no evidence of dysarthria or articulation errors (Weiner, Neubecker, Bret, & Hynan, 2008).

Spoken language is grammatical, though errors of grammar and spelling are common in written language (Blanken, Dittman, Haas, & Wallesch, 1987; Irigaray, 1967). Content of language is noticeably affected and characterized by tangentiality and an increase in the number of "empty words," such as "thing" and "it." Because AD patients often forget what they just heard or thought, their oral discourse contains more sentence fragments and repetitiousness and is less cohesive than the discourse of healthy peers (Bayles, Tomoeda, & Boone, 1985; Bayles, Tomoeda, Kaszniak, Stern, & Eagans, 1985; Tomoeda & Bayles, 1993). Moreover, mildly demented AD patients pause more frequently and have a slower speech rate (Gayraud, Lee, & Barkat-Defradas, 2011). Mild dysnomia is common and when a naming error occurs, it is usually semantically related to the target word (e.g., "lime" for "lemon" and "sharp" for "saw") (Bayles & Tomoeda, 1983a). Performance on tests of receptive vocabulary reveal that vocabulary gradually shrinks over time. Performance on tests of verbal fluency show significant deficits, compared to healthy elders, that worsen as the disease progresses (De Araujo et al., 2011; Henry, Crawford, & Phillips, 2004; Perry et al., 2000; Small & Bäckman, 1998).

Language Use. Writing is more affected than oral language: written discourse contains intrusions, perseverations, and more spatial–mechanical disturbances than that of healthy peers (Appell, Kertesz, & Fisman, 1982; Croisile, 1999; Groves-Wright, Neils-Strunjas, Burnett, O'Neill, 2004; Horner, Heyman, Dawson, & Rogers, 1988; Kertesz, Appell, & Fisman, 1986).

Although individuals with mild Alzheimer's dementia generally comprehend what they hear and read, they quickly forget it (Bayles, Tomoeda, & Trosset, 1992). These individuals are also able to answer most questions and define words (Bayles & Tomoeda, 1993). However, they often miss the point of a joke and may be confused by sarcasm. Some mildly demented individuals exhibit logorrhea (Gus-

Table 4–2. Linguistic Communication Symptoms Listed in Order of Prevalence from Most to Least Frequent

Most Frequent
Word-finding problems
Difficulty naming objects
Difficulty writing a letter
Impaired comprehension of instructions
Difficulty sustaining a conversation
Problem completing sentences
Tendency to repeat ideas
Reading comprehension problems
Production of meaningless sentences
Decrease in talkativeness
Inappropriate topics
Socially inappropriate utterances
Tendency to interpret literally
Failure to recognize humor
Increase in talkativeness
Least Frequent

Source: Bayles & Tomoeda (1991).

tafson, Hagberg, & Ingvar, 1978; Obler & Albert, 1985), perhaps from disinhibition associated with frontal lobe damage.

Table 4–2 presents the linguistic communication symptoms of Alzheimer's patients with mild dementia (Bayles & Tomoeda, 1991) listed in order of prevalence, from most to least frequent, as reported by 99 primary caregivers of AD patients. The most commonly reported symptom was word finding difficulty. The least prevalent was an increase in talkativeness.

Discourse Sample of Mild AD Patient. The following discourse sample is typical of early-stage AD patients. The individual who pro-duced this sample was instructed to explain what is happening in the Norman Rockwell picture entitled, *Easter Morning*. Rockwell portrays a man sitting in the family living room clad in pajamas and looking sheepish because he is not going to church with his wife and three children on Easter Sunday. Rather, he is staying home to read the newspaper, drink coffee, and smoke cigarettes. His wife and children are lined up behind him ready to go out the door.

Sample: Description of the Easter Morning Picture by Individual with Early-Stage AD. It's evidently snowing outside of the window. And it's the mother I guess and the two girls and the boy, they are dressed like going to church, because they each have bibles in their hands. And this lazy goof . . . he sits in the chair and he's got his slipper this way and his eyes go over there. His hair looks like hell. Pardon me. And whatever he's got on, it's ridiculous. And he, he, he is a good person to do that because he can do it. You know. Get his eyes over. And so, eh, he wants to stay home and see the funny papers and the newspapers and I love that Norman Rockwell anyway. And, eh, he's got his eyes almost out of sight. You know. But yet you can get him, he's a terrific guy. And so all these little darlings get to go to church. That's the way I see it because they each have a bible in their hand and, eh, he's looking to see what he can see. And it looks like he's saying, "thank God I don't have to go." Eh, so that's about it.

Notice that the utterances are generally grammatically correct; however, compared with neurologically normal adults, this mild AD patient is a less efficient communicator. Also, she did not express the gist of the picture, namely, that the wife is angry with her husband for staying home and he is feeling sheepish and guilty. The volume of discourse produced is not necessarily less than what a healthy elder would produce, but contains fewer ideas. Early-stage AD patients tend to repeat ideas as did this woman who repeated mention of the father's eyes, going to church, and holding bibles. This phenomenon of *ideational perseveration* occurs more in mild and moderate patients than in severe patients, because by the severe stage, individuals with AD have fewer ideas (Tomoeda, Bayles, Trosset, Azuma, & McGeagh, 1996).

Table 4–3. Middle Stage AD Scores

ABCD Mental Status Test	1.3–7.7
Mini-Mental State Examination	8–15
Clinical Dementia Rating Scale	2
Global Deterioration Scale	4–6

Middle Stage

Many physicians and neuropsychologists define the middle stage of Alzheimer's disease, when individuals have moderately severe dementia, by mental status. Those individuals scoring below 16 on the MMSE are recognized as being in the middle stage of the disease; however, no hard and fast rule exists for defining the difference between the early and middle stage.

Mental Status

In mid-stage AD, the patient changes most dramatically, becoming increasingly dependent on others for survival. Disorientation worsens and includes confusion about place as well as time, although orientation to self is intact. Table 4–3 shows the average scores of mid-stage individuals on widely used mental status tests.

Motor Function

Motor function in mid-stage AD patients remains good, but restlessness is common.

Memory

Many changes occur in memory in mid-stage AD including worsening of episodic memory, attenuation of memory span, encoding and retrieval deficits, and degradation of semantic memory. Mid-stage patients have difficulty focusing attention, are easily distracted, and can be difficult to engage in activities. Visual-perceptual and visual-constructive deficits are apparent and, in fact, AD patients perform inferiorly to healthy peers on virtually all executive function and cognitive-communication tests.

Continence

During the latter portion of mid-stage AD, incontinence of bladder becomes a problem.

Activities of Daily Living

With supervision and environmental support, most mid-stage AD patients can carry out basic ADLs. In contrast, instrumental ADLs, such as taking messages and managing finances are problematic. It is in this stage that driving becomes an issue. Although the mid-stage AD patient can manipulate the controls and mechanically drive a car, problems with attention, judgment, and memory make them dangerous to themselves and others.

Definitions

Activities of daily living (ADLs): Activities routinely performed in the course of an average day such as feeding, bathing, dressing, and grooming.

Instrumental activities of daily living (IADLs): Activities related to independent living such as preparing meals, managing inances, shopping, doing housework, and using the telephone.

Linguistic Communication

Speech. Speech is fluent, though often slower and halting, and filled with more silent pauses that occur outside syntactic boundaries (Gayraud et al., 2011) and on more frequently occurring words.

Form of Language. The form of language remains generally intact but content is prominently affected (Bayles et al., 1992). Oral discourse contains fewer nouns relative to verbs (Blanken et al., 1987; Fung, Chertkow, & Templeman, 2000; Robinson, Rossor, & Cipolotti, 1999), is less cohesive (Critchley, 1964), and can be described as "empty." Performance on vocabulary tests indicates loss of vocabulary and greater degradation of conceptual knowledge (Bayles et al., 1992; Hier, Hagenlocker, & Shindler, 1985; Tomoeda & Bayles, 1993). Mid-stage AD patients are significantly impaired relative to healthy peers in generating exemplars of a category (Bayles et al., 1989; Bayles & Tomoeda, 1983b; Hodges, Salmon, & Butters, 1990; Huff, Corkin, & Growdon, 1986) and naming on confrontation (Bayles et al., 1992). Written language is replete with errors. Mid-stage patients exhibit diminished comprehension of written and spoken language (Bayles, 1982; Cummings, Benson, Hill, & Read, 1985; Faber-Langendoen et al., 1998; Horner, Dawson, Heyman, & McGorman-Fish, 1992; Kempler, Almor, Tyler, Anderssen, & Macdonald, 1998; Rochon, Waters, & Caplan, 2000), although most do well at the word and phrase level. The mechanics of reading are spared, but comprehension is impaired and that which is comprehended is rapidly forgotten.

Language Use. Word-finding difficulties are more obvious in spontaneous speech and on confrontation and generative naming tests (Bayles & Tomoeda, 1983b; Benson, 1979; Kirshner, Webb, & Kelly, 1984; Salmon, Butters, & Chan, 1999; Weiner et al., 2008). Ideational repetition (Bayles et al., 1985) is frequent in conversation and when individuals are asked to describe a picture or object. Mid-stage patients

have poor sensitivity to context (Tomoeda et al., 1996) and may miss the point of jokes. Also, they have a tendency to interpret nonliteral language literally. Although able to perform the mechanics of reading aloud, comprehend written language at the word level, and follow simple commands, mid-stage patients have serious difficulty defining words and repeating phrases (Bayles & Tomoeda, 1993). In terms of writing, mid-stage patients make many spelling errors and mechanical distortions (Neils-Strunjas, Groves-Wright, Mashima, & Harnish, 2006) and their narratives are less complex.

Discourse Samples of Moderately Demented AD Patients

Sample 1: Task: Description of the Easter Morning Picture. Yeah, well, this man is, knows that he is, is in the wrong place here. So, but he's hiding away and, and these other people, I don't know whether this boy is ready to do it or not but this man is doing it from someplace over here, but it won't do it. And, ah, these, these, two children are evidently are just very excellent that they are both the same person. And, this man I don't know, would rather . . . He gets his too. And uh, oh, he's got this thing, worried because it's going to have a . . . going up there, you can see it. (Subject points to the cigarette smoke in the picture). And all this stuff is just a mess. Darn fools got anybody. Darn fools got them walking in it. They want to, I don't think they do. I don't want to go in this place. I don't know what he's for. He's looks like he's getting a ten paper. Here's some more paper. Here's some more, my God! Look at it. He has to be worn down before he can do anything, 'cause these people don't want to work, work anything with him. Don't you think that's about right?

Sample 2: Task: Individual Is Describing a Marble. Literally speaking, a marble. And the white is uh, is, uh, is the harder part. Well, it's a, I'd say cassium. The colored part, I don't know. Associated rocks. This is, uh, this is of the granitic nature. The whole thing. When you say cassium you're, you're talking about the hardest part of a, of a, of a rock. Well, there's some design to it. Some reason how it took that shape. But, uh, that doesn't mean a whole lot, exactly, the way someone de-, designed it.

As is apparent from these language samples, moderately demented AD patients produce discourse that expresses significantly fewer ideas than those with mild dementia. They are increasingly less concise and more repetitious. Intentions are often forgotten resulting in many sentence fragments. As did the mildly demented patient, the individual who produced this discourse failed to state the gist of the Rockwell picture. The intention to describe remains, but word sequences often have little apparent meaning. Furthermore, there is a lack of self-monitoring and self-correction.

Late Stage

During the late stage, AD patients often become disoriented for person as well as place and time. Their MMSE scores range from 0 to 9 (Folstein, Folstein, & McHugh, 1975); on the Clinical Dementia Rating Scale, they score 3 (Hughes et al., 1982). Intellect is devastated by a global failure of working and declarative memory systems and individuals are unable to carry out basic ADLs. There is incontinence of bladder and, later, bowel. Motor impairment may be present and, in the very late stage, many are nonambulatory.

Linguistic Communication

Speech is typically fluent but generally slower and more halting. In many patients, the form of language remains intact (Bayles, Tomoeda, Cruz, & Mahendra, 2000; Mayhew, Acton, Yauk, & Hopkins, 2001), although meaningful output is greatly reduced (Appell et al., 1982). Some individuals are mute, others exhibit palilalia (repetition of phrases, words, or syllables that tend to increase in speed at the end of an utterance) (Appell et al., 1982), echolalia (Irigaray, 1967), or jargon (Obler & Albert, 1984); however, other advanced patients can

contribute to a conversation, state their name, and retain aspects of social language (Kim & Bayles, 2007). Reading comprehension is severely impaired, though some can read single words aloud (Bayles et al., 2000; Bayles & Tomoeda, 1994). Virtually all late-stage patients are unable to express themselves in writing.

Communicative Abilities of Late-Stage AD Patients. As part of an NIH-supported longitudinal study of individuals with AD, Bayles and colleagues evaluated communication skills, using the Functional Linguistic Communication Inventory (FLCI) (Bayles & Tomoeda, 1994), of 49 late-stage patients for whom there were data about continence and ability to walk. The FLCI evaluates greeting and naming, question answering, writing, sign comprehension and object-to-picture matching, word reading and comprehension, ability to reminisce, follow commands, pantomime, gesture, and converse. Study results revealed that AD patients who were *incontinent only for bladder* had more communication skills than individuals who were bladder and bowel incontinent. They were able to respond appropriately when greeted and to a closing comment and compliment. Several of them could recognize the written form of their name, state their spouse's name, recognize a common object from a line drawing, follow a one-step command, and even correct misinformation about themselves.

None of the individuals who were *incontinent for both bladder and bowel* were able to contribute to a conversation. Neither could they state their spouse's name, follow a one-step command, or provide relevant information about a common object. The most limited language was observed in individuals who were bowel and bladder incontinent *and* bedridden; however, contrary to what was expected, given previous characterizations of the verbal ability of late-stage AD patients (Reisberg et al., 1984; Reisberg, Ferris, De Leon, & Crooke, 1982), *82% of the study participants produced language during the evaluation.*

The incontinent but ambulatory patients produced more words than those who were incontinent and nonambulatory. Of the 10 individuals who were incontinent but ambulatory, one AD participant produced 252 words and another produced a single word. Of the 17 individuals who were incontinent and nonambulatory, three individuals were nonverbal, two produced a single word, and one produced 131 words, of which 82 were different words.

The following are examples of answers provided by severely demented study participants to questions such as, "Where would you like to go on a trip?" and "What is your favorite food?"

"Right now I think I'd like to see Hawaii."

"Fruit of all kind is all right with me; I love fruit."

"I don't think I ought to go anywhere because I'm in bad shape."

"I eat a lot of things now."

Discourse Samples of Severely Demented AD Patients

Sample 1: Task: Description of a Button.

Examiner: Tell me all about this [button].

Patient: Well, it's a button, with two holes in it for . . . for sewing on thread. That's the only . . .

Examiner: Can you tell me anything else?

Patient: Uh, that's the only thing I can see.

Sample 2: Task: Description of a Nail.

Examiner: Tell me about this [nail].

Patient: That's a shingle nail. That's for tack on shingles and tack on roofing, and to tack on uh, uh, it's, er a plasterboard.

Examiner: Can you describe it to me?

Patient: You mean this nail? Yeah, it's long, short, small. That's uh, that about all . . .

As you can see, meaningful verbal output has diminished dramatically; however, grammar is generally intact. Without a context, listeners often have difficulty understanding what the AD patient is saying.

Summary of Important Points

- AD is the most common cause of dementia.
- The near epic number of affected individuals worldwide is a global concern.
- Three stages of AD are recognized: a preclinical phase, MCI (no dementia), and frank dementia.
- The key diagnostic criterion for diagnosis of dementia is the presence of multiple cognitive deficits sufficient to interfere with communicative function as well as social and occupational functioning.
- The onset of the disease is gradual and progressive in nature, spanning many years.
- AD begins in brain areas important to episodic memory and spreads to areas important to working and declarative memory. Procedural memory is spared until late in the disease course.
- The characteristic morphologic changes in the brain are neuritic plaques and neurofibrillary tangles with areas of granulovacuolar degeneration and atrophy.
- The greatest risk factor for AD is age.
- AD rarely affects individuals younger than 60 years, but for every decade thereafter, the number of individuals with AD doubles.
- A small number of individuals develop familial AD in their 40s, an autosomal dominant form of the disease.
- A type of cholesterol-carrying protein has been found to be a major risk factor for late-onset AD; namely, the type 4 allele of apolipoprotein E.
- Chronic sleep deprivation results in neural waste accumulating in the brain that may contribute to likelihood of AD.
- Higher education and a socially active and cognitively stimulating life appear to reduce the risk of AD.
- A diagnosis of AD reduces life expectancy to one-half that for healthy individuals of a similar age.

- Several types of cognitive deficits appear early, but the best known early symptom is a deficit in episodic memory.
- Because of the relation of communication to cognition, communicative function is affected early and is increasingly being recognized as an important early symptom of neurodegenerative disease.
- Communicative ability gradually deteriorates over the disease course. In the early stages of Alzheimer's dementia, individuals are verbally fluent and able to comprehend most of what they read and hear, but rapidly forget recently acquired information. By end-stage disease, individuals are intellectually devastated and language output is greatly diminished and often nonsensical.
- Semantics and pragmatics are affected early; phonology and syntax are generally preserved well into the disease course.
- Longer hesitations and a slower speech rate are common in the MCI phase.
- Writing is more affected than oral language.
- Considerable variability exists in the ability of late-stage AD patients to communicate—some are mute, others produce some meaningful language.

References

Ahlskog, J. E., Geda, Y. E., Graff-Radford, N. R., & Petersen, R. C. (2011). Physical exercise as a preventive or disease-modifying treatment of dementia and brain aging. *Mayo Clinic Proceedings, 86,* 976–884.

Albert, M. S., DeKosky, S. T., Dickson, D., Dubois, B., Feldman, H. H., Fox, N. C., . . . Phelps, C. H. (2011). The diagnosis of mild cognitive impairment due to Alzheimer's disease: Recommendations from the National Institute on Aging–Alzheimer's Association workgroups on diagnostic guidelines for Alzheimer's disease. *Alzheimer's and Dementia, 7,* 270–279.

Alzheimer's Association. (2018). Alzheimer's disease facts and figures. *Alzheimer's and Dementia, 14,* 367–429.

Alzheimer's Disease International. (2016). *World Alzheimer's Report 2016: Improving healthcare for people living with dementia.* London, UK: Author.

Appell, J., Kertesz, A., & Fisman, M. (1982). A study of language functioning in Alzheimer's patients. *Brain and Language, 17,* 73–91.

Bäckman, L., Small, B. J., & Fratiglioni, L. (2001). Stability of the preclinical episodic memory deficit in Alzheimer's disease. *Brain, 124,* 96–102.

Ballard, C., O'Brien, J., Morris, C. M., Barber, R., Swann, A., Neill, D., & McKeith, I. (2001). The progression of cognitive impairment in dementia with Lewy bodies, vascular dementia and Alzheimer's disease. *International Journal of Geriatric Psychiatry, 16,* 499–503.

Bayles, K. A. (1982). Language function in senile dementia. *Brain and Language, 16,* 265–280.

Bayles, K. A. (1991). Alzheimer's disease symptoms: Prevalence and order of appearance. *Journal of Applied Gerontology, 10,* 419–430.

Bayles, K. A., Salmon, D. P., Tomoeda, C. K., Jacobs, D., Caffrey, J. T., Kaszniak, A. W., & Tröstor, A. I. (1989). Semantic and letter category naming in Alzheimer's patients: A predictable difference. *Developmental Neuropsychology, 5,* 335–347.

Bayles, K. A., & Tomoeda, C. K. (1983a). Confrontation naming impairment in dementia. *Brain and Language, 19,* 98–114.

Bayles, K. A., & Tomoeda, C. K. (1983b). Confrontation naming and generative naming abilities of dementia patients. In R. Brookshire (Ed.), *Clinical aphasiology conference proceedings 1983* (pp. 304–315). Minneapolis, MN: BRK Publications.

Bayles, K. A., & Tomoeda, C. K. (1991). Caregiver report of prevalence and appearance order of linguistic symptoms in Alzheimer's patients. *The Gerontologist, 31,* 210–216.

Bayles, K. A., & Tomoeda, C. K. (1993). *Arizona Battery for Communication Disorders of Dementia.* Austin, TX: Pro-Ed.

Bayles, K. A., & Tomoeda, C. K. (1994). *Functional Linguistic Communication Inventory.* Austin, TX: Pro-Ed.

Bayles, K. A., Tomoeda, C. K., & Boone, D. R. (1985). A view of age-related changes in language function. *Developmental Neuropsychology, 1,* 231–264.

Bayles, K. A., Tomoeda, C. K., Cruz, R. F., & Mahendra, N. (2000). Communication abilities of individuals with late-stage Alzheimer's disease. *Alzheimer's Disease and Associated Disorders, 14,* 176–181.

Bayles, K. A., Tomoeda, C. K., Kaszniak, A. W., Stern, L. Z., & Eagans, K. K. (1985). Patterns of perseveration of dementia patients. *Brain and Language, 25,* 102–116.

Bayles, K. A., Tomoeda, C. K., & Trosset, M. W. (1992). Relation of linguistic communication abilities of Alzheimer's patients to stage of disease. *Brain and Language, 42,* 454–472.

Benson, D. F. (1979). Neurologic correlates of anomia. In H. Whitaker & H. A. Whitaker (Eds.), *Studies in neurolinguistics* (pp. 298–328). New York, NY: Academic Press.

Blanken, G., Dittmann, J., Haas, J., & Wallesch, C. (1987). Spontaneous speech in senile dementia and aphasia: Implications for a neurolinguistic model of language production. *Cognition, 27,* 247–274.

Braak, H., Braak, E., & Bohl, J. (1993). Staging of Alzheimer-related cortical destruction. *European Neurology, 33*, 403–408.

Braak, H., & Del Tredici, K. (2011). The pathological process underlying Alzheimer's disease in individuals under thirty. *Acta Neuropathologica, 121*, 171–181.

Braak, H., Thal, D. R., Ghebremedhin, E., & Del Tredici, K. (2011). Stages of the pathologic process in Alzheimer disease: Age categories from 1 to 100 years. *Journal of Neuropathology and Experimental Neurology, 11*, 960–969.

Breitner, J. C. S., Gatz, M., Bergem, A. L. M., Christian, J. C., Mortimer, J. A., Mcclearn, G. E., . . . Radebaugh, T. S. (1993). Use of twin cohorts for research in Alzheimer's disease. *Neurology, 43*, 261–267.

Cohen, D., Eisdorfer, C., & Leverenz, J. (1982). Alzheimer's disease and maternal age. *Journal of the American Geriatrics Society, 30*, 656–659.

Collie, A., & Maruff, P. (2000). The neuropsychology of preclinical Alzheimer's disease and mild cognitive impairment. *Neuroscience and Biobehavioral Reviews, 24*, 365–374.

Corder, E. H., Saunders, A. M., Strittmatter, W. J., Schmechel, D. E., Gaskell, P. C., Small, G. W., . . . Pericak-Vance, M. A. (1993). Gene dose of apolipoprotein e type 4 allele and the risk of Alzheimer's disease in late onset families. *Science, 261*, 921–923.

Critchley, M. (1964). The neurology of psychotic speech. *British Journal of Psychiatry, 110*, 353–364.

Croisile, B. (1999). Agraphia in Alzheimer's disease. *Dementia and Geriatric Cognitive Disorders, 10*, 226–230.

Cummings, J., Benson, F., Hill, M., & Read, S. (1985). Aphasia in dementia of the Alzheimer type. *Neurology, 35*, 394–397.

De Araujo, N. B., Barca, M. L., Engedal, K., Coutinho, E. S. F., Deslandes, A. C., & Laks, J. (2011). Verbal fluency in Alzheimer's disease, Parkinson's disease, and major depression. *Clinics (Sao Paulo, Brazil), 66*, 623–627.

Elias, M. F., Beiser, A., Wolf, P. A., Au, R., White, R. F., & D'Agostino, R. B. (2000). The preclinical phase of Alzheimer disease: A 22-year prospective study of the Framingham cohort. *Archives of Neurology, 57*, 808–813.

Etgen, T., Sander, D., Huntgeburth, U., Poppert, H., Förstl, H., & Bickel, H. (2010). Physical activity and incident cognitive impairment in elderly persons: the INVADE study. *Archives of Internal Medicine, 170*, 186–193.

Evans, D. A., Beckett, L. A., Field, T. S., Feng, L., Albert, M. S., Bennett, D. A., . . . Mayeux, R. (1997). Apolipoprotein epsilon4 and incidence of Alzheimer disease in a community population of older persons. *Journal of the American Medical Association, 277*, 822–824.

Faber-Langendoen, K., Morris, J. C., Knesevich, J. W., LaBarge, E., Miller, J. P., & Berg, L. (1998). Aphasia in senile dementia of the Alzheimer type. *Annals of Neurology, 23*, 365–370.

Fabrigoule, C., Lafont, S., Letenneur, L., Rouch, I., & Dartigues, J. F. (1996). WAIS similarities subtest performance as predictors of dementia in elderly community residents. *Brain and Cognition, 30*, 323–326.

Farkas, T., Ferris, S. H., Wolf, A. P., De Leon, M. J., Christmas, D. R., Reisberg, B., . . . Reivich, M. (1982). (18F) F2-deoxy-2-fluoro-D-glucose as a tracer in positron emission tomographic study of senile dementia. *American Journal of Psychiatry, 139*, 352–353.

Ferris, S. H., & Farlow, M. (2013). Language impairment in Alzheimer's disease and benefits of acetylcholinesterase inhibitors. *Clinical Interventions in Aging, 8*, 1007–1014.

Fisher, N., Rourke, B., Bieliauskas, L., & Giordani, B. (1996). Neuropsychological subgroups of patients with Alzheimer's disease. *Journal of Clinical and Experimental Neuropsychology, 18*, 349–370.

Fleminger, S., Oliver, D., Lovestone, S., Rabe-Hesketh, S., & Giora, A. (2003). Head injury as a risk factor for Alzheimer's disease: The evidence 10 years on; a partial replication. *Journal of Neurology and Neurosurgery, 74*, 857–862.

Folstein, M. F., Folstein, S. E., & McHugh, P. R. (1975). "Mini-Mental State": A practical method for grading the mental state of patients for the clinician. *Journal of Psychiatric Research, 12*, 189–198.

Frisoni, G. B., Pievani, M., Testa, C., Sabattoli, F., Bresciani, L., Bonetti, M., . . . Thompson, P. M. (2007). The topography of grey matter involvement in early and late onset Alzheimer's disease. *Brain, 130*, 720–730.

Fujimori M., Imamura T., Yamashita H., Hirono N., Ikejiri Y., Shimomura T., & Mori, E. (1998). Age at onset and visuocognitive disturbances in Alzheimer disease. *Alzheimer's Disease and Associated Disorders, 12*, 163–166.

Fung, T., Chertkow, H., & Templeman, F. (2000). Pattern of semantic memory impairment in dementia of Alzheimer's type. *Brain and Cognition, 43*, 200–205.

Galton, C., Patterson, K., Xuereb, J., & Hodges, J. (2000). Atypical and typical presentations of Alzheimer's disease: A clinical neuropsychological, neuroimaging and pathological study of 13 cases. *Brain, 123*, 484–498.

Gatz, M., Reynolds, C. A., Fratiglioni, L., Johansson, B., Mortimer, J. A., Berg, S., . . . Pedersen, N. L. (2006). Role of genes and environments for explaining alzheimer disease. *Archives General Psychiatry, 63*, 168–174.

Gayraud, F., Lee, H.-R., & Barkat-Defradas, M. (2011). Syntactic and lexical context of pauses and hesitations in the discourse of Alzheimer's patients and healthy elderly subjects. *Clinical Linguistics and Phonetics, 25*, 198–209.

Grady, C., Haxby, J., Horwitz, B., Sundaram, M., Berg, G., Schapiro, M., . . . Rapoport, S. I. (1988). Longitudinal study of the early neuropsychological and cerebral metabolic changes in dementia of the Alzheimer type. *Journal of Clinical and Experimental Neuropsychology, 10*, 576–596.

Grober, E., Lipton, R., Hall, C., & Crystal, H. (2000). Memory impairment on free and cued selective reminding predicts dementia. *Neurology, 54*, 827–832.

Groves-Wright, K., Neils-Strunjas, J., Burnett, R., & O'Neill, M. J. (2004). A comparison of verbal and written language in Alzheimer's disease. *Journal of Communication Disorders, 37*, 109–130.

Gustafson, L., Hagberg, B., & Ingvar, D. (1978). Speech disturbances in presenile dementia related to local cerebral blood flow abnormalities in the dominant hemisphere. *Brain and Language, 5*, 103–118.

Haxby, J. V., Grady, C. L., Duara, R., Schlageter, N., Berg, G., & Rapoport, S. I. (1986). Neocortical metabolic abnormalities precede non-memory cognitive defects in early Alzheimer-type dementia. *Archives of Neurology, 43*, 882–885.

Haxby, J. V., Grady, C. L., Koss, E., Holtz, B., Heston, L., Shapiro, M., . . . Rapoport, S. I. (1990). Longitudinal study of cerebral metabolic asymmetries and associated neuropsychological patterns in early dementia of the Alzheimer type. *Archives of Neurology, 47*, 753–760.

Hebert, L. E., Scherr, P. A., Beckett, L. A., Albert, M. S., Pilgrim, D. M., Chown, M. J., ... Evans, D. A. (1995). Age-specific incidence of Alzheimer's disease in a community population. *Journal of the American Medical Association, 273*, 1354–1359.

Hebert, L. E., Weuve, J., Scherr, P. A., & Evans, D. A. (2013). Alzheimer disease in the United States (2010–2050) estimated using the 2010 census. *Neurology, 80*, 1778–1783.

Henry, J. D., Crawford, J. R., & Phillips, L. H., (2004). Verbal fluency performance in dementia of the Alzheimer's type: A meta-analysis. *Neuropsychologia, 42*, 1212–1222.

Hier, D., Hagenlocker, K., & Shindler, A. (1985). Language disintegration in dementia: Effects of etiology and severity. *Brain and Language, 25*, 117–133.

Hodges, J. (1998). The amnestic prodrome of Alzheimer's disease. *Brain, 121*, 1601–1602.

Hodges, J., Salmon, D., & Butters, N. (1990). Differential impairment of semantic and episodic memory in Alzheimer's and Huntington's diseases: A controlled prospective study. *Journal of Neurology, Neurosurgery and Psychiatry, 53*, 1089–1095.

Hoffmann, I., Nemeth, D., Dye, C.D., Pákáski, M., Irinyi, M., & Kálmán, J. (2010). Temporal parameters of spontaneous speech in Alzheimer's disease. *International Journal of Speech-Language Pathology, 12*, 1.

Horner, J., Dawson, D., Heyman, A., & McGorman-Fish, A. (1992). The usefulness of the Western Aphasia Battery for differential diagnosis of Alzheimer dementia and focal stroke syndromes: Preliminary evidence. *Brain and Language, 42*, 77–88.

Horner, J., Heyman, A., Dawson, D., & Rogers, H. (1988). The relationship of agraphia to the severity of dementia in Alzheimer's disease. *Archives of Neurology, 45*, 760–763.

Howieson, D. B., Dame, A., Camicioli, R., Sexton, G., Payami, H., & Kaye, J. A. (1997). Cognitive markers preceding Alzheimer's dementia in the healthy oldest old. *Journal of the American Geriatrics Society, 45*, 584–589.

Huff, F., Corkin, S., & Growdon, J. (1986). Semantic impairment and anomia in Alzheimer's disease. *Brain and Language, 28*, 235–249.

Hughes, C. P., Berg, L., Danziger, W. L., Coben, L. A., & Martin, R. L. (1982). A new clinical scale for the staging of dementia. *British Journal of Psychiatry, 140*, 566–572.

Irigaray, L. (1967). Approche psycho-linguistique du langage des dements. *Neuropsychologia, 5*, 25–52.

Jack Jr., C. R., Petersen, R. C., O'Brien, P. C., & Tangalos, E. G. (1992). MR-based hippocampal volumetry in diagnosis of Alzheimer's disease. *Neurology, 42*, 183–188.

Jacobs, D., Sano, M., Dooneief, G., & Marder, K. (1995). Neuropsychological detection and characterization of preclinical Alzheimer's disease. *Neurology, 45*, 957–962.

Jacobs, D., Sano, M., Marder, K., & Bell, K. (1994). Age at onset of Alzheimer's disease: Relation to pattern of cognitive dysfunction and rate of decline. *Neurology, 44*, 1215–1220.

Jagger, C., Clarke, M., & Stone, A. (1995). Predictors of survival with Alzheimer's disease: A community-based study. *Psychological Medicine, 25*, 171–177.

Jarrold, W., Peintner, B., Wilkins, D., Vergryi, D., Richey, C., Gorno-Tempini, M. L., & Ogar, J. (2014). Aided diagnosis of dementia type through computer-based analysis of spontaneous speech. *Proceedings of Computational Linguistics and Clinical Psychology*, (Baltimore, MDO), pp. 27–37.

Johnson, S. C., Saykin, A. J., Flashman, L. A., & Riordan, H. J. (1998). Reduction of hippocampal formation in Alzheimer's disease and correlation with memory: A meta-analysis. *Journal of the International Neuropsychological Society, 4*, 22.

Katzman, R. (1993). Education and the prevalence of dementia and Alzheimer's disease. *Neurology, 43*, 13–20.

Kawas, C. H., & Katzman, R. (1999). Epidemiology of dementia and Alzheimer disease. In R. D. Terry, R. Katzman, K. L. Bick, & S. S. Sisodia (Eds.), *Alzheimer disease* (pp. 95–116). Philadelphia, PA: Lippincott Williams & Wilkins.

Kempler, D., Almor, A., Tyler, L., Andersen, E., & Macdonald, M. (1998). Sentence comprehension deficits in Alzheimer's disease: A comparison of off-line vs. on-line sentence processing. *Brain and Language, 64*, 297–316.

Kertesz, A., Appell, J., & Fisman, M. (1986). The dissolution of language in Alzheimer's disease. *Canadian Journal of Neurological Science, 13*, 415–418.

Khachaturian, Z. S., & Radebaugh, T. S. (1998). AD: Where are we now? Where are we going? *Alzheimer Disease and Associated Disorders, 12*, 24–28.

Kim, E. S., & Bayles, K. A. (2007). Communication in late-stage Alzheimer's disease: Relation to functional markers of disease severity. *Alzheimer's Care Quarterly, 8*, 43–52.

Kirshner, H., Webb, W., & Kelly, M. (1984). The naming disorder of dementia. *Neuropsychologia, 22*, 23–30.

Knopman, D. S., DeKosky, S. T., Cummings, J. L., Chui, H., Corey-Bloom, J., Relkin, N., . . . Stevens, J. C. (2001).

Practice parameters: diagnosis of dementia (an evidence-based review). Report of the Quality Standards Subcommittee of the American Academy of Neurology. *Neurology, 56*, 1143–1153.

Kokmen, E., Chandra, V., & Schoenberg, B. S. (1988). Trends in incidence of dementing illness in Rochester, Minnesota, in three quinquennial periods, 1960–1974. *Neurology, 38*, 975–980.

Krasuski, J. S., Alexander, G. E., Horwitz, B., Daly D. M., Murphy, D. G., Rapoport, S. I., & Shapiro, M. B. (1998). Volumes of medial temporal lobe structures in patients with Alzheimer's disease and mild cognitive impairment (and in healthy controls). *Biological Psychiatry, 42*, 60–68.

Li, Y., Li, Y., Li, X., Zhang, S., Zhao, J., Zhu, X., Tian, G. (2017). Head injury as a risk factor for dementia and Alzheimer's disease: A systematic review and meta-analysis of 32 observational studies. *PLoS One, 12*(1), e0169650. doi: 10.1371/journal.pone.0169650.

Lin, A. L., & Doraiswamy, P. M. (2015). When Mars versus Venus is not a cliché: Gender differences in the neurobiology of Alzheimer's disease. *Frontiers in Neurology, 5*, 288.

Lopez, O. L., Mcdade, E., Riverol, M., & Becker, J. T. (2011). Evolution of the diagnostic criteria for degenerative and cognitive disorders. *Current Opinion in Neurology, 24*, 532–541.

Lovestone, S. (1999). Early diagnosis and the clinical genetics of Alzheimer's disease. *Journal of Neurology, 246*, 69–72.

Mander, B. A., Marks, S. M., Vogel, J. W., Rao, V., Lu, B., Saletin, J. M., . . . Walker, M. P. (2015). Beta-amyloid disupts human NREM slow waves and related hippocampus-dependent memory consolidation. *Nature Neuroscience, 18*, 1051–1057.

Martin, A., Brouwers, P., Lalonde, F., Cox, C., Teleska, P., Fedio, P., . . . Chase, T. N. (1986). Towards a behavioral typology of Alzheimer's patients. *Journal of Clinical and Experimental Neuropsychology, 8*, 594–610.

Masur, D. M., Sliwinski, M., Lipton, R. B., Blau, A. D., & Crystal, H. A. (1994). Neuropsychological prediction of dementia and the absence of dementia in healthy elderly persons. *Neurology, 44*, 1427–1432.

Mayeux, R., Ottman, R., Maestre, G., Ngai, C., Tang, M. X., Ginsberg, H., . . . Shelanski, M. (1995). Synergistic effects of traumatic head injury and apolipoprotein-e4 in patients with Alzheimer's disease. *Neurology, 45*, 555–557.

Mayeux, R., Stern, Y., & Spanton, S. (1985). Heterogeneity in dementia of the Alzheimer type: Evidence of subgroups. *Neurology, 35*, 453–461.

Mayhew, P. A., Acton, G. J., Yauk, S., & Hopkins, B. A. (2001). Communication from individuals with advanced DAT: Can it provide clues to their sense of self-awareness and well-being? *Geriatric Nursing, 22*, 106–110.

McGonigal, G., Thomas, B., McQuade, C., Starr, J. M., MacLennan, W. J., & Whalley, L. J. (1993). Epidemiology of Alzheimer's presenile dementia in Scotland, 1974–88. *British Medical Journal, 306*, 680–683.

McKhann, G. M., Knopman, D. S., Chertkow, H., Hyman, B. T., Jack Jr., C. R., Kawas, C. H., . . . Phelps, C. H. (2011). The diagnosis of dementia due to Alzheimer's disease: Recommendations from the National Institute on Aging–Alzheimer's Association workgroups on diagnostic guidelines for Alzheimer's disease. *Alzheimer's and Dementia, 7*, 263–269.

Morris, R. G. M. (1996). Attentional and executive dysfunction. In R. G. M. Morris (Ed.), *The cognitive neuropsychology of Alzheimer-type dementia* (pp. 49–70). New York, NY: Oxford University Press.

Myers, R. H., Schaefer, E. J., Wilson, P. W. F., D'Agostino, R., Ordovas, J. M., Espino, A., . . . Wolf, P. A. (1996). Apolipoprotein E epsilon 4 association with dementia in a population-based study: The Framingham study. *Neurology, 46*, 673–677.

National Institute on Aging. (2008). *Alzheimer's disease: Unraveling the mystery.* (NIH Publication 08-3782). Silver Spring, MD: Alzheimer's Disease Education and Referral (ADEAR) Center.

Neils-Strunjas, J., Groves-Wright, K., Mashima, P., & Harnish, S. (2006). Dysgraphia in Alzheimer's disease: A review for clinical and research purposes. *Journal of Speech Language Hearing Research, 49*, 1313–1330.

Obler, L. K., & Albert, M. L. (1984). Language in aging. In M. L. Albert (Ed.), *Clinical neurology of aging* (pp. 245–252). New York, NY: Oxford University Press.

Obler, L. K., & Albert, M. L. (1985). Historical notes: Jules Séglas on language in dementia. *Brain and Language, 24*, 314–325.

Paillard, T., Rolland, Y., & de Souto Barreto, P. (2015). Protective effects of physical exercise in Alzheimer's disease and Parkinson's disease: A narrative review. *Journal of Clinical Neurology, 11*, 212–219.

Pappolla, M. A., Bryant-Thomas, T. K., Herbert, D., Pacheco, J., Fabra Garcia, M., Manjon, M., . . . Refolo, L. M. (2003). Mild hypercholesterolemia is an early risk factor for the development of Alzheimer amyloid pathology. *Neurology, 61*, 199–205.

Pase, M. P., Himali, J.J., Grima, N.A., Beiser, A.S., Satizabal, C.L., Aparicio, H.J., . . . Seshadri, S. (2017). Sleep architecture and the risk of incident dementia in the community. *Neurology, 89*, 1244–1250.

Pearlson, G. D., Harris, G. J., Powers, R. E., Barta, P. E., Camargo, E. E., Chase, G. A., . . . Tune, L. E. (1992). Quantitative changes in mesial temporal volume, regional cerebral blood flow, and cognition in Alzheimer's disease. *Archives of General Psychiatry, 49*, 402–408.

Perry, R., Watson, P., & Hodges, J. (2000). The nature and staging of attention dysfunction in early (minimal and mild) Alzheimer's disease: Relationship to episodic and semantic memory impairment. *Neuropsychologia, 38*, 252–271.

Perry, R. J., & Hodges, J. R. (2000). Relationship between functional and neuropsychological performance in early

Alzheimer disease. *Alzheimer Disease and Associated Disorders, 14*, 1–10.

Plassman, B. L., Welsh, K. A., Helms, M., Brandt, J., Page, W. F., & Breitner, J. C. S. (1995). Intelligence and education as predictors of cognitive state in late life: A 50-year follow-up. *Neurology, 45*, 1446–1450.

Rainville, C., Fabrigoule, C., Amieva, H., & Dartigues, J. F. (1998). Problem-solving deficits in patients with dementia of the Alzheimer's type on a tower of London task. *Brain and Cognition, 37*, 135.

Reisberg, G., Ferris, S. H., Anand, R., De Leon, M. J., Schneck, M. K., Buttinger, C., & Borenstein, J. (1984). Functional staging of dementia of the Alzheimer type. *Annals of the New York Academy of Sciences, 435*, 481–483.

Reisberg, B., Ferris, S. H., De Leon, M. J., & Crooke, T. (1982). The global deterioration scale for assessment of primary degenerative dementia. *American Journal of Psychiatry, 139*, 1136–1139.

Robinson, G., Rossor, M., & Cipolotti, L. (1999). Selective sparing of verb naming in a case of severe Alzheimer's disease, *Cortex. 35*, 443–450.

Rochon, E., Waters, G. S., & Caplan, D. (2000). The relationship between measures of working memory and sentence comprehension in patients with Alzheimer's disease. *Journal of Speech, Language, and Hearing Research, 43*, 395–413.

Sando, S. B., Melquist, S., Cannon, A., Hutton, M., Sletvold, O., Saltvedt, I., . . . Aasly, J. (2008). Risk-reducing effect of education in Alzheimer's disease. *International Journal of Geriatric Psychiatry, 23*, 1156–1162.

Salmon, D., Butters, N., & Chan, A. (1999). The deterioration of semantic memory in Alzheimer's disease. *Canadian Journal of Experimental Psychology, 53*, 108–116.

Satt, A., Hoory, R., Konig, A., Aalten, P., & Robert, P. H. (2014, September). *Speech-based automatic and robust detection of very early dementia.* Paper presented at Interspeech, Singapore.

Schoenberg, B. S., Anderson, D. W., & Haeren, A. F. (1985). Severe dementia: Prevalence and clinical features in a biracial U.S. population. *Archives of Neurology, 42*, 740–743.

Selkoe, D. J. (2000). The genetics and molecular pathology of Alzheimer's disease: Roles of amyloid and the presenilins. *Neurologic Clinics, 18*, 903–922.

Sharp, E. S., & Gatz, M. (2011). Relationship between education and dementia: An updated systematic review. *Alzheimer Disease and Associated Disorders, 25*, 289–304.

Shively S., Scher, A., Perl, D., Diaz-Arrastia, R. (2012). Dementia resulting from traumatic brain injury: What is the pathology? *Archives of Neurology, 69*, 1245–1251.

Singh-Manoux, A., Hillsdon, M., Brunner, E., & Marmot, M. (2005). Effects of physical activity on cognitive functioning in middle age: Evidence from the Whitehall II prospective cohort study. *American Journal of Public Health, 95*, 2252–2258.

Small, B. J., & Bäckman, L. (1998). Predictors of longitudinal changes in memory, visuospatial, and verbal functioning in very old demented adults. *Dementia and Geriatric Cognitive Disorders, 9*, 258–266.

Soininen, H., Laulumaa, B., Helkala, E. L., Hartikainen, P., & Riekkinen, P. J. (1992). Extrapyramidal signs in Alzheimer's disease: A 3-year follow-up study. *Journal of Neural Transmission, 4*, 107–119.

Solan, M. (2017, September 8). Can getting quality sleep help prevent Alzheimer's disease? [Harvard Health Blog post].Retrieved from https://www.health.harvard.edu/blog/waking-up-to-alzheimers-can-getting-qualitysleep-help-prevent-the-disease-201709081 2293

Stern, R. G., Mohs, R. C., Davidson, M., Schmeidler, J., Silverman, J., Kramer-Ginsberg, E.,. . . Davis, K. L. (1994). A longitudinal study of Alzheimer's disease: Measurement, rate and predictors of cognitive deterioration. *American Journal of Psychiatry, 151*, 390–396.

Stern, Y., Albert, M., Brandt, J., Jacobs, D. M., Tang, M. X., Marder, K., . . . Bylsma, F. F. (1994). Utility of extrapyramidal signs and psychosis as predictors of cognitive and functional decline, nursing home admission and death in Alzheimer's disease: Prospective analyses from the Predictors Study. *Neurology, 44*, 2300–2307.

Stern, Y., Mayeux, R., Sano, M., & Hauser, W. (1987). Predictors of disease course in patients with probable Alzheimer's disease. *Neurology, 37*, 1649–1653.

Szatloczki, G., Hoffmann, I., Vinczem V., Kalman, J., & Pakaski, M. (2015). Speaking in Alzheimer's disease, is that an early sign? Importance of changes in language abilities in Alzheimer's disease. *Frontiers in Aging Neuroscience, 7*, 195.

Tjalling, J. H., Deeg, D. J. H., Beekman, A. T. F., van Tilburg, T. G., Stek, M. L., Jonker, C., Schoevers, R. A. (2014). Feelings of loneliness, but not social isolation, predict dementia onset: results from the Amsterdam Study of the Elderly (AMSTEL). *Journal of Neurology, Neurosurgery and Psychiatry, 85*, 135–142.

Tomoeda, C. K., & Bayles, K. A. (1993). Longitudinal effects of Alzheimer's disease on discourse production. *Alzheimer Disease and Associated Disorders, 7*, 223–236.

Tomoeda, C. K., Bayles, K. A., Trosset, M. W., Azuma, T., & McGeagh, A. (1996). Cross-sectional analysis of Alzheimer disease effects on oral discourse in a picture description task. *Alzheimer Disease and Associated Disorders, 10*, 204–215.

Van Duijn, C. M., Hofman, A., & Kay, D. W. K. (1991). Risk factors for Alzheimer's disease: A collaborative reanalysis of case-control studies. *International Journal of Epidemiology, 20*, S1.

Van Hoesen, G. (1997). Ventromedial temporal lobe anatomy, with comments on Alzheimer's disease and temporal injury. *Journal of Neuropsychiatry and Clinical Neurosciences, 9*, 331–341.

Weiner, M. F., Neubecker, K. E., Bret, M. E., & Hynan, L. S. (2008). Language in Alzheimer's disease. *Journal of Clinical Psychiatry, 69,* 1223–1227.

Weuve, J., Kang, J. H., Manson, J. E., Breteler, M. M. B., Ware, J. H., & Grodstein, F. (2004). Physical activity including walking and cognitive function in older women. *Journal of the American Medical Association, 292,* 1454–1461.

Wilson, R. S., Bennet, D. A., Gilley, D. W., Beckett, L. A., Schneider, J. A., & Evans, D. A. (2000). Progression of parkinsonian signs in Alzheimer's disease. *Neurology, 54,* 1284–1289.

Wilson, R. S., Krueger, K. R., Arnold, S. E., Schneider, J. A., Kelly, J. F., Barnes, L. L., . . . Bennett, D. A. (2007). Loneliness and risk of Alzheimer disease. *Archives of General Psychiatry, 64,* 234–240.

World Health Organization. (2017, November 27). Dementia: Fact sheet. Retrieved from http://www.who.int/mediacentre/factsheets/fs362/en/

Xie, J., Brayne, C., & Matthews, F. E. (2008). Survival times in people with dementia: Analysis from population-based cohort study with 14-year follow-up. *British Medical Journal, 336,* 258–262.

5

Dementia and Down Syndrome

Introduction

Down syndrome (DS), the most common cause of intellectual disability in the United States, is a genetic disorder associated with three copies of chromosome 21. Affected individuals have intelligence quotients ranging from 30 to 70, with an average of 50 (Vicari, 2004). In the United States, the incidence of DS is approximately one in 792 live births (de Graaf, Buckley, & Skotko, 2015; Hartley et al., 2015) and the estimated prevalence is 271,000 (Presson et al., 2013). Worldwide, the prevalence approximates 5.8 million people (Hanney et al., 2012).

Mortality rates for individuals with DS differ from those of the general population. After the age of 35 years, the rate doubles every 6.4 years compared with every 9.6 years for people without DS. However, life expectancy has improved dramatically since the 1900s when it was nine to 11 years, and the 1980s when it was 25 years; nonetheless, it remains below that of the general population. A baby born with DS today can expect to live to 60 years of age (Bittles & Glasson, 2004; National Down Syndrome Society, 2017; Strauss & Eymann, 1996) because of better medical care and improved quality of life (Brown & Faragher, 2014). Some researchers believe that the life expectancy of individuals with DS will continue to increase (Bittles, Bower, Hussain & Glasson, 2007; Glasson et al., 2002).

Common Features of People with DS

Common features of people with DS include:

- Almond-shaped eyes with an epicanthal fold
- Flat nasal bridge
- Shorter limbs
- Poor muscle tone
- Single transverse palmar crease
- Intellectual disability

Risk of Developing Alzheimer's Disease

Individuals with DS are at higher risk for developing Alzheimer's disease (AD) as compared to the typically developing population (Ballard, Mobley, Hardy, Williams, & Corbett, 2016). In fact, virtually all people with DS have the neuropathological and neurochemical abnormalities that define AD by the time they reach their 30s (Figure 5–1) and approximately 70% will develop AD in their lifetime (Hartley et al., 2015). Recall that the *neuropathological* features necessary for diagnosis of AD are neuritic plaques and neurofibrillary tangles in sufficient numbers (Khachaturian, 1985; Mirra et al., 1991; National Institute on Aging, 1997). Within the neuritic plaque is beta-amyloid that is derived from the processing of amyloid

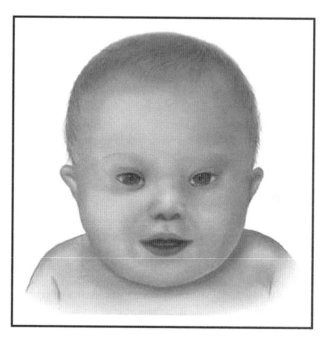

Figure 5–1. A drawing of the facial features of Down syndrome. (Courtesy of Centers for Disease Control and Prevention, National Center on Birth Defects and Developmental Disabilities.)

precursor protein (APP). APP is located on chromosome 21, the chromosome that is triplicated in individuals with DS. This triplication likely accounts for the overexpression of beta-amyloid in individuals with DS (Ness et al., 2012) that begins even in childhood (Leverenz & Raskind, 1998).

Other factors also raise the risk of AD in people with DS, among them accelerated aging that in females is marked in part by the earlier advent of menopause (Hogervorst, 2013; Horvath et al., 2015). Associated with menopause is reduction in endogenous estradiol that also heightens the risk of AD (Patel et al., 2004; Schupf et al., 2003). In addition, those individuals with DS who have one or two apolipoprotein E (APOE) 4 alleles are at even greater risk.

Although AD is the most common cause of dementia in DS, dementia can also result from other causes, among them Lewy body disease (Bodhireddy, Dickson, Mattiace, & Weidenheim, 1994; Prasher, Airuehia, & Carey, 2010). When Lewy body disease is present, irritability,

apathy, and psychotic symptoms may be early features (Simard & Van Reekum, 2001). As for disease duration, Margallo-Lana and colleagues (2007) found the mean survival period of those individuals with DS who were diagnosed with dementia at age 55 to average 3.5 years.

Prevalence of Dementia in DS

Whereas AD pathology is virtually omnipresent in individuals with DS, dementia is not. Researchers have yet to understand why some adults with DS develop AD before the age of 50 and others do not (Devenny, Krinsky-McHale, Sersen, & Silverman, 2000). As in the general population, the prevalence of dementia in individuals with DS increases with age, particularly after age 35 (Strydom et al., 2010) when AD pathology accelerates. Although variation exists regarding age of dementia onset, it most commonly manifests between the ages of 46 and 56 years (Head, Powell, Gold,

& Schmitt, 2012; Silverman, Zigman, Krinsky-McHale, Ryan, & Schupf, 2013) and is greatest in individuals over age 60 (Margallo-Lana et al., 2007), varying between 26% and 50% (Janicki & Dalton, 2000; Strydom, Livingston, King, & Hassiotis, 2007).

Diagnosing Dementia in Individuals with DS

The diagnosis of dementia in individuals with DS is challenging because mental impairment is an inherent feature of DS. Clinicians must tease apart those cognitive deficits associated with DS and normal aging from those caused by AD or other dementia-producing diseases. Furthermore, subtle symptoms of cognitive decline are difficult to recognize if individuals have not developed many skills, or when the environment demands little of them (Sheehan et al., 2015). Adding to the confusion is the lack of a gold standard for making a diagnosis. For these reasons, individuals with DS who have developed dementia are typically diagnosed later in the course of the disease compared to the general population; thus shortening the window for offering pharmacologic and psychosocial interventions (Sheehan et al., 2015).

Symptoms of dementia in DS include:

- Cognitive changes
  - Episodic memory deficits
  - Executive dysfunction
  - Selective inattention
  - Disorientation
- Changes in affect
  - Irritability
  - Depression
  - Sleep disturbance
  - Anxiety
  - Apathy/disinterest
- Behavioral change
  - Personality change
  - Increased dependence
- Neurologic signs
  - Aphasia
  - Apraxia

- Gait disturbance
- Social isolation
- Hallucinations
- Seizures

Clinicians should take into account more than change in memory when evaluating this population because of numerous reports in the literature of individuals with DS presenting with prefrontal lobe symptoms rather than the more typical episodic memory deficits (Adams & Oliver, 2010; Ball et al., 2006; Krinsky-Mchale, Devenny, Kittler, & Silverman, 2008; Lott & Head, 2001; Stanton & Coetzee, 2004; Zigman, Silverman, & Wisniewski, 1996). Commonly reported early signs include indifference, apathy, depression, uncooperativeness, and deficits in selective attention. Many individuals with DS also experience attention deficit hyperactivity disorder (ADHD) (Ekstein, Glick, Weill, Kay, Berger, 2011) that likely impacts the presentation of behavior-related early symptomology (Ballard et al., 2016).

The course of cognitive deterioration in DS with dementia mirrors that of individuals with AD who do not have DS (Adams & Oliver, 2010; Nelson, Orme, Osann, & Lott, 2001; Prasher et al., 2003). The following guidelines can help clinicians better recognize the presence of dementia in DS adults (Alyward, Burt, Thorpe, Lai, & Dalton, 1995):

- First, obtain a baseline of cognitive and behavioral functioning by the time the individual is 25 years of age.
- Use standardized instruments and assess cognition, health, and functional skills.
- Periodically thereafter, but especially by the time the individual has reached the age of 40, assessments should be readministered and family and caregivers interviewed about possible changes in cognitive function and behavior.
- If change is reported, the individual should be referred to a physician to evaluate whether the cause of mental and/or behavioral decline is treatable.

■ When early AD is suspected, the individual should be periodically evaluated, ideally every 6 months but at least annually.

A Study of the Cognitive-Communication Profiles of DS Adults with and without Dementia

Moss, Tomoeda, and Bayles (2000) investigated the relation of age to neuropsychological test performance in 22 nondemented DS adults and two with dementia and compared their performance to individuals with mild and moderate AD. The average chronologic age of the individuals with DS was 42.9 years (ranging 32–65 years) and their average mental age was 5.5 years. The Arizona Battery for Communication Disorders of Dementia (ABCD) (Bayles & Tomoeda, 1993), comprising 14 subtests of 5 constructs, was administered to study participants. An inverse correlation was obtained between ABCD total score and chronologic age ($r = -.57$, $p = .002$); that is, older age in the DS group (demented and nondemented) was associated with lower mental age and lower performance on the ABCD. The two oldest individuals with DS (ages 62 and 65 years) had the lowest mental ages and ABCD overall score and met the diagnostic criteria for dementia in DS.

Comparison of Performance of DS Readers with DS Nonreaders

Because study participants with DS were heterogeneous in cognitive development, their performance data were grouped by mental age and whether they could read at the single-word level. The nondemented adults with DS who could read ($n = 13$) had higher scores on ABCD subtests that did not involve reading than DS adults who could not read ($n = 9$). For nine of the 14 subtests, the scores of the readers were significantly higher (Mental Status, Story Retelling– Immediate, Comparative Questions, Word Learning–Free Recall, Word Learning–Total Recall, Word Learning

Recognition, Repetition, Object Description, and Story Retelling–Delayed). Differences between the readers and nonreaders were particularly noticeable on the three components of the Word Learning subtest in which the ability to read can aid performance, although reading is not required. Thus, Moss et al. (2000) cautioned that the scores of nonreaders on the Word Learning subtest likely did not accurately reflect their ability to encode and remember verbal stimuli.

Comparison of Nondemented Adults with DS with Individuals with Mild AD

The nondemented adults with DS had lower scores than AD patients on two measures of linguistic comprehension and two measures of visuospatial construction ability. The only subtest on which the nondemented DS subjects had higher scores than the AD patients was Story Retelling–Delayed, an episodic memory test.

Comparison of Demented DS Individuals with AD Subjects

The construct scores of the two DS adults with dementia were compared with those of mild and moderate AD patients in the ABCD standardization study and with the group of nondemented DS adults with mental ages of six years or less. The demented DS individuals scored lower on all five ABCD constructs than individuals with AD, and they scored lower on episodic memory and linguistic expression than the nondemented DS adults with mental ages of six years or less.

Language and Communication Skills of Adults with DS

Premorbid Language

Individuals with DS commonly have impaired language abilities (Chapman, Hesketh, & Kistler, 2002; Laws & Bishop, 2003). Compared with nondemented individuals of similar age in the general population, they use simpler grammar, perform poorer on tests of language, and have a shorter mean length of utterance (Rondal, 1988; Rondal & Lambert, 1983; Sabsay & Kernan, 1993). Overall, morphosyntax and phonology have been identified as areas of weakness and semantics and pragmatics as areas of strength (Martin, Klusek, Estigarribia, & Roberts, 2009; Rondal & Comblain, 1996, 2002).

Witecy and Penke (2017) reported that the receptive language skills of adults with DS are impaired for a variety of grammatical structures likely because, as results of their study indicate, syntax learning plateaus in adolescence. As to whether receptive language skills are maintained after adolescence, results are mixed. Some investigators report that receptive language skills are maintained after adolescence unless there is a diagnosis of AD (Iacono, Torr, & Wong, 2010; Rondal & Comblain, 1996, 2002; Witecy & Penke, 2017); other investigators report loss of receptive language skills with age (Chapman et al., 2002; Couzens, Cuskelly, & Haynes, 2011). An issue in interpreting results of studies of receptive language skills is determining whether decline represents the effect of aging or aging plus the onset of AD.

Even though the percentage of individuals with DS who learn to read has not been firmly established, many acquire literacy with instruction (Byrne, MacDonald & Buckley, 2002; Kay-Raining Bird, Cleave, & McConnell, 2000; Kay-Raining Bird, Cleave, White, Pike, & Helmkay, 2008).

Language Change in Dementia

Iacono and colleagues (2010) conducted a cross-sectional study of the effect of AD on language in individuals with DS. They administered a comprehensive battery of language and cognitive tests to 55 individuals with DS, 10 of whom had a diagnosis of AD or signs of early AD. As age increased, scores on all measures decreased. Also, deficits in expressive language were present earlier than previously reported by Cooper and Collacott (1995). Roeden and Zitman (1997) reported progressive declines in receptive and expressive language over 4.5 years in 28 individuals with DS, 14 of whom had dementia. Likewise, the communication skills of four individuals with DS were reported by caregivers who participated in a study by Rasmussen and Sobsey (1994). The four individuals were confirmed as having AD pathology at postmortem examination. In a case study of confrontation naming in an individual with DS and dementia, Kledaras, McIlvane, and Mackay (1989) reported significant longitudinal decline over a 20-month period. The types of naming errors made by the individual were like those of individuals with AD: naming items related to the target (visually and/or semantically) or the category of the target item, rather than the item. Verbal intrusions appear more numerous in DS adults with early AD and precede memory decline (Kittler, Krinsky-McHale & Devenny, 2006). Kittler and colleagues attribute intrusions to compromised executive function and disinhibition.

Cognitive and Behavioral Measures Appropriate for Individuals with DS

Several standardized cognitive and behavioral measures have been developed for use with adults with intellectual impairment. Table 5–1 contains descriptions of commonly used measures. The CAMDEX-R was modified for use with people with DS and is called the Cambridge Examination for Mental Disorders of Older People with Down's Syndrome and Others with Intellectual Disabilities (CAMDEX-DS) (Ball et al., 2004). It is composed of an informant interview, direct assessment of the individual with DS, and recommendations for post-diagnosis intervention. Emphasis is placed on establishing change from the individual's previous best level of function.

The Dementia Screening Questionnaire for Individuals with Intellectual Disabilities (DSQIID) is a dementia screening tool with

Table 5–1. Measures of Cognitive Function and Behavior Commonly Used with Adults with Down Syndrome

Observer Rating Scales of Cognitive Function

Modified CAMDEX Informant Interview (Roth, Huppert, Mountjoy, & Tym, 1998)

- Includes an informant interview, client interview, and an objective examination of cognitive function
- Has demonstrated validity and reliability (Ball et al., 2004)

Dementia Questionnaire for Persons with Mental Retardation (Evenhuis, 1992)

- Comprises 50 questions that respondents answer "normally yes," "sometimes," or "normally no"
- Provides a summary of cognitive scores and a summary of social scores
- A cutoff score is provided for diagnosis of dementia in people with differing levels of intellectual disability
- Has good sensitivity (.92) and specificity (.92)

Dementia Scale for Down Syndrome (Gedye, 1995)

- Contains questions in three categories: early-, middle-, and late-stage dementia
- Places emphasis on change in function
- Distinguishes between new and typical behaviors
- Diagnosis is based on reaching a global numerical threshold at each level of severity
- Has good sensitivity (.85) and specificity (.89)

Measures of Functional and Vocational Abilities

- Scales of Independent Behavior (Thase, Liss, Smeltzer, & Maloon, 1982)
- Vineland Adaptive Behavior Scales (Sparrow, Balla, & Cicchetti, 1984)
- Disability Assessment Schedule (Holmes, Shah, & Wing, 1982)

Neuropsychologic Batteries

Cambridge Examination for Mental Disorders of Older People with Down's Syndrome and Others with Intellectual Disabilities (CAMDEX-DS) (Ball et al., 2004)

Neuropsychologic Assessment of Dementia in Individuals with Intellectual Disability (Prasher, 2009)

Severe Impairment Battery (Saxton, McGonigle, Swihart, & Boller, 1993)

strong psychometric properties for adults with intellectual disabilities (Deb, Hare, Prior, & Bhaumik, 2007). Sensitivity and specificity are reported to be 0.92 and 0.97, respectively, for the DS population, making it both valid and reliable for application to this population (Moriconi, Schlamb, & Harrison, 2015).

Another battery that was recently administered to adults with DS, to evaluate the test's criterion validity, is the Severe Impairment Battery (SIB) (Saxton, McGonigle, Swihart, & Boller, 1993). The SIB was developed to assess cognitive function in individuals with advanced dementia. Hutchinson and Oakes (2011) gave the SIB to 37 adults with DS whose caregivers completed the Dementia Questionnaire for Mentally Retarded Persons (DMR). The latter served as the criterion measure. The correlation of the SIB total score with the DMR sum of cognitive scores was .73, a value that indicates good concurrent criterion validity.

Deb and Braganza (1999) compared several measures used to screen for dementia, among them the widely used Mini-Mental State Examination (Folstein, Folstein, & McHugh, 1975), and reported it as unreliable because it could not be used in almost half of the study sample because of literacy issues.

Summary of Important Points

- Clinicians need to be mindful of the high incidence of AD in individuals with DS, particularly those older than 50 years.
- To detect dementia, clinicians need to obtain a profile of cognitive abilities when the individual with DS is in young adulthood. This profile can serve as a baseline that will facilitate later detection of cognitive decline.
- Standardized measures of cognition and language, as well as functional abilities, should be used.
- Clinicians should identify whether the individual can read and take that into account when selecting and interpreting test performance.
- When the individual with DS reaches the age of 40 years, periodic evaluations and interviews of family about possible changes in function should be started.
- When using the ABCD with DS adults, attention should be paid to their performance on episodic memory tests. If the individual's score is equal to or less than the average of AD subjects in the standardization sample, consider the possibility of dementia.
- If a change in function is detected in individuals with DS, refer the individual to a neurologist and include information about the nature of the change with your referral.
- When dementia is apparent, continue to periodically reevaluate the individual and provide counseling to family about accommodations that will enable the individual to function maximally and have quality of life.

References

Adams, D., & Oliver, C. (2010). The relationships between acquired impairments of executive function and behaviour change in adults with Down syndrome. *Journal of Intellectual Disability Research, 54*, 393–405.

Alyward, E., Burt, D., Thorpe, L., Lai, F., & Dalton, A. J. (1995). *Diagnosis of dementia in individuals with intellectual disability: Report of the AAMR-IASSID Working Group for Establishment of Criteria for the Diagnosis of Dementia in Individuals with Intellectual Disability.* Washington, DC: American Association on Mental Retardation.

Ball, S. L., Holland, A. J., Hon, J., Huppert, F. A., Treppner, P., & Watson, P. C. (2006). Personality and behaviour changes mark the early stages of Alzheimer's disease in adults with Down's syndrome: Findings from a prospective population-based study. *International Journal of Geriatric Psychiatry, 21*, 661–673.

Ball, S. L., Holland, A. J., Huppert, F. A., Treppner, P., Watson, P., & Hon, J. (2004). The modified CAMDEX informant interview is a valid and reliable tool for use in the diagnosis of dementia in adults with Down's syndrome. *Journal of Intellectual Disability Research, 48*, 611–620.

Ballard, C., Mobley, W., Hardy, J., Williams, G., & Corbett, A. (2016). Dementia in Down's syndrome. *The Lancet Neurology, 15*, 622–636.

Bayles, K. A., & Tomoeda, C. K. (1993). *Arizona Battery for Communication Disorders of Dementia.* Austin, TX: Pro-Ed.

Bittles, A. H., Bower, C., Hussain, R., & Glasson, E. J. (2007). The four ages of Down syndrome. *European Journal of Public Health, 17*, 221–225.

Bittles, A. H., & Glasson, E. J. (2004). Clinical, social, and ethical implications of changing life expectancy in Down syndrome. *Developmental Medicine and Child Neurology, 46*, 282–286.

Bodhireddy, S., Dickson, D. W., Mattiace, L., & Weidenheim, K. M. (1994). A case of Down's syndrome with diffuse Lewy body disease and Alzheimer's disease. *Neurology, 44*, 159–161.

Brown, R. I., & Faragher, R. M. (2014). Quality of life in the wider world challenges from the field of intellectual and developmental disabilities. In R. I. Brown & R. M. Faragher (Eds.), *Quality of life and intellectual disability: knowledge application to other social and educational challenges.* New York, NY: Nova Science Publishers.

Byrne, A., MacDonald, J., & Buckley, S. (2002). Reading, language and memory skills: A comparative longitudinal study of children with Down syndrome and their mainstream peers. *British Journal of Educational Psychology, 72,* 513–529.

Chapman, R. S., Hesketh, L. J., & Kistler, D. J. (2002). Predicting longitudinal change in language production and comprehension in individuals with Down syndrome: Hierarchical linear modeling. *Journal of Speech, Language, and Hearing Research, 45,* 902–915.

Cooper, S. A., & Callacott, R. A. (1995). The effect of age on language in people with Down's syndrome. *Journal of Intellectual Disability Research, 39,* 197–200.

Couzens, D., Cuskelly, M., & Haynes, M. (2011). Cognitive development and Down syndrome: Age-related change on the Stanford-Binet test (4th ed.). *American Journal on Intellectual and Developmental Disabilities, 116,* 181–204.

de Graaf, G., Buckley, F., & Skotko, B. G. (2015). Estimates of the live births, natural losses, and elective terminations with Down syndrome in the United States. *American Journal of Medical Genetics Part A, 167,* 756–767.

Deb, S., & Braganza, J. (1999). Comparison of rating scales for the diagnosis of dementia in adults with Down's syndrome. *Journal of Intellectual Disability Research, 43,* 400–407.

Deb, S., Hare, M., Prior, L., & Bhaumik, S. (2007). Dementia screening questionnaire for individuals with intellectual disabilities. *British Journal of Psychiatry, 190,* 440–444.

Devenny, D. A., Krinsky-McHale, S. J., Sersen, G., & Silverman, W. P. (2000). Sequence of cognitive decline in dementia in adults with Down's syndrome. *Journal of Intellectual Disability Research, 44,* 654–665.

Ekstein, S., Glick, B., Weill, M., Kay, B., & Berger, I. (2011). Down syndrome and attention-deficit/hyperactivity disorder (ADHD*). Journal of Child Neurology, 26,* 1290–1295.

Evenhuis, H. M. (1992). Evaluation of a screening instrument for dementia in ageing mentally retarded persons. *Journal of Intellectual Disability Research. 36,* 337–447.

Folstein, M. F., Folstein, S. E., & McHugh, P. R. (1975). "Mini-mental state." A practical method for grading the cognitive state of patients for the clinicians. *Journal of Psychiatric Research, 12,* 189–198.

Gedye, A. (1995). Dementia Scale for Down's Syndrome. Vancouver, BC: Gedye Research and Consulting.

Glasson, E. J., Sullivan, S. G., Hussain, R., Petterson, B. A., Montgomery, P. D., & Bittles, A. H. (2002). The changing survival profile of people with Down's syndrome: Implications for genetic counselling. *Clinical Genetics, 62,* 390–393.

Hanney, M., Prasher, V., Williams, N., Jones, E. L., Aarsland, D., Corbett, A., . . . Johnson, T. (2012). Memantine for dementia in adults older than 40 years with Down's syndrome (MEADOWS): A randomised, double-blind, placebo-controlled trial. *The Lancet, 379,* 528–536.

Hartley, D., Blumenthal, T., Carillo, M., DiPaolo, G., Esralew, L., Gardiner, K., . . . Wisniewski, T. (2015). Down syndrome and Alzheimer's disease: Common pathways, common goals. *Alzheimer's and Dementia, 11,* 700–709.

Head, E., Powell, D., Gold, B., & Schmitt, F. (2012). Alzheimer's disease in Down syndrome. *European Journal of Neurodegenerative Diseases, 1,* 353–364.

Hogervorst, E. (2013). Effects of gonadal hormones on cognitive behaviour in elderly men and women. *Journal of Neuroendocrinology, 25,* 1182–1195.

Holmes, N., Shah, A., & Wing, L. (1982). The Disability Assessment Schedule: A brief screening device for use with the mentally retarded. *Psychological Medicine, 12,* 879–890.

Horvath, S., Garagnani, P., Bacalini, M. G., Pirazzini, C., Salvioli, S., Gentilini, D.,...Franceschi, C. (2015). Accelerated epigenetic aging in Down syndrome. *Aging Cell, 14,* 491–495.

Hutchinson, N., & Oakes, P. (2011). Further evaluation of the criterion validity of the Severe Impairment Battery for the assessment of cognitive functioning in adults with Down syndrome. *Journal of Applied Research in Intellectual Disabilities, 24,* 172–180.

Iacono, T., Torr, J., & Wong, H.Y. (2010). Relationships amongst age, language and related skills in adults with Down syndrome. *Research in Developmental Disabilities, 31,* 568–576.

Janicki, M. P., & Dalton, A. J. (2000). Prevalence of dementia and impact on intellectual disability services. *Mental Retardation, 38,* 276–288.

Kay-Raining Bird, E., Cleave, P. L., & McConnell, L. (2000). Reading and phonological awareness in children with Down syndrome: A longitudinal study. *American Journal of Speech-Language Pathology, 9,* 319–330.

Kay-Raining Bird, E., Cleave, P. L., White, D., Pike, H., & Helmkay, A. (2008). Written and oral narratives of children and adolescents with Down syndrome. *Journal of Speech, Language, and Hearing Research, 51,* 436–450.

Khachaturian, Z. S. (1985). Diagnosis of Alzheimer's disease. *Archives of Neurology, 421,* 1097–1106.

Kittler, P., Krinsky-McHale, S. J., & Devenny, D. A. (2006). Verbal intrusions precede memory decline in adults with Down syndrome. *Journal of Intellectual Disability Research, 50,* 1–10.

Kledaras, J. B., McIlvane, W. J., & Mackay, H. A. (1989). Progressive decline of picture naming in an ageing Down syndrome man with dementia. *Perceptual and Motor Skills, 69,* 1091–1100.

Krinsky-McHale, S. J., Devenny, D. A., Kittler, P., & Silverman, W. (2008). Selective attention deficits associated with mild cognitive impairment and early stage Alzheimer's disease in adults with Down syndrome. *American Journal of Mental Retardation, 113,* 369–386.

Laws, G., & Bishop, D. V. M. (2003). A comparison of language abilities in adolescents with Down syndrome and children with specific language impairment. *Journal of Speech, Language, and Hearing Research, 46,* 1324–1339.

Leverenz, J. B., & Raskind, M. A. (1998). Early amyloid deposition in the medial temporal lobe of young Down syndrome patients: A regional quantitative analysis. *Experimental Neurology, 150,* 296–304.

Lott, I. T., & Head, E. (2001). Down syndrome and Alzheimer's disease: A link between development and aging. *Mental Retardation and Developmental Disabilities Research Reviews, 7,* 172–178.

Margallo-Lana, M. L., Moore, P. B., Kay, D. W. K., Perry, R. H., Reid, B. E., Berney, T. P., & Tyrer, S. P. (2007). Fifteen-year follow-up of 92 hospitalized adults with Down's syndrome: Incidence of cognitive decline, its relationship to age and neuropathology. *Journal of Intellectual Disability Research, 51,* 463–477.

Martin, G. E., Klusek, J., Estigarribia, B., & Roberts, J. (2009). Language characteristics of individuals with Down syndrome. *Topics in Language Disorders, 29,* 112–113.

Mirra, S. S., Heyman, A., McKeel, D., Sumi, S. D., Crain, B. J., Brownlee, L. M., . . . Berg, L. (1991). The Consortium to Establish a Registry for Alzheimer's Disease (CERAD). Part II. Standardization of the neuropathologic assessment of Alzheimer's disease. *Neurology, 41,* 479–486.

Moriconi, C., Schlamb, C., & Harrison, B. (2015). Down syndrome and dementia: Guide to identification, screening, and management. *Journal for Nurse Practitioners, 11,* 812–818.

Moss, S. E., Tomoeda, C. K., & Bayles, K. A. (2000). Comparison of the cognitive-linguistic profiles of Down syndrome adults with and without dementia to individuals with Alzheimer's disease. *Journal of Medical Speech-Language Pathology, 8,* 69–81.

National Down Syndrome Society. (2017, November 15). Down syndrome fact sheet. Retrievedfrom http://www.ndss.org/about-down-syndrome/down-syndrome-facts/

National Institute on Aging & Reagan Institute Working Group on Diagnostic Criteria for the Neuropathological Assessment of Alzheimer's disease. (1997). Consensus recommendations for the post mortem diagnosis of Alzheimer's disease. *Neurobiology of Aging, 18,* 1–2.

Nelson, L. D., Orme, D., Osann, K., & Lott, I. T. (2001). Neurological changes and emotional functioning in adults with Down syndrome. *Journal of Intellectual Disability Research, 45,* 450–456.

Ness, S., Rafii, M., Aisen, P., Krams, M., Silverman, W. P., & Manji, H. (2012). Down's syndrome and Alzheimer's disease: Towards secondary prevention. *Nature reviews, Drug Discovery. 11,* 655–656.

Patel, B. N., Pang, D., Stern, Y., Silverman, W., Kiline, J. K., Mayeux, R., & Schupf, N. (2004). Obesity enhances verbal memory in postmenopausal women with Down syndrome. *Neurobiology of Aging, 25,* 159–166.

Prasher, V. P., Airuehia, E., & Carey, M. (2010). The first confirmed case of Down syndrome with dementia with Lewy bodies. *Journal of Applied Research in Intellectual Disabilities, 23,* 296–300.

Prasher, V. P., Cumella, S., Natarajan, K., Rolfe, E., Shah, S., & Haque, M. S. (2003). Magnetic resonance imaging, Down's syndrome and Alzheimer's disease research

and clinical implications. *Journal of Intellectual Disability Research, 47,* 90–100.

Presson, A. P., Partyka, G., Jensen, K. M., Devine, O. J., Rasmussen, S. A., McCabe, L. L., & McCable, E. R. (2013). Current estimate of Down syndrome population prevalence in the United States. *Journal of Pediatrics, 163,* 1163–1168.

Rasmussen, D. E., & Sobsey, D. (1994). Age, adaptive behaviour, and Alzheimer disease in Down syndrome: Cross-sectional and longitudinal analysis. *American Journal on Mental Retardation, 99,* 151–165.

Roeden, J. M., & Zitman, F. G. (1997). A longitudinal comparison of cognitive and adaptive changes in participants with Down's syndrome and an intellectually disabled control group. *Journal of Applied Research in Intellectual Disabilities, 10,* 289–302.

Rondal, J. A. (1988). Language development in Down's syndrome: A life-span perspective. *International Journal of Behavioural Development, 11,* 21–36.

Rondal, J. A., & Comblain, A. (1996). Language in adults with Down syndrome. *Down Syndrome Research and Practice, 4,* 3–14.

Rondal, J. A., & Comblain, A. (2002). Language in ageing persons with Down syndrome. *Down Syndrome Research and Practice, 8,* 1–9.

Rondal, J. A., & Lambert, J. L. (1983). The speech of mentally retarded adults in a dyadic communication situation: Some formal and informative aspects. *Psychologic Belgica, 23,* 49–56.

Roth, M., Huppert, F., Mountjoy, C., & Tym, E. (1998). *CAMDEX-R: The Cambridge Examination for Mental Disorder of the Elderly* (Rev. Ed.). Cambridge, UK: Cambridge University Press.

Sabsay, S., & Kernan, K. T. (1993). On the nature of language impairment in Down syndrome. *Topics in Language Disorders, 13,* 20–35.

Saxton, J., McGonigle, K. L., Swihart, A. A., & Boller, F. (1993). Severe Impairment Battery (SIB). London, UK: Thames Valley Test Company.

Schupf, N., Pang, D., Patel, B. N., Silverman, W., Schubert, R., Lai, F., . . . Mayeux, R. (2003). Onset of dementia is associated with age at menopause in women with Down's syndrome. *Annals of Neurology, 54,* 433–438.

Sheehan, R., Sinai, A., Bass, N., Blatchford, P., Bohnen, I., Bonell, S., . . . Strydom, A. (2015). Dementia diagnostic criteria in Down syndrome. *International Journal of Geriatric Psychiatry, 30,* 857–863.

Silverman, W. P, Zigman, W. B, Krinsky-McHale, S. J, Ryan, R., & Schupf, N. (2013). Intellectual disability, mild cognitive impairment, and risk for dementia. *Journal of Policy and Practice in Intellectual Disabilities, 10,* 245–251.

Simard, M., & Van Reekum, R. (2001). Dementia with Lewy bodies in Down's syndrome. *International Journal of Geriatric Psychiatry, 16,* 311–320.

Sparrow, S. S., Balla, D. A., & Cicchetti, D. V. (1984). Vineland Adaptive Behavior Scales. Circle Pines, MN: American Guidance Service.

Stanton, L. R. & Coetzee, R. H. (2004). Down's syndrome and dementia. *Advances in Psychiatric Treatment, 10,* 50–58.

Strauss, D., & Eymann, R.K. (1996). Mortality of people with mental retardation in California with and without Down syndrome. *American Journal of Mental Retardation, 100,* 643–653.

Strydom, A., Livingston, G., King, M., & Hassiotis, A. (2007). Prevalence of dementia in intellectual disability using different diagnostic criteria. *British Journal of Psychiatry, 191,* 150–157.

Strydom, A., Shooshtari, S., Lee, L., Raykar, V., Torr, J., Tsiouris, J., . . . Maaskant, M. (2010). Dementia in older adults with intellectual disabilities: Epidemiology, pre-

sentation, and diagnosis. *Journal of Policy and Practice in Intellectual Disabilities, 7,* 96–110.

Thase, M. E., Liss, L., Smeltzer, D., & Maloon, J. (1982). Clinical evaluation of dementia in Down's syndrome: A preliminary report. *Journal of Mental Deficit Research, 26,* 239–244.

Vicari, S. (2004). Memory development and intellectual disabilities. *Acta Paediactrica. 93,* 60–63.

Witecy, B., & Penke, M. (2017). Language comprehension in children, adolescents, and adults with Down syndrome. *Research in Developmental Disabilities, 62,* 184–196.

Zigman, W. B., Silverman, W., & Wisniewski, H. M. (1996). Aging and Alzheimer's disease in Down syndrome: Clinical and pathological changes. *Mental Retardation and Developmental Disabilities Research Reviews, 2,* 73–79.

6

Vascular Dementia

Introduction

Cerebrovascular disease competes with Lewy body disease and frontotemporal pathology as the second most common cause of dementia (Doody et al., 2001; Jellinger, 2007; Korczyn, 2016; Lobo et al., 2000; McKeith et al., 2005; Rockwood et al., 2000; Román, 2002, 2003). According to a report from the American Heart Association, the prevalence of vascular dementia (VaD) doubles every 5.3 years (Gorelick et al., 2011) and is nine times higher in individuals who have suffered a stroke. Within a year after stroke, 25% of stroke victims develop dementia (Alagiakrishnan, 2017).

In the 1970s and 1980s, the term "multi-infarct dementia" (Hachinski, Lassen, & Marshall, 1974) was commonly used to characterize cognitive impairment caused by vascular disease. Today, that term is out of favor because multiple infarctions are not the sole cause of vascular-related cognitive impairment. The reality is that diverse vascular pathologies can eventuate in dementia. Thus, in 2011 the American Heart and American Stroke Associations endorsed the term "vascular cognitive impairment" (VCI) to refer to the breadth of cognitive impairments, from mild to severe dementia, that are caused by any type of vascular pathology (Dichgans & Leys, 2017; Gorelick et al., 2011).

Neuropathology

The myriad pathophysiologic processes associated with VCI include (Rosenberg, 2016; Sachdev et al., 2014):

- *Large vessel disease or atherothromboembolic disease*
  - Multiple infarcts, cortical and subcortical
  - Single strategically located infarct

- *Small vessel disease associated with multiple infarcts*
  - Multiple small lacunar infarcts especially in white matter (Figure 6–1)
  - Ischemic white matter change
  - Dilatation of perivascular spaces
  - Cortical microinfarcts and microhemorrhages

- *Hemorrhage*
  - Intracerebral hemorrhage
  - Multiple cortical and subcortical microbleeds
  - Subarachnoid hemorrhage

- *Hypoperfusion*
  - Hippocampal sclerosis
  - Laminar cortical sclerosis
  - Incomplete white matter infarcts
  - Border zone infarcts
  - Diffuse hypoxic–ischemic encephalopathy

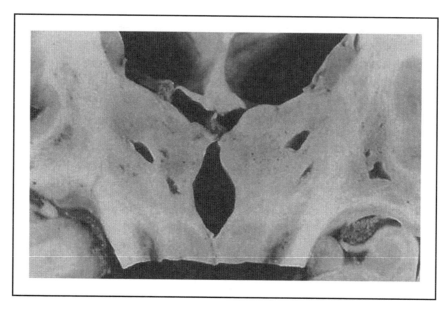

Figure 6–1. Lacunar state in a patient who suffered from a stepwise cognitive decline. There are at least seven lacunes of varying sizes in this plane section of the thalamus and posterior putamen. Other planes of section in this case showed additional lacunes with very little focal vascular disease elsewhere in the brain. (Courtesy of Cambridge University Press, 2014.)

Definitions (Blumenfeld, 2002)

Infarct: An area of dead or dying tissue due to inadequate blood supply.

Ischemic: The process in which there is inadequate blood supply to a region of the brain for enough time to cause infarction (death) of brain tissue.

Lacunar: Lacunes are small, deep ischemic infarcts that resemble small lakes or cavities when the brain is examined on pathologic section.

Dilatation: The action of being expanded or the state of being expanded.

Subarachnoid: The fluid-filled space between the arachnoid membrane of the brain and the pia mater.

Hypoperfusion: Decreased blood flow.

Sclerosis: Abnormal hardening of tissue or an increase in connective tissue.

Laminar: Thin layer of tissue.

Border zones: The junction between two main arterial territories.

Granular: Describes types of cells found both in cortex and throughout the body.

Hypoxic: Deprived of oxygen at the tissue level.

Encephalopathy: A term for any diffuse disease of the brain that alters brain function or structure (see http://www.ninds.nih.gov/disorders/encephalopathy/encephalopathy.htm).

Diagnostic Criteria

Three criteria are recommended for diagnosing cognitive impairment associated with vascular disease (Sachdev et al., 2014):

1. Subjective evidence in the form of concern by the patient or an informant of a change in cognitive ability.
2. Objective evidence of cognitive impairment, preferably from a neuropsychological examination.
3. Evidence of vascular pathology from clinical tests and neuroimaging that is sufficient to account for neurocognitive impairments.

Diagnosing Vascular Cognitive Impairment

A variety of classification systems for possible and probable vascular cognitive impairment have been developed over the years. The following is the current system (Sachdev et al., 2014):

Possible VCI is diagnosed if the clinical criteria are met but neuroimaging data are unavailable, or when there is an absence of a clear temporal relationship between the neurocognitive syndrome and a stroke or vascular problem.

Probable VCI is diagnosed if one of the following is present; otherwise, *possible* vascular neurocognitive disorder should be diagnosed:

1. Neuroimaging evidence of significant parenchymal injury attributed to cerebrovascular disease.
2. The neurocognitive syndrome is related in time to one or more documented cerebrovascular events.
3. Both clinical and genetic (e.g., cerebral autosomal dominant arteriopathy with subcortical infarcts and leukoencephalopathy) evidence of cerebrovascular disease are present.

Risk Factors for VaD

Researchers have identified numerous risk factors for VCI, some associated with aging and genetics and others that reflect lifestyle choices.

Aging

As a result of normal aging, cerebral blood flow is reduced, producing a state of chronic cellular hypoxia in the brain (Iadecola, Park, & Capone, 2009). Without well-regulated and regular cerebral blood flow, the functional integrity of the brain becomes compromised and can result in cell death (Enciu, Constantinescu, Popescu, Muresanu, & Popescu, 2011; Moskowitz, Lo, & Iadecola, 2010). These natural events, together with oxidative stress, inflammation, and endothelial malfunction, create a foundation for the development of vascular disease, stroke, and dementia. The reality is that after age 55 years, the incidence of stroke doubles with each decade. When hypertension, diabetes, obesity, high cholesterol, or other chronic conditions are added to the effects of aging, the risk for stroke and VCI greatly increases.

Hypertension

Hypertension deserves particular attention as a risk factor because so many individuals with VCI have a history of hypertension that is untreated or poorly controlled. In fact, *untreated or undertreated hypertension is the single most important risk factor for VCI and the most common modifiable risk factor for stroke* (Jack, 2010; Sharp et al., 2011). Moreover, not only does it increase the likelihood of cerebrovascular disease and stroke (European Society of Hypertension, 2003), it also increases the likelihood of the cognitive impairment (Elias, Wolf, d'Agostino, Cobb, & White, 1993; Kilander, Andrén, Nyman, Lind, Boberg, & Lithell, 1998) associated with VaD and AD (Sharp et al., 2011; Swan et al., 1998).

Family History

Individuals with a first-degree relative (parent or sibling) with a history of stroke are themselves at greater risk for stroke. Additionally, individuals who have had a stroke are nine times more likely to develop VCI (Acee, 2012). Of those who have suffered a stroke, only 39% survive longer than 5 years (Acee, 2012).

Ethnicity and Gender

According to epidemiologic data, prevalence of stroke is higher in black populations than white, and is more common in Asia than in Western Europe and the United States. No gender differences in VCI were reported in two large studies, one by Andersen et al. (1999) and the other by Xing et al. (2012), although women had an increased risk of AD.

Diabetes Mellitus (Type 2)

Data from longitudinal studies show a relationship between type 2 diabetes mellitus (DM) and accelerated cognitive decline and the development of VCI (Allen, Frier, & Strachan, 2004; Peila, Rodriguez, & Launeer, 2002; Umegaki, 2014). Luchsinger, Tang, Stern, Shea, and Mayeux (2001) followed 1,262 individuals for an average of 4.3 years and reported that those who had diabetes were three times more likely to develop stroke-associated dementia than those without it.

Lifestyle

According to a recent report from the Lancet Commission on Dementia Prevention (Livingston et al., 2017), nine modifiable risk factors are linked to dementia: low level of education, midlife hearing loss, physical inactivity, high blood pressure, type 2 diabetes, obesity, smoking, depression, and social isolation. Lifestyle choices can increase the risk of VCI, among

them unhealthy, high fat diets (Morris, Tangney, Wang, Sacks, Barnes, et al., 2015; Morris, Tangney, Wang, Sacks, Bennett, et al., 2015), lack of physical exercise, alcohol abuse, and smoking (Ouldred & Bryant, 2010). Unhealthy diets frequently produce obesity, which is associated with greater cognitive decline (Profenno, Porteinsson, & Faraone, 2010). Cournot and colleagues (2006) studied the relation of body mass index to cognitive function in a prospective study of healthy, middle-aged men and women. Cognitive function was evaluated at the beginning of the study and again 5 years later. After controlling for age, sex, education level, blood pressure, diabetes, and other psychosocial covariables, higher body mass index at baseline was related to lower cognitive scores and was associated with greater cognitive decline after 5 years (Cournot et al., 2006).

Aerobic exercise promotes blood flow to the brain and improves cognitive function (Baker et al., 2010). Even six months of regular exercise can produce an increase in the volume of the hippocampus, important in episodic memory formation and fact learning. Then too, aerobic exercise increases brain-derived neurotrophic factor, which nourishes neurons (Whiteman et al., 2014). The current NIH recommendation for adults 65 years or older is 150 min (2 hr 30 min) of physical activity each week. Being as physically active as you are capable is emphasized and aerobic exercise is recognized as being particularly beneficial. The scientific evidence shows that older men and women, who are more active, have lower rates of heart disease, high blood pressure, stroke, type 2 diabetes, colon cancer, breast cancer, and a higher level of cardiorespiratory and muscular fitness as well as healthier body mass and composition (World Health Organization Report and Physical Activity Guidelines Advisory Committee, 2010).

Stress can also damage the brain and increase the risk for VCI (Andel et al., 2012; Belkic, Landsbergis, Schnall, & Baker, 2004; Eller et al., 2009). Jobs associated with low job control, high job demands, and low social support at work are those that are most stressful (Andel et al., 2012).

In summary, the risk of stroke and/or VCI increases as a function of the number of risk factors that an individual has. Management of hypertension and healthy lifestyle choices significantly reduce the risk of stroke and, therefore, VCI.

Vascular Pathology May Be a Trigger for Alzheimer's Dementia

Research shows that Alzheimer's disease (AD) and cerebrovascular disease share risk factors and possibly a common etiology (Santos et al., 2017). Many investigators theorize that vascular disease may trigger dementia in individuals with AD pathology (de la Torre, 2004; Jellinger & Attems, 2010; Nagy et al., 1997; Pluta & Ulamek, 2008; Scheibel, Duong, & Jacobs, 1989; Snowdon et al., 1997). Consider the findings from the now famous "nun study." Several hundred sisters over age 75 who shared a similar lifestyle consented to extensive neuropsychological evaluation and postmortem examination of their brains (Snowdon et al., 1997). About one-third of those with AD pathology at post mortem examination were *not* demented according to results of a clinical neuropsychological examination that occurred prior to their deaths. What differentiated the nuns with AD pathology *and* dementia from those with AD pathology who were *not* demented was the *presence of neurovascular lesions*. AD pathology and the presence of cerebral infarcts appear to have an "additive effect on the odds of developing dementia" (Schneider, Wilson, Bienias, Evans, & Bennett, 2004).

Findings from other autopsy studies also suggest a synergistic relation between vascular disease and AD with the rate of co-occurrence of the two pathologies ranging from 20% to 60% (Erkinjuntti & Gauthier, 2009; Jellinger, 2002; Korczyn, 2005; Lee, Olichney, Hansen, Hofstetter, & Thal, 2000; Román & Kalaria, 2006; Zarei et al., 2009). Researchers now know that midlife vascular risk factors such as high blood pressure, diabetes, high cholesterol, and obesity are associated with elevated levels of the protein fragments (amyloid) that characterize AD (Gottesman et al., 2017). As a result, many physicians now screen for neurovascular damage through neuroimaging when evaluating patients at risk for dementia.

Comparison of Effects of Cortical and Subcortical Pathologies on Cognition and Communicative Function

Cortical Pathologies

The effects of cortical pathologies are as follows:

- In those with focal cortical lesions, one or more focal cognitive syndromes (e.g., aphasia, spatial neglect) may be present. However, their overall cognitive performance may be insufficient to meet dementia criteria.
- Individuals with large vessel disease that significantly damages left perisylvian cortex typically exhibit aphasia (Erkinjuntti, 1987; Erkinjuntti, Haltia, Palo, Sulkava, & Paetau, 1988).
- Individuals whose perisylvian pathology is insufficient to produce aphasia, nonetheless, have communication disorders secondary to executive function deficits that make them less efficient processors of linguistic information.
- If a stroke is strategically located and involves the distributions of the posterior or anterior cerebral arteries, basal ganglia, and thalamus, then language and memory are disrupted and the risk of dementia increases (Bain, 2006).
- Poststroke changes in thinking and perception that are associated with VCI include trouble speaking or understanding speech, vision loss, disorientation, and confusion (Gorelick et al., 2011).
- If damage is to fronto-subcortical circuits, particularly the circuit involving the dorsolateral prefrontal cortex, then executive dysfunction and psychomotor slowing are likely (Breteler et al., 1994; Fukuda, Kobayashi, Okada, & Tsunematsu, 1990; Hom & Reitan,

1990; Kertesz & Clydesdale, 1994; Selnes & Vinters, 2006; Tatemichi et al., 1994; Traykov et al., 2002; Wolfe, Linn, Babikian, Knoefel, & Albert, 1990).

Subcortical Pathologies

The effects of subcortical pathologies are as follows:

- Infarctions in subcortical sites, as a result of small vessel disease, can cause procedural memory deficit in individuals with VCI (Esiri, Wilcock, & Morris, 1997).
- Patients with subcortical disease often have a stepwise course of cognitive decline because of recurrent subcortical ischemic strokes.
- Individuals with subcortical ischemic disease frequently have dysarthria, motor weakness, gait disturbance, bulbar signs, deficits in executive functioning (Babikian & Ropper, 1987; Erkinjuntti, 2005; Ishii, Nishihara, & Imamura, 1986; Román, 1987), and alterations in the melody, pitch, and rate of articulation (Powell, Cummings, Hill, & Benson, 1988).
- Individuals with left dorsolateral frontal lobe damage from vascular disease often have deficits in language formulation and comprehension (Damasio & Anderson, 1993).
- The learning function deficit that exists in VCI is typically the consequence of impairment in executive control, unlike in individuals with AD whose learning deficit is secondary to episodic memory impairment that prevents the encoding of new information (Graham, Emery, & Hodges, 2004).

VCI Compared with AD

- Compared with patients with AD, patients with VCI have poorer verbal fluency, more perseverative behavior, and often exhibit apathy earlier in the course of the disease (Acee, 2012).
- A primary difference that typically distinguishes the two groups is *episodic memory function*. In individuals with AD, episodic

memory is dramatically impaired because of disease pathology in the basal forebrain and hippocampal complex. In VCI patients, "memory problems" are typically secondary to attentional and executive function deficits resulting from disruption of corticosubcortical prefrontal circuitry (Benedet, Montz, & Delgado-Bolton, 2012).

- As would be expected, individuals with both vascular and AD pathology generally have more cognitive impairment (Neal, 2012; Schneider et al., 2004; Song, Kim, Kim, Eah, & Lee, 2007; Vermeer et al., 2003; White, 2009) than those with either VCI or AD.
- Both groups of patients exhibit slowed thinking, "absent mindedness," difficulty with organization and complex problem solving, and word retrieval problems (UCSF Memory and Aging Center, 2010).
- The progression of VCI is less predictable than that of AD (World Health Organization, 2007). Some individuals with VCI exhibit relatively stable cognitive functioning with subsequent vascular events headlining a sudden decline in cognitive function (Barnes, Covinsky, Kuller, Lopez, & Yaffe, 2007), whereas AD is characterized by a progressive deterioration in cognition (World Health Organization, 2007).
- To the degree that the cognitive impairments are similar in individuals with VCI and those with AD, so also are the effects on communicative functioning.

Observations from Course-of-Disease Studies

Lechner, Bertha, and Ott (1988) conducted a 5-year prospective study of 94 patients with VCI and reported cognitive impairment in 77 of the 94 patients at the onset of stroke. Depression and loss of motivation and attention also typified the clinical picture. These same cognitive disturbances remained at follow-up but were more pronounced. The annual mortality rate ranged between 7% and 13% over the 5 years of the study. By the end of the study,

43% of study subjects had died, two-thirds from cardiovascular events. In six patients, the symptoms of dementia resolved with recovery from a strategic infarct (an infarct in a brain area that affects many cognitive functions).

Results of other course-of-disease studies have shown that the prevalence of depression ranges from 14% to 64% in VCI (Ballard & Oyebode, 1995; Burns, Jacoby, & Levy, 1990; Lyketsos et al., 2000; Starkstein, Jorge, Mizrahi, & Robinson, 2005) and the prevalence of psychosis ranges from 15% to 60% (Ballard & Oyebode, 1995; Engelborghs et al., 2005; Leroi, Voulgari, Breitner, & Lyketsos, 2003).

Desmond et al. (2000) also conducted a study of the course of cognitive decline in 453 patients who were 60 years or older and had been hospitalized with acute ischemic stroke. Patients were given a neuropsychological examination 3 months poststroke. One hundred nineteen patients, or 26.3% of the sample, were demented 3 months poststroke. Of these patients, 57% had dementia that was directly attributable to stroke or vascular disease, 38.7% had dementia due to the co-occurrence of stroke and AD, and 4.2% had dementia for other reasons such as alcohol abuse.

Similar epidemiologic studies were conducted in Finland by Pohjasvaara et al. (1998) and in Spain by Barba et al. (2000). Results of these studies, together with those from the Desmond study (Desmond, 2000), strongly suggest that between one-quarter and one-third of elderly individuals who suffer a stroke meet the criteria for dementia within 3 months.

Summary: Effects of VCI on Cognitive and Communicative Functioning

Differentiating the cognitive profiles associated with the myriad types of neurovascular disease is extremely challenging because, as previously noted, the vascular pathology present is generally not the only neuropathology. In fact, pure VCI is rare (Jellinger & Attems, 2010; Korczyn, 2002). As yet, clinicians and researchers lack well-defined cognitive and communicative function profiles. Nonetheless, regardless of the type of vascular etiology there are common problems notably: mental slowness, emotional lability, personality change, depression, and dysexecutive syndrome (McVeigh & Passmore, 2006; Wallin, Sjögren, Edman, Blennow, & Regland, 2000).

Conclusion

Much remains to be understood about the effects of the various vascular pathologies on cognitive and communicative function. Researchers are challenged by the sheer number of possible combinations of pathology and the high rate of co-occurrence of pathologies. Linguistic communication is a cognitive enterprise that depends on all aspects of memory, perception, and executive function. Deficits in virtually every aspect of cognition can have a communication consequence. Clinicians are advised to comprehensively assess clients at risk for VCI to define deficits and retained abilities that can form the basis for therapeutic intervention to improve function and quality of life.

Summary of Important Points

- Cerebrovascular disease competes with Lewy body disease and frontotemporal pathology as the second-most common cause of dementia.
- The term "vascular cognitive impairment" (VCI) is the preferred term for referring to individuals with cognitive impairment resulting from cerebrovascular disease.
- The term, "multi-infarct" dementia is out of favor because cognitive impairment and dementia can be caused by many other kinds of vascular pathology.
- VCI is the loss of cognitive function sufficient to interfere with activities of daily living that can result from large vessel or atherothromboembolic disease, small vessel disease associated with multiple infarcts, hemorrhage, or hypoperfusion.

- The diagnosis of probable VCI requires evidence of a concern about change in cognitive function, objective evidence of cognitive impairment, and neuroimaging evidence of vascular pathology.
- Among the many risk factors, hypertension is the single most important, especially when untreated for long periods of time. The incidence and prevalence of vascular disease increase with age and tend to be higher in men.
- Family history is another VCI risk factor, with an increased risk of stroke for individuals with a first-degree relative with a history of stroke.
- Prevalence of stroke is higher in black populations than white.
- Individuals who have had a stroke are nine times more likely to develop VCI.
- Although women have an increased risk for AD, there does not appear to be a gender effect for VCI.
- Diabetes (type 2) is a risk factor for stroke-associated dementia, as well as poor lifestyle choices including unhealthy diet, lack of physical exercise, alcohol abuse, obesity, smoking, and stress.
- Vascular pathology and AD pathology frequently co-occur.
- Moreover, vascular pathology appears to deleteriously interact with AD pathology to produce earlier and more severe cognitive impairment and shorter length of survival.
- In individuals with cerebrovascular disease, risk of developing dementia is increased if lesions are multiple, bilateral, and located in fronto-subcortical and limbic structures.
- Although much is understood about the type of linguistic communication deficit an individual can have with pathology in a particular region of the brain, the frequency of co-occurrence of AD, vascular disease, and Lewy body disease make it impossible to specify a "typical" linguistic communication deficit profile for the various types of vascular disease.
- Clinicians are encouraged to comprehensively assess the cognitive and communicative function of individuals at risk for VCI.

References

Acee, A. M. (2012). Type 2 diabetes and vascular dementia: Assessment and clinical strategies of care. *Medsurg Nursing, 21*, 349–353.

Alagiakrishnan, K. (2017, December 1). Vascular dementia. *Medscape*. Retrieved from https://emedicine.medscape.com/article/292105-overview

Allen, K., Frier, B., & Strachan, M. (2004). The relationship between type II diabetes and cognitive dysfunction. Longitudinal studies and their methodological limitations. *European Journal of Pharmacology, 490*, 169–175.

Andel, R., Crowe, M., Hahn, E. A., Mortimer, J. A., Pedersen, N. L., Fratiglioni, L., . . . Gatz, M. (2012). Work-related stress may increase the risk of vascular disease. *Journal of American Geriatric Society, 60*, 60–67.

Andersen, K., Launer, L. J., Dewey, M. E., Letenneur, L., Ott, A., Copeland, J. R. M., . . . Hofman, A. (1999). Gender differences in the incidence of AD and vascular dementia. *Neurology, 53*, 1992–1997.

Babikian, V., & Ropper, A. H. (1987). Binswanger's disease: A review. *Stroke, 18*, 2–12.

Bain, L. J. (2006). A review of the "state of the art" on mild cognitive impairment: The fourth annual conference. *Alzheimer's Dementia, 2*, 246–256.

Baker, L. D., Frank, L. L., Foster-Schubert, K., Green, P. S., Wilkinson, C. W., & McTiernan, A. (2010). Aerobic exercise improves cognition for older adults with glucose intolerance, a risk factor for Alzheimer's disease. *Journal of Alzheimers Disease, 22*, 569–579.

Ballard, C., & Oyebode, F. (1995). Psychotic symptoms in patients with dementia. *International Journal of Geriatric Psychiatry, 10*, 743–752.

Barba, R., Martinez-Espinosa, S., Rodriguez-Garcia, E., Pondal, M., Vivancos, J., & del Ser, T. (2000). Poststroke dementia: Clinical features and risk factors. *Stroke, 31*, 1494–1501.

Barnes, D., Covinsky, K., Kuller, L., Lopez, O., & Yaffe, K. (2007). Predicting an individual's risk of developing dementia: The cardiovascular health cognition study. *Alzheimer's and Dementia, 3*, S166.

Belkic, K. L., Landsbergis, P. A., Schnall, P. L., & Baker, D. (2004). Is job strain a major source of cardiovascular disease risk? *Scandinavian Journal of Work, Environment, and Health, 30*, 85–128.

Benedet, M. J., Montz, R., & Delgado-Bolton, R. C. (2012). Alzheimer's disease and vascular dementia: Neuropsychological differentiation in clinical practice. *Clinical Gerontologist, 35*, 88–104.

Blumenfeld, H. (2002). *Neuroanatomy through clinical cases*. Sunderland, MA: Sinauer Associates.

Breteler, M. M., Van Swieten, J. C., Bots, M. L., Grobbee, D. E., Claus, J. J., Van den Hout, J. H., . . . Hofman, A. (1994). Cerebral white matter lesions, vascular risk factors, and cognitive function in a population-based study: The Rotterdam study. *Neurology, 44*, 1246–1252.

Burns, A., Jacoby, R., & Levy, R. (1990). Psychiatric phenomena in Alzheimer's disease. III: Disorders of mood. *British Journal of Psychiatry, 157,* 81–86, 92–94.

Cournot, M., Marquié, J. C., Ansiau, D., Martinaud, C., Fonds, H., Ferriéres, J., & Ruidavets, J. B. (2006). Relation between body mass index and cognitive function in healthy middle-aged men and women. *Neurology, 67,* 1208–1214.

Damasio, A. R., & Anderson, S. W. (1993). The frontal lobes. In K. H. Heilman & E. Valenstein (Eds.), *Clinical neuropsychology* (pp. 409–460). New York, NY: Oxford University Press.

de la Torre, J. C. (2004). Is Alzheimer's disease a neurodegenerative or a vascular disorder? Data, dogma, and dialectics. *Lancet Neurology, 3,* 184–190.

Desmond, D. W., Moroney, J. T., Paik, M. C., Sano, M., Mohr, J. P., Aboumatar, S., . . . Stern,Y. (2000). Frequency and clinical determinants of dementia after ischemic stroke. *Neurology, 54,* 1124–1131.

Dichgans, M., & Leys, D. (2017) Vascular cognitive impairment. *Circulation Research, 120,* 573–591.

Doody, R. S., Stevens, J. C., Beck, C., Dubinsky, R. M., Kaye, J. A., Gwyther, L., . . . Cummings, J. L. (2001). Practice parameter: Management of dementia (an evidence-based review). Report of the Quality Standards Subcommittee of the American Academy of Neurology. *Neurology, 56,* 1154–1166.

Elias, M. F., Wolf, P. A., d'Agostino, R. B., Cobb, J., & White, L. R. (1993). Blood pressure level is inversely related to cognitive functioning: The Framingham study. *American Journal of Epidemiology, 138,* 353–364.

Eller, N. H., Netterstrøm, B., Gyntelberg, F., Kristensen, T. S., Nielsen, F., Steptoe, A., & Theorell, T. (2009). Work-related psychosocial factors and the development of ischemic heart disease: A systematic review. *Cardiology in Review, 17,* 83–97.

Enciu, A.-M., Constaninescu, S. N., Popescu, L. M., Muresanu, D. F., & Popescu, B. O. (2011). Neurobiology of vascular dementia. *Journal of Aging Research, 2011,* 1–11.

Engelborghs, S., Maertens, K., Nagels, G., Vloeberghs, E., Mariën, P., Symons, A., . . . de Deyn, P. P. (2005). Neuropsychiatric symptoms of dementia: Cross-sectional analysis from a prospective, longitudinal Belgian study. *International Journal of Geriatric Psychiatry, 20,* 1028–1037.

Erkinjuntti, T. (1987). Types of multi-infarct dementia. *Acta Neurologica Scandinavica, 75,* 391–399.

Erkinjuntti, T. (2005). Vascular cognitive impairment. In A. Burns, J. O'Brien, & D. Ames (Eds.), *Dementia* (3rd ed., pp. 529–545). London, UK: Hodder Arnold.

Erkinjuntti, T., & Gauthier, S. (2009). The concept of vascular cognitive impairment. *Frontiers of Neurology and Neuroscience, 24,* 79–85.

Erkinjuntti, T., Haltia, M., Palo, J., Sulkava, R., & Paetau, A. (1988). Accuracy of the clinical diagnosis of vascular dementia: A retrospective clinical and post-mortem neuropathological study. *Journal of Neurology, Neurosurgery, and Psychiatry, 51,* 1037–1044.

Esiri, M. M., Wilcock G. K., & Morris, J. H. (1997). Neuropathological assessment of the lesions of significant in vascular dementia. *Journal of Neurology, Neurosurgery, and Psychiatry, 63,* 749–753.

European Society of Hypertension. (2003). European Society of cardiology guidelines for the management of arterial hypertension guidelines committee. *Journal of Hypertension, 21,* 1011–1053.

Fukuda, H., Kobayashi, S., Okada, K., & Tsunematsu, T. (1990). Frontal white matter lesions and dementia in lacunar infarction. *Stroke, 21,* 1143–1149.

Gorelick, P. B., Scuteri, A., Black, S. E., Decarli, C., Greenberg, S., Iadecola, C., . . . Seshadri, S. (2011). American Heart Association Stroke Council, Council on Epidemiology and Prevention, Council on Cardiovascular Nursing, Council on Cardiovascular Radiology and Intervention, and Council on Cardiovascular Surgery and Anesthesia. Vascular contributions to cognitive impairment and dementia: A statement for healthcare professionals from the American Heart Association/American Stroke Association. *Stroke, 42,* 2672–2713.

Gottesman, R. F., Schneider, A. L. C., Zhou, Y., Coresh, J., Green, E., Gupta, N., . . . Mosley, T. H. (2017). Association between midlife vascular risk factors and estimated brain amyloid deposition. *Journal of American Medical Association, 317,* 1443.

Graham, N. L., Emery, T., & Hodges, J. R. (2004). Distinctive cognitive profiles in Alzheimer's disease and subcortical vascular dementia. *Journal of Neurology, Neurosurgery, and Psychiatry, 75,* 61–71.

Hachinski, V. C., Lassen, N. A., & Marshall, J. (1974). Multi-infarct dementia: A cause of mental deterioration in the elderly. *Lancet, 2,* 207–210.

Hom, J., & Reitan, R. M. (1990). Generalized cognitive function after stroke. *Journal of Clinical and Experimental Neuropsychology, 12,* 644–654.

Iadecola, C., Park, L., & Capone, C. (2009). Threats to the mind. *Stroke, 40,* S40–S44.

Ishii, N., Nishihara, Y., & Imamura, T. (1986). Why do frontal lobe symptoms predominate in vascular dementia with lacunes? *Neurology, 36,* 340–345.

Jack, V. T. (2010). Reducing the global burden of stroke: INTERSTROKE. *Lancet, 376,* 74–75.

Jellinger, K. A. (2002). Alzheimer disease and cerebrovascular pathology: An update. *Journal of Neural Transmission, 109,* 813–836.

Jellinger, K. A. (2007). The enigma of vascular cognitive disorder and vascular dementia. *Acta Neuropathologica, 113,* 349–388.

Jellinger, K. A., & Attems, J. (2010). Is there pure vascular dementia in old age? *Journal of the Neurological Sciences, 299,* 150–154.

Jouvent, E., & Chabriat, H. (2014). Conventional imaging of lacunar infarcts. In L. Pantoni & P. Gorelick (Eds.), *Cerebral Small Vessel Disease* (pp. 129–138). Cambridge, UK: Cambridge University Press.

Kertesz, A., & Clydesdale, S. (1994). Neuropsychological deficits in vascular dementia vs Alzheimer's disease. Frontal lobe deficits prominent in vascular dementia. *Archives of Neurology, 51*, 1226–1231.

Kilander, L., Andrén, B., Nyman, H., Lind, L., Boberg, M., & Lithell, H. (1998). Atrial fibrillation is an independent determinant of low cognitive function: A cross-sectional study in elderly men. *Stroke, 29*, 1816–1820.

Korczyn, A. D. (2002). Mixed dementia—the most common cause of dementia. *Annals of the New York Academy of Sciences, 977*, 129–134.

Korczyn, A. D. (2005). The underdiagnosis of the vascular contribution to dementia. *Journal of the Neurological Sciences, 229–230*, 3–6.

Korczyn, A. D. (2016). What is new in vascular dementia? *BMC Medicine, 14*, 175.

Lechner, H., Bertha, G., & Ott, E. (1988). Results of a five-year prospective study of 94 patients with vascular and multi-infarct dementia. In J. S. Meyer, H. Lechner, J. Marshall, & J. F. Toole (Eds.), *Vascular and multiinfarct dementia* (pp. 101–111), Mount Kisco, NY: Future Publishing.

Lee, J. H., Olichney, J. M., Hansen, L. A., Hofstetter, C. R., & Thal, L. J. (2000). Small concomitant vascular lesions do not influence rates of cognitive decline in patients with Alzheimer disease. *Archives of Neurology, 57*, 1474–1479.

Leroi, I., Voulgari, A., Breitner, J. C., & Lyketsos, C. G. (2003). The epidemiology of psychosis in dementia. *American Journal of Geriatric Psychiatry, 11*, 83–91.

Livingston, G., Sommerlad, A., Orgeta, V., Costafreda, S. G., Huntley, J., Ames, D., ... Mukadam, N. (2017) Dementia prevention, intervention, and care. *The Lancet, 17*, 31363–31366.

Lobo, A., Launer, L. J., Fratiglioni, L., Andersen, K., di Carlo, A., Breteler, M. M., . . . Hofman, A. (2000). Prevalence of dementia and major subtypes in Europe: A collaborative study of population-based cohorts. Neurologic diseases in the elderly research group. *Neurology, 54*, S4–S9.

Luchsinger, J. A., Tang, M. X., Stern, Y., Shea, S., & Mayeux, R. (2001). Diabetes mellitus and risk of Alzheimer's disease and dementia with stroke in a multiethnic cohort. *American Journal of Epidemiology, 154*, 635–641.

Lyketsos, C. G., Steinberg, M., Tschanz, J. T., Norton, M. C., Steffens, D. C., & Breitner, J. C. S. (2000). Mental and behavioral disturbances in dementia: Findings from the cache county study on memory in aging. *American Journal of Psychiatry, 157*, 708–714.

McKeith, I. G., Dickson, D. W., Lowe, J., Emre, M., O'Brien, J. T., Feldman, H., . . . Yamada, M. (2005). Diagnosis and management of dementia with Lewy bodies: Third report of the DLB consortium. *Neurology, 65*, 1863–1872.

McVeigh, C., & Passmore, P. (2006). Vascular dementia: Prevention and treatment. *Clinical Interventions in Aging, 1*, 229–235.

Morris, M. C., Tangney, C. C., Wang, Y., Sacks, F. M., Barnes, L. L., Bennett, D. A., & Aggarwal, N. T. (2015a). MIND diet slows cognitive decline with aging. *Alzheimers Dementia, 11*, 1015–1022.

Morris, M. C., Tangney, C. C., Wang, Y., Sacks, F. M., Bennett, D. A., & Aggarwal, N. T. (2015b). MIND diet associated with reduced incidence of Alzheimer's disease. *Alzheimers Dementia, 11*, 1007–1014.

Moskowitz, M. A., Lo, E. H., & Iadecola, C. (2010). The science of stroke: Mechanisms in search of treatments. *Neuron, 67*, 181–198.

Nagy, Z., Esiri, M. M., Jobst, K. A., Morris, J. H., King, E. M., Mcdonald, B., . . . Smith, A. D. (1997). The effects of additional pathology on the cognitive deficit in Alzheimer disease. *Journal of Neuropathology and Experimental Neurology, 56*, 165–170.

Neal, J. W. (2012). Vascular dementia: Why pathology is still important. *Reviews in Clinical Gerontology, 22*, 35–51.

Ouldred, E., & Bryant, C. (2010). Vascular risk factors and dementia. *British Journal of Cardiac Nursing, 5*, 240–246.

Peila, R., Rodriguez, B. L., & Launeer, L. J. (2002). Type 2 diabetes. APOE gene and the risk for dementia and related pathologies. The Honolulu-Asia aging study. *Diabetes, 51*, 1256–1262.

Pluta, R., & Ulamek, M. (2008). Brain ischemia and ischemic blood-brain barrier as etiological factors in sporadic Alzheimer's disease. *Neuropsychiatric Disease and Treatment, 4*, 855–864.

Pohjasvaara, T., Erkinjuntti, T., Ylikoski, R., Hietanen, M., Vataja, R., & Kaste, M. (1998). Clinical determinants of poststroke dementia. *Stroke, 29*, 75–81.

Powell, A. L., Cummings, J. L., Hill, M. A, & Benson, D. F. (1988). Speech and language alterations in multi-infarct dementia. *Neurology, 38*, 717–719.

Profenno, L. A., Porteinsoon, A. P., & Faraone S. V. (2010). Meta-analysis of Alzheimer's disease risk with obesity, diabetes, and related disorders. *Biological Psychiatry, 67*, 505–512.

Rockwood, K., Wenzel, C., Hachinski, V., Hogan, D. B., MacKnight, C., & Mcdowell, I. (2000). Prevalence and outcomes of vascular cognitive impairment. *Neurology, 54*, 447–451.

Román, G. C. (1987). Senile dementia of the Binswanger type. A vascular form of dementia in the elderly. *Journal of the American Medical Association, 258*, 1782–1788.

Román, G. C. (2002). Vascular dementia may be the most common form of dementia in the elderly. *Journal of Neurological Sciences, 15*, 203–204.

Román, G. C. (2003). Stroke, cognitive decline and vascular dementia: The silent epidemic of the 21st century. *Stroke, 22*, 161–164.

Román, G. C., & Kalaria, R. N. (2006). Vascular determinants of cholinergic deficits in Alzheimer disease and vascular dementia. *Neurobiology of Aging, 27*, 1769–1785.

Rosenberg, J. (2016). Vascular cognitive impairment: Biomarkers in diagnosis and molecular targets in therapy. *Journal of Cerebral Blood Flow Metabolism, 36*, 4–5.

Sachdev, P., Kalaria, R., O'Brien, J., Skoog, I., Alladi, S., Black, S. E., ... Scheltens, P. (2014). Diagnostic criteria for vascular cognitive disorders: A VASCOG statement. *Alzheimer's Disease and Associated Disorders, 28*, 206–218.

Santos, C. Y., Snyder, P. J., Wu, W.-C., Zhang, M., Echeverria, A., & Alber, J. (2017). Pathophysiologic relationship between Alzheimers disease, cerebrovascular disease, and cardiovascular risk: A review and synthesis. *Alzheimer's and Dementia: Diagnosis, Assessment and Disease Monitoring, 7*, 69–87.

Scheibel, A. B., Duong, T., & Jacobs, R. (1989). Alzheimer's disease as a capillary dementia, *Annals of Medicine, 21*, 103–107.

Schneider, J. A., Wilson, R. S., Bienias, J. L., Evans, D. A., & Bennett, D. A. (2004). Cerebral infarctions and the likelihood of dementia from Alzheimer's disease pathology. *Neurology, 62*, 1148–1155.

Selnes, O. A., & Vinters, H. V. (2006). Vascular cognitive impairment. *Nature Clinical Practice Neurology, 2*, 538–547.

Sharp, S. I., Aarsland, D., Day, S., Sønnesyn, H., Alzheimer's Society Vascular Dementia Systematic Review Group, & Ballard, C. (2011). Hypertension is a potential risk factor for vascular dementia: A systematic review. *International Journal of Geriatric Psychiatry, 26*, 661–669.

Snowdon, D. A., Greiner, L. H., Mortimer, J. A., Riley, K. P., Greiner, P. A., & Markesbery, W. R. (1997). Brain infarction and the clinical expression of Alzheimer disease: The nun Study. *The Journal of the American Medical Association, 277*, 813–817.

Song, I. U., Kim, J. S., Kim Y. I., Eah, K. Y., & Lee, K. S. (2007). Clinical significance of silent cerebral infarctions in patients with Alzheimer disease. *Cognitive Behavioral Neurology, 20*, 93–98.

Starkstein, S. E., Jorge, R., Mizrahi, R., & Robinson, R. G. (2005). The construct of minor and major depression in Alzheimer's disease. *American Journal of Psychiatry, 162*, 2086–2093.

Swan, G. E., Decarli, C., Miller, B. L., Reed, T., Wolf, P. A., Jack, L. M., & Carmelli, D. (1998). Association of midlife blood pressure to late life cognitive decline and brain morphology. *Neurology, 51*, 986–993.

Tatemichi, T. K., Desmond, D. W., Stern, Y., Paik, M., Sano, M., & Bagiella, E. (1994). Cognitive impairment after stroke: Frequency, patterns, and relationship to function abilities. *Journal of Neurology, Neurosurgery, and Psychiatry, 57*, 202–207.

Traykov, L., Baudic, S., Thibaudet, M. C., Rigaud, A. S., Smagghe, A., & Boller, F. (2002). Neuropsychological deficit in early subcortical vascular dementia: Comparison to Alzheimer's disease. *Dementia and Geriatric Cognitive Disorders, 22*, 445–454.

UCSF Memory and Aging Center. (2010). *Vascular dementia*. Retrieved from https://memory.ucsf.edu/vascular-dementia

Umegaki, H. (2014). Type 2 diabetes as a risk factor for cognitive impairment: Current insights. *Clinical Interventions in Aging, 9*, 1011–1019.

Vermeer, S. E., Prins, N. D., den Heijer, T., Hofman, A., Koudstaal, P. J., & Breteler, M. M. (2003). Silent brain infarcts and the risk of dementia and cognitive decline. *New England Journal of Medicine, 348*, 1215–1222.

Wallin, A., Sjögren, M., Edman, A., Blennow, K., & Regland, B. (2000). Symptoms, vascular risk factors and blood-brain barrier function in relation to CT white-matter changes in dementia. *European Neurology, 44*, 229–235.

White, L. (2009). Brain lesions at autopsy in older Japanese-American men as related to cognitive impairment and dementia in the final years of life: A summary report from the Honolulu-Asia aging study. *Journal of Alzheimers Disease, 18*, 713–725.

Whiteman, A., Young, D. E., He, X., Chen, T. C., Wagenaar, R. C., & Stern, C. (2014). Interaction between serum BDNF and aerobic fitness predicts recognition memory in healthy young adults. *Behavioral Brain Research, 259*, 302–312.

Wolfe, N., Linn, R., Babikian, V. L., Knoefel, J. E., & Albert, M. L. (1990). Frontal systems impairment following multiple lacunar infarcts. *Archives of Neurology, 47*, 129–132.

World Health Organization. (2010). *Global recommendations on physical activity for health*. Retrieved from http://www.who.int/dietphysicalactivity/global-PA-recs-2010.pdf

World Health Organization. (2007). *The ICD-10 Classification of Mental and Behavioural Disorders: Clinical descriptions and diagnostic guidelines*. 10th revision. World Health Organization, Geneva. Retrieved December 4, 2017, from http://www.who.int/classifications/icd/en/bluebook.pdf

Xing, Y., Wei, C., Changbiao, C., Zhou, A., Fang, L., Wu, L., ... Jia, J. (2012). Stage-specific gender differences in cognitive and neuropsychiatric manifestations of vascular dementia. *American Journal of Alzheimer's Disease and Other Dementias, 27*, 433–438.

Zarei, M., Damoiseaux, J. S., Morgese, C., Beckman, C. H. F., Smith, S. M., Matthews, P. M., . . . Barkhof, F. (2009). Regional white matter integrity differentiates between vascular dementia and Alzheimer disease. *Stroke, 40*, 773–779.

7

Parkinson's Disease and Dementia

Parkinsonism and Parkinson's Disease (PD)

Parkinsonism is a syndrome characterized by resting tremor, muscle rigidity, and slowness of movement. It is associated with several neurological conditions and neurodegenerative diseases, among them Alzheimer's disease (AD), Lewy body disease (LBD), multiple system atrophy, progressive supranuclear palsy, and cortical–basal ganglionic degeneration. However, the vast majority of individuals with the movement disorders of parkinsonism have idiopathic Parkinson's disease (PD), named for James Parkinson, the English neurologist who described it in 1817. In addition to the characteristic movement disorders, PD is associated with cognitive impairment, and a significant percentage of patients develop frank dementia.

Incidence and Prevalence

With advancing age, the incidence and prevalence of PD increase (de Rijk et al., 1995; Morens et al., 1996; Reeve, Simcox, & Turnbull, 2016). Appearance of the disease before the age of 40 is unusual, and men are one and a half times more likely to have the disease than women (Fall et al., 1996; Kuopio, Marttila, Helenius, & Rinne, 1999; Mayeux et al., 1995; Parkinson's Disease Foundation, 2017). The overall incidence rate in individuals 40 years

and older is 37.75 per 100,000 person years for women and 61.21 for men (Hirsch, Jette, Frolkis, Steeves, & Pringsheim, 2016).

Within North America, approximately a million individuals carry the PD diagnosis and 60,000 new cases are diagnosed yearly (Parkinson's Disease Foundation, 2017), though many more go undiagnosed. With the growth in the elderly population, these figures are expected to double by the year 2040. The cost of the disease in the United Stated is estimated to be nearly $25 billion annually as a result of lost income from the inability to work, treatment, and social security payments.

Symptoms of PD: Motor, Affective, Cognitive

Common initial complaints of individuals with PD are aching pains, paresthesia (a sensation of burning or tingling in the absence of external stimulation), numbness, and coldness. These complaints are followed by the appearance of one or more of the classic *motor symptoms*: slowness of movement, rigidity, postural instability, and rest tremor. Often motor symptoms develop first on one side of the body. Changes in gait and arm swing can also appear early, before postural instability is noted. The degree of arm swing during walking becomes asymmetric. Another common symptom is the lack of expressive movement in the face, a condition known as masked facies, or hypomimia. Other symptoms include drooling, changes in rate of blinking, and micrography (tiny writing).

In addition to the movement disorders, individuals with PD can present with *behavioral and affective symptoms*, among them apathy, sleep disorders, excessive daytime sleepiness, delusions, constipation, and difficulty swallowing (Chaudhuri & Schapira, 2009). The speech-language pathologist may be the first professional to see an individual who is in the early stage of PD because of swallowing difficulty or changes in voice and speech that include soft speech and dysarthria.

Depression is common in individuals with PD and is the result of endogenous and exogenous factors; namely, altered brain chemistry because of disease pathology and the knowledge of having a chronic disease. Between 35% and 50% of individuals with PD develop

depression (Arun, Bharath, Pal, & Singh, 2011; Chaudhuri & Schapira, 2009). Usually it is mild, but in 5% to 7% of cases, it is severe. Its appearance is more common in younger female patients in the early stage of illness (Wengel, Bohac, & Burke, 2005). Clinicians need to be aware of the high frequency of depression because its presence can impact memory, disrupt executive function, cause a misdiagnosis of dementia, and severely diminish quality of life (Menza et al., 2009). If suspected, clinicians should refer the patient to a neurologist or psychiatrist for treatment.

Subtle changes in *cognition* also occur early (Biundo, Weis, & Antonini, 2016; Cooper, Sagar, Jordan, Harvey, & Sullivan, 1991; Lees & Smith, 1983; Litvan et al., 2011). Between 20% and 50% of PD patients have mild cognitive impairment (PD-MCI) (Pedersen, Larsen, Janvin, Larsen, Aarsland, & Hugdahl, 2006; Tysnes, & Alves,

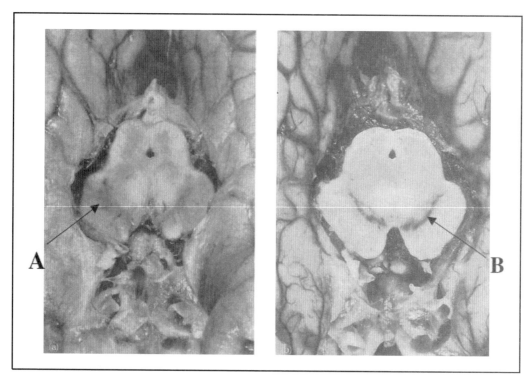

Figure 7–1. A. The substantia nigra in a case of idiopathic Parkinson's disease. **B.** Normally pigmented mesencephalon. (From Esiri & Morris, 2004; arrows added)

2013). Commonly reported are deficits in the various memory systems, attention, executive function; processing speed; and visuospatial function. Consensus criteria now exist for detecting mild cognitive impairment in individuals with PD and are listed later in this chapter.

Neuropathology of PD

Given the varied symptomatology, it is unsurprising that PD is considered a *multisystem* neurodegenerative disorder that affects the central and peripheral nervous systems. When half or more dopaminergic cells in the substantia nigra disappear, as a result of alpha-synuclein pathology, parkinsonian symptoms develop (Lozano & Kalia, 2005). Alpha-synuclein is a protein that normally occurs in the brain and body. It is found in the presynaptic terminals of neurons in the brain and has a role in the release of neurotransmitters that relay signals between neurons. When unregulated, this protein impairs synaptic dopamine release, an effect that is thought to eventuate in the death of nigrostriatal neurons (Longhena, Faustini, Missale, Pizzi, Spano, & Bellucci, 2017). The result is movement disorders. Because alpha-synuclein attacks neuron terminals, PD is considered a "synaptopathy," which is a disease characterized by synapse defects (Brose, O'Connor, & Skehel, 2010; Lepeta et al., 2016). Alpha-synuclein is also a major constituent of Lewy bodies: abnormal clumps of protein that collect in the nerve cells of people with PD. They are named after Frederich Lewy, the neurologist who discovered them. These aggregations of proteins interfere with synaptic transmission (Braak & Braak, 2000; Hirsh, 2000; Takahashi & Wakabayashi, 2005). Figure 7–1A is a picture of the brain of an individual with idiopathic PD; Figure 7–1B is a picture of a normal brain. Note the widespread distribution of Lewy bodies.

Other changes in the brains of people with PD include widespread cortical atrophy and thinning of the neocortex, particularly in the temporoparietal area and subcortex (Biundo et al., 2016). PD patients with exclusive Lewy body pathology are rare, approximately a third of those who come to autopsy (Colosimo, Hughes, Kilford, & Lees, 2003; Kotzbauer et al., 2012). Because PD pathology is so diffuse and varied, many cognitive domains are affected, making it difficult to attribute the various cognitive deficits to a specific pathology in a specific brain area or system.

Risk Factors

Many factors appear to influence development of the disease: age, heredity, sex, and exposure to toxins. The primary and undisputed risk factor is age. As previously noted, young adults rarely experience the disease and most people develop the disease in their 60s (Van Den Eeden et al., 2003).

A number of gene mutations have been identified, but they appear to be responsible for only a small number of individuals with PD. Having a first degree relative (father, mother, sister, brother) with the disease increases one's chances; nonetheless, the risk is small unless many family relatives have the disease.

Toxin exposure can lead to PD (Campdelacreu, 2014; Fitzmaurice et al., 2013), particularly exposure to carbon monoxide, herbicides, and pesticides. In fact, pesticides can destroy dopaminergic neurons (Wirdefeldt, Adami, Cole, Trichopoulos, & Mandel, 2011). Results of a systematic review and meta-analytic studies of pesticide exposure and the development of PD (van der Mark et al., 2012) revealed a positive association between exposure to herbicides and insecticides but not fungicides. Other environmental variables that are associated with PD are rural living (Koller et al. 1990; Wong, Gray, Hassanein, & Koller, 1991), consumption of well water (Koller et al., 1990; Wong et al., 1991), and exposure to certain metals (Gorell et al., 1997). For example, parkinsonism has been reported in individuals with high exposure to manganese and lead (Kwakye, Paoliello, Mukhopadhyay,

Bowman, & Aschner, 2015), and researchers have documented higher than normal levels of iron, copper, and zinc in the substantia nigra of individuals with PD (Qureshi, Qureshi, Memon, & Parvez, 2006). Aluminum has received considerable attention as a causative agent because it is often present in drinking water and is a known neurotoxin that can induce formation of neurofibrillary tangles. Results of a 15-year follow-up study revealed that cognitive decline over time was greater in individuals with a higher daily intake of aluminum from drinking water or geographic exposure (Rondeau, Jacqmin-Gadda, Commenges, Helmer, & Dartigues, 2009).

Diagnostic Criteria for PD

Criteria exist for distinguishing clinically possible from clinically probable and clinically definite PD. Clinically *possible* idiopathic PD requires the presence of one of the following: resting or postural tremor, rigidity, or bradykinesia. Clinically *probable* idiopathic PD requires any two of the four cardinal features: resting tremor, rigidity, bradykinesia, or impaired postural reflexes. Alternatively, asymmetric resting tremor, rigidity, or bradykinesia are sufficient. Clinically *definite* idiopathic PD requires any combination of three of the four cardinal features. Alternatively, two of these features are sufficient with one of the first three (tremor, ridigity, bradykinesia) displaying asymmetry.

Cognition: Continuum from Normal to Dementia

Mild cognitive impairment (MCI) is a transitional state between normal cognition and dementia and is common in the early stages of PD (Biundo et al., 2016; Yang, Tang, & Guo, 2016). Thus, clinicians are keenly interested in detecting mild cognitive impairment early to enable those with the disease to build cognitive reserve. As the disease progresses, the degree

of cognitive impairment increases and if individuals have the disease long enough, they typically develop dementia (Aarsland & Kurz, 2010). Many individuals develop dementia within 6 to 10 years of disease onset (Dubois et al., 2007). In 2012, the following criteria were provided for the diagnosis of PD-MCI (Litvan et al., 2012).

Diagnostic Criteria PD-MCI

The criteria for PD-MCI include: (a) a diagnosis of PD; (b) a report of gradual decline in cognitive ability by either the patient, knowledgeable informant, or clinician; and (c) subnormal performance on normed neuropsychological tests of the following cognitive domains: attention/working memory, executive function, episodic memory, visuoperceptual and visuospatial function, and language. Two levels of neuropsychological evaluation were recommended. Level I permits the use of a global cognitive assessment or fewer than two tests in each of the five cognitive domains, whereas Level II requires the use of more than one test in each of the domains. PD-MCI is diagnosed when any two (or more) impaired test scores are 1 to 2 standard deviations below normative data but the examinee is nonetheless able to carry out activities of daily living. Additionally, a below normal performance on the neuropsychological tests cannot be attributed to delirium, stroke, depression, metabolic abnormalities, drug side-effects, severe anxiety, or head trauma.

A red flag for PD-MCI is rapid eye movement behavior disorder (RBD). During rapid eye movement sleep (REM sleep) in healthy individuals, movement is inhibited. When that inhibition does not occur, many motor behaviors can occur during dreaming, among them limb twitching, flailing of arms and legs, even hopping out of bed. RBD has been characterized as dreamers "acting out" their dreams. In a study by Boot and colleagues (2012), RBD was associated with a 2.2-fold increased risk of PD-MCI over the next 4 years.

Diagnostic Criteria for Parkinson's Disease with Dementia (PDD)

The Task Force of the Movement Disorder Society specified diagnostic criteria for PDD (Dubois et al., 2007). These criteria are essentially the same as those established by the American Psychiatric Association (2013) for dementia with the addition of the criterion that the individual must have been clinically diagnosed with PD:

- Evidence of significant cognitive decline from a previous level of performance in at least two of the core cognitive domains: attention/working memory, language, executive function, visual perceptual-motor function, and social cognition.
- The examinee must require assistance in the execution of the instrumental activities of daily living, such as paying bills or managing medications.
- The cognitive deficits do not occur exclusively in the context of delirium.
- The cognitive deficits are not better explained by another mental disorder.

Prevalence of PDD

In a review of 24 studies in which PDD was differentiated from dementia with Lewy bodies, 31% of PD patients were found to have dementia (Rodnitzky, 2017). Among all individuals with dementia, PDD accounts for approximately 4% of cases (Aarsland et al., 2008). Although estimates of the incidence of dementia vary significantly, there is no dispute that the longer individuals have the disease, the more likely they are to develop dementia. Foltynie, Brayne, Robbins, and Barker (2004) reported that 50% of those in their longitudinal study had dementia at the 8-year follow-up. Janvin, Aarsland, and Larsen (2005) documented a higher conversion rate after 8 years in a community-based population: at baseline, the conversion rate was 26%, 52% at 4 years, and 78% at 8 years. An even higher rate was

observed by Hobson and Meara (2015) in their 16-year follow-up study. By 16 years, 90% of those with mild cognitive impairment had evolved to dementia.

Reid, Hely, Morris, Loy, and Halliday (2011) observed that conversion to dementia occurs around the age of 70 years regardless of time of disease onset. This may account for the numerous reports of higher prevalence of dementia in patients who are diagnosed when they are older (Matilla & Rinne, 1976; Mayeux et al., 1992; Reid, 1992) and the shorter time period between diagnosis and conversion to dementia. It is widely known that those who developed the disease at an earlier age typically have longer survival and later onset of dementia. When dementia does develop, death frequently occurs within 3 years (Kempster, O'Sullivan, Holton, Revesz, & Lees, 2010). Factors that increase the risk for developing dementia are older age, greater severity of parkinsonism, history of hallucinations, and MCI at first evaluation (Hobson & Meara, 2015; Levy et al., 2002).

Nature of Cognitive Impairment

As previously noted, cognitive deficits occur early in a range of cognitive domains (Litvan et al., 2011). Those cognitive deficits most commonly observed are in attention, executive function, memory, visuoperceptual and visuomotor skills, and language (Dubois & Pillon, 1997; Galtier, Nieto, & Barroso, 2016; Girotti et al., 1988; Hobson & Meara, 2015; Stern, Richards, Sano, & Mayeux, 1993; Watson & Leverenz, 2010).

Attention/Executive Function

Impaired vigilance and fluctuating attention occur in the majority of PD patients without dementia (Mamikonyan et al., 2009; Muslimovic, Post, Speelman, & Schmand, 2005). These nondemented PD patients often have deficits on tasks like Trail Making, which requires the examinee to draw a line between a sequence of numbers and letters (A then 1, B then 2, C then 3, and so on), and other measures of divided attention, planning, response inhibition, and mental flexibility (Aarsland, Bronnick, Larsen, Tysnes, & Alves, 2009; Janvin et al., 2006; Siegert, Weatherall, Taylor, & Abernethy, 2008).

The executive function deficits of individuals with PD are particularly apparent on tasks requiring generation of information, such as naming exemplars in a category (a.k.a., verbal fluency or generative naming) (Aarsland, Andersen, Larsen, Lolk, & Kragh-Sorensen, 2003; Azuma, Cruz, Bayles, Tomoeda, & Montgomery, 2003; Bom de Araujo et al., 2011; Cahn-Weiner, Grace, Ott, Fernandez, & Friedman, 2002; Dadgar, Khatoonabadi, & Bakhtiyari, 2013; Henry & Crawford, 2004). In semantic or letter category naming, individuals must hold an instruction in mind while searching long-term memory for as many exemplars of items in the category as possible in a limited time period, usually a minute. Common semantic category fluency tasks include naming animals, birds, methods of transportation, and fruits; common letter fluency tasks include naming words that begin with the letters F, A, and S.

Particularly characteristic of PD is slowness in the processing of information, a condition called bradyphrenia (Rippon & Marder, 2005). Reaction time is also slower than that of healthy elders (Camicioli, Wieler, de Frias, & Martin, 2008; de Frias, Dixon, Fisher, & Camicioli, 2007). Slowness is particularly apparent in tasks that involve problem solving, sequencing, shifting sets, and planning (Bondi, Kaszniak, Bayles, & Vance, 1993; Emre, 2003; Lees & Smith, 1983; Owen et al., 1992; Taylor, Saint-Cyr, & Lang, 1986).

Severity of executive function deficits appears to differ between those nondemented PD patients who experience visual hallucinations and those who do not (Imamura, Wada-Isoe, Kitayama, & Nakashima, 2008). Imamura and colleagues compared executive function performance on a variety of tests (verbal fluency, Stroop, digit span, counting backward, and speeded recitations of months and letter counts) in these two groups and those with hallucinations had executive dysfunction that was similar in severity to that of PDD subjects.

Memory

Memory for recall of recently presented verbal and nonverbal material can be disrupted early in the disease course. Ultimately, all forms of memory (working, declarative and nondeclarative, and prospective) are impacted in individuals with dementia (Helkala, Laulumaa, Soininen, & Riekkinen, 1989; Litvan, Mohr, Williams, Gomez, & Chase, 1991; Pillon, Deweer, Agid, & Dubois, 1993; Stern et al., 1993). Smith, Souchay, and Moulin (2011) report deficits in prospective memory ("delayed execution of actions to be performed in the future"), especially in time-based tasks requiring examinees to be aware of the passing of time. This finding is related to other reports that time estimation is consistently impaired in people with PD (Koch et al., 2008; Wearden et al., 2008). Whereas the deficits in working memory are attributed to damage to the prefrontal cortex, the episodic and procedural learning and memory deficits are attributed to basal ganglia pathology (Harrington, Haaland, Yeo, & Marder, 1990; Hochstadt, Nakano, Lieberman, & Friedman, 2006; Stefanova, Kostic, Ziropadja, Markovic, & Ocic, 2000).

Results of a longitudinal study of cognitive function in individuals with PD indicate that three cognitive factors primarily account for the dementia: progressive worsening of visuospatial memory, verbal memory, and working memory (Johnson & Galvin, 2011). The most precipitous decline in patients with PD in the Johnson and Galvin study was on measures of visuospatial function. They emphasized that "PD takes a heavy toll on visuospatial abilities regardless of the status in other cognitive domains" (Johnson & Galvin, p. 105).

Visuoperceptual/Visuospatial Function Deficits

Individuals with PD have myriad visual system impairments that are linked to their dopamine deficiency (Bodis-Wollner, 2002; Rodnitzky, 1998). When given dopaminergic therapy, they improve. The most frequently reported diminished functions are with:

- Visual acuity (Archibald, Clarke, Repka, Claro, Loupe, & Reich, 1996; Mosimann, & Burn, 2011)
- Navigating everyday environments (Archibald et al., 2011; Urwyler et al., 2014)
- Visuospatial construction, orientation, and memory (Antal, Bandini, Kéri, & Bodis-Wollner, 1998; Garcia-Diaz et al., 2014)
- Space perception (Ramirez-Ruiz, Junque, Marti, Valldeoriola, & Tolosa, 2007)
- Object perception (Barnes, Boubert, Harris, Lee, & David, 2003)
- Visuospatial orientation (Davidsdottir, Cronin-Golomb, & Lee, 2005; Galtier, Nieto, Barroso, & Lorenzo, 2009; Kemps, Szmalec, Vandierendonck, & Crevits, 2005)
- Color discrimination (Bertrand et al., 2012; Büttner et al., 1993, 1995)
- Contrast sensitivity (Bulens, Meerwaldt, & van der Wildt, 1988; Regan & Maxner, 1987; Silva et al., 2005; Struck, Rodnitzky, & Dobson, 1990)
- Facial recognition and recognition of emotion (Bruna, Roig, Junque, & Vendrell, 2000; Hipp, Diederich, Pieria & Vaillant, 2014)

Additionally, visual hallucinations are common in PD, although auditory, olfactory, and tactile hallucinations are also reported (Chaudhury, 2010). Researchers report that disconnections of brain areas that subserve attention and visual processing may contribute to visual hallucinations in PD (Hepp et al., 2017). Visuoperceptual and visuomotor deficits also are present and exacerbated by executive function deficits (Levin et al. 1991; Stern, Mayeux, Rosen, & Ilson, 1983).

Communicative Function of PD Patients without and with Dementia

According to Krysiak (2011), 89% of PD patients have speech and language disorders, though few receive treatment for them. The speech of affected individuals is softer, less precise, and hypokinetic dysarthria is common. True language disorders involving loss of linguistic knowledge are uncommon. On the other hand, language performance problems are common and typically reflect deficits in cognitive processes rather than loss of linguistic knowledge. Normal linguistic communication requires linguistic knowledge (knowledge of phonology, syntax, semantics, pragmatics) *and* integrity of cognitive abilities such as attention, perception, and memory.

An individual can have a communication disorder without a language deficit, and in nondemented PD (NPD) patients that generally is the case. A diminished performance on neuropsychological tasks that involve language, such as semantic category naming, typically reflect deficits in executive function and working memory rather than loss of linguistic knowledge (Bayles, 1990). Hochstadt et al. (2006) administered tests of sentence comprehension, verbal working memory span, and cognitive set switching to 41 PD patients. Although impairment was evident on sentences containing relative clauses, it was attributed to observed deficits in cognitive set switching, verbal working memory, and articulatory rehearsal.

Some investigators have reported data showing that NPD patients are challenged in the comprehension of nonliteral language (Berg, Björnram, Hartelius, Laakso, & Johnels, 2003; Monetta & Pell, 2007; Monetta, Cheang, & Pell, 2008), irony, and making correct inferences from discourse. Monetta, Grindrod, and Pell (2009) engaged NPD subjects in a story interpretation task and observed impairment in interpreting the "intended" meaning of ironic remarks, the severity of which was correlated with scores on verbal fluency and verbal working memory span. Performance on verbal fluency tests and tests of nonliteral language comprehension have been reported to be worse in PD patients with depression compared to both those who are not depressed and healthy peers (Tremblay, Monchi, Hudon, Macoir, & Monetta, 2012). Tremblay and colleagues recommend taking into account the presence of depressive symptoms when evaluating language abilities in this population.

When the performance of 31 NPD patients on the Western Aphasia Battery (WAB) was compared to that of 20 healthy adults, the Aphasia Quotient (AQ) score was significantly lower (Liu et al., 2015). The PD patients had particular difficulty on the subtests for spontaneous speech, repetition, writing, praxis, and construction. However, not all the NPD patients performed similarly. Seventeen were found to score at least 2 standard deviations below the mean AQ of the healthy controls. Liu and colleagues reported that the language performance of these individuals was not accounted for by cognitive status. They concluded that language disability in PD applied only to a subset of PD patients, namely those with later age of onset. These individuals experience faster motor deterioration, more severe motor symptoms, and rapid cognitive impairment.

Scientists have linked language performance deficits in individuals with PD to deficits in the functioning of the circuitry that connects frontal lobes and basal ganglia that are not involved in controlling motor function. Although language processing has historically been considered the province of neocortical regions, principally Broca's and Wernicke's areas and adjacent cortex, evidence has accumulated that subcortical regions modulate linguistic function (Lieberman, 2000, 2002). Some of the evidence supporting this interpretation comes from studies of language processing of individuals with PD (Chenery, Angwin, & Copland, 2008).

The circuitry that runs from the cortex to the striatum and back to the cortex is known to be involved in planning, dual task performance, mood, and motor control (Brainard &

Doupe, 2000; Cools, Barker, Sahakian, & Robbins, 2001; Mesulam, 1990; Monchi, Petrides, Petre, Worsley, & Dagher, 2001). Cortico-striato-cortical circuitry is also important in speech production and sentence comprehension (Caplan & Waters, 1999; Copland, 2003; Copland, Chernery, & Murdock, 2000; Friederici, Kotz, Werheid, Hein, & von Cramon, 2003; Grossman, 1999; Grossman et al., 2001; Stowe, Paans, Wijers, & Zwarts, 2004). Chenery et al. (2008) advanced the hypothesis that brain circuits and dopamine act to enhance or suppress the meanings of lexically ambiguous words that require processing of sentence context. In fact, they hypothesized the existence of an integrated basal ganglia thalamocortical circuit that links striatum and inferior frontal cortex. Furthermore, they argued that disruption of this circuitry, as a result of PD and subsequent dopaminergic dysregulation, accounts for the impaired performance of individuals with PD in processing ambiguous word pairs that rely on contextual processing and suppression of unintended meanings. Finally, because PD subjects with poor working memory show impaired metaphor processing, they acknowledged that working memory capacity may also influence lexical ambiguity resolution.

In summary, memory, attention, and the ability to modulate the processing of linguistic information as well as age of disease onset appear to play a key role in the language processing deficits seen on various linguistically oriented neuropsychological tasks. Variability in the language performance profiles of NPD patients likely results from differences in the degree and type of pathology and the possible co-occurrence of vascular disease and AD.

A Study of Communicative Function in Demented PD Patients

Bayles et al. (1997) conducted a study of the effect of idiopathic PD on language function in 74 individuals with PD and 32 normal elderly control subjects. Individuals with PD were subdivided according to performance on the

Mini-Mental State Examination (MMSE) (Folstein, Folstein, & McHugh, 1975). PD patients with MMSE scores of 27 to 30 were classified as nondemented ($n = 42$), those with MMSE scores of 24 to 26 were defined as questionably demented ($n = 25$), and those with MMSE scores 16 to 23 were designated as mildly demented ($n = 7$). All study participants were given 15 linguistic communication tasks to assess linguistic competence and performance. The four measures of linguistic competence were semantic judgment, semantic correction, syntactic judgment, and syntactic correction. The 11 measures of linguistic performance were:

1. Repetition of phrases
2. Confrontation naming
3. Definitions
4. Generative naming—fruits
5. Generative naming—animals
6. Following commands
7. Picture description
8. Reading comprehension of words
9. Reading comprehension of sentences
10. Comparative questions
11. Object description

The only measures on which the *questionably demented* PD participants achieved significantly lower scores than normal control participants were the generative naming tests. *Mildly demented* PD participants performed significantly poorer than both the control and nondemented PD groups on six tasks: confrontation naming, generative naming—fruits, generative naming—animals, definitions, repetition, and semantic correction. The mildly demented PD participants had significantly lower scores than the questionably demented PD participants on five of the six aforementioned tasks, the exception being generative naming—fruits. Based on these findings, Bayles and colleagues (1997) concluded that although individuals with PD and mild dementia performed more poorly on some linguistic communication tasks, their performance was more indicative of working memory and executive function problems rather than a language competence (knowledge) problem. Indeed, mildly demented PD patients did not perform significantly more poorly than healthy elders on 9 of the 15 tasks.

Individuals with PD and Dementia Compared with Individuals with AD on the ABCD

The Arizona Battery for Communication Disorders of Dementia (ABCD) (Bayles & Tomoeda, 1993)—which comprises 14 subtests that measure linguistic comprehension, linguistic expression, verbal memory, visuospatial function, and mental status—was administered to eight PD patients with dementia, 62 nondemented PD patients, 86 AD patients, and 86 age-matched normal elders. The eight PD patients with mild dementia had scores similar to those of mildly demented AD patients on most subtests. For the five subtests on which significant differences were observed (object description, comparative questions, generative naming, and figure copying), mildly demented AD patients obtained *better* scores than the demented PD patients; however, mildly demented PD patients obtained higher scores than the mildly demented AD patients on word learning total recall.

Discourse Sample of PD Patient with Dementia

The following is a sample of the discourse produced by a PD patient with dementia on the object description test. It is similar to that produced by AD patients. The sentences are grammatically sound but content is aberrant and reflects disordered perception and thinking.

Examiner: Tell me about this [marble].
Subject: It's like candy and it's nearly as light. You can feel it. It's light. Some liquid in it. It hasn't been used. That's the way it looks to me. Orange color, or orange-colored candy.

Orange-colored candy that you put in your mouth. That's all I can think of.

Examiner: What does it mean, "To advise"?

Subject: Oh, asking questions. I was able to ask me questions.

Examiner: What does it mean, "To predict"?

Subject: There's moisture on a big plant object.

Relation of PDD, Dementia with Lewy Bodies, and AD

Scientists are working to unravel the puzzle of how and why PD with dementia (PDD), Lewy body disease (LBD), and AD are related. The fact is, the pathology associated with each disorder commonly occurs in the others. Indeed, PDD and LBD are conceptualized as different points on a continuum of conditions that share alpha-synuclein pathology (Compta et al., 2011). As previously noted, the alpha-synuclein protein is a key component of the Lewy bodies that proliferate in the brains of individuals diagnosed with PDD or dementia with Lewy bodies (DLB). The term "Lewy body diseases" is used to refer to both PDD and DLB. The apparent single difference between PDD and DLB is the temporal sequence of symptom appearance. PD is diagnosed when motor symptoms precede cognitive symptoms by a year; LBD is diagnosed when cognitive symptoms precede motor symptoms.

What adds to the difficulty of the puzzle is the fact that the amyloid-beta and tau pathologies of AD commonly occur in both PD and LBD; moreover, Lewy bodies are very common in the brains of individuals with AD. In fact, if sufficiently profuse, the affected individual is said to have a Lewy body variant of AD (Hansen, Masliah, Galask, & Terry, 1993; Mrak & Griffin, 2007). The dementia associated with PD is likely caused by Lewy body pathology in brainstem, limbic, and neocortical regions (Compta et al., 2011). On the other hand, PDD may be the result of AD pathology in the brains of individuals with PD. Matilla and colleagues reported that 40% to 50% of PDD cases meet the neuropathologic criteria for AD pathology (Matilla, Rinne, Helenius, Dickson, & Roytta, 2000). In many individuals with PDD, the amyloid-beta and tau pathologies coexist with Lewy body pathology (Sabbagh et al., 2009) along with progressive deficits in dopamine and acetylcholine. Recognition that these diseases are related and frequently coexist enables clinicians to better understand the symptomatology of the dementia patients they treat. It also indicates the need for caution in predicting clinical course.

Summary of Important Points

- Parkinsonism is a syndrome associated with resting tremor, muscle rigidity, and slowness of movement.
- Idiopathic PD is a disease that includes parkinsonism.
- Many disorders are associated with parkinsonism, among them AD, LBD, multiple system atrophy, and cortical–basal ganglionic degeneration.
- Some common behavioral and affective symptoms that present early in PD are changes in mood, apathy, sleep, excessive daytime sleepiness, delusions, voice weakness, difficulty swallowing, and constipation.
- Depression is common in individuals with PD and can diminish cognitive functioning resulting in a misrepresentation of cognitive function.
- Subtle changes in cognition can occur early in attention, executive function, memory, visuospatial processing, and language.
- PD is a multisystem disorder affecting both the central and peripheral nervous systems.
- The defining pathology of PD is a loss of dopaminergic neurons in the substantia nigra pars compacta and the widespread presence of neuronal Lewy bodies (due to alpha-synuclein pathology) as well as cortical atrophy and thinning.
- Risk factors include age, which is the most important, as well as heredity, sex, and exposure to toxins.

- Most genetic parkinsonism occurs in individuals younger than age 50 years.
- Diagnostic criteria exist for diagnosing the disease and staging cognitive status.
- To evaluate cognitive status, clinicians should use standardized neuropsychological tests related to core cognitive abilities.
- Hypokinetic dysarthria is common.
- Loss of linguistic knowledge is not a major contributor to the language disabilities of PD patients.
- The communicative functioning of nondemented PD patients is affected by cognitive deficits in attention, the visual system, memory and executive function, as well as motor system impairment.
- Individuals with later onset have more severe communication problems.
- The basal ganglia appear to have a role in language processing and a subset of individuals with PD have more pronounced problems in processing language than other patients.
- The longer an individual has PD, the greater the likelihood of developing dementia.
- Three cognitive factors primarily account for the dementia in PD: progressively worsening visuospatial memory, verbal memory, and working memory.
- PD and LBD are both Lewy body spectrum disorders. PD is diagnosed when motor symptoms precede cognitive symptoms; LBD is diagnosed when cognitive symptoms precede motor symptoms.

References

Aarsland, D., Andersen, K., Larsen, J. P., Lolk, A., & Kragh-Sorensen, P. (2003). Prevalence and characteristics of dementia in Parkinson disease: An 8-year prospective study. *Archives of Neurology, 60*, 387–392.

Aarsland, D., Bronnick, K., Larsen, J. P., Tysnes, O. B., & Alves, G. (2009). Cognitive impairment in incident, untreated Parkinson disease: The Norwegian Park West study. *Neurology, 72*, 1121–1126.

Aarsland, D., & Kurz, M. W. (2010). The epidemiology of dementia associated with Parkinson's disease. *Brain Pathology, 20*, 633–639.

Aarsland, D., Rongve, A., Nore, S., Skogseth, R., Skulstad, S., Ehrt, U., . . . Ballard, C. (2008). Frequency and case

identification of dementia with Lewy bodies using the revised consensus criteria. *Dementia and Geriatric Cognitive Disorders, 26*, 445–452.

American Psychiatric Association. (2013). *Diagnostic and statistical manual of mental disorders* (5th ed.). Arlington, VA: American Psychiatric Publishing.

Antal, A., Bandini, F., Kéri, S., & Bodis-Wollner, I. (1998). Visuo-cognitive dysfunctions in Parkinson's disease. *Clinical Neuroscience, 5*, 147–152.

Archibald, N. K., Clarke, M. P., Mosimann, U. P., & Burn, D. J. (2011). Visual symptoms in Parkinson's disease and Parkinson's disease dementia. *Movement Disorders, 26*, 2387–2395.

Arun, M. P., Bharath, S., Pal, P. K., & Singh, G. (2011). Relation of depression, disability and quality of life in Parkinson's disease: A hospital-based case-control study. *Neurology Indian, 59*, 185–189.

Azuma, T., Cruz, R. F., Bayles, K. A., Tomoeda, C. K., & Montgomery, E. B. Jr. (2003). A longitudinal study of neuropsychological change in individuals with Parkinson's disease. *International Journal of Geriatric Psychiatry, 18*, 1115–1120.

Barnes, J., Boubert, L., Harris, J., Lee, A., & David, A. S. (2003). Reality monitoring and visual hallucinations in Parkinson's disease. *Neuropsychologia, 41*, 565–574.

Bayles, K. A. (1990). Language and communication in Parkinson's disease. *Alzheimer's Disease and Associated Disorders, 4*, 171–180.

Bayles, K. A., & Tomoeda, C. K. (1993). *Arizona Battery for Communication Disorders of Dementia*. Austin, TX: Pro-Ed.

Bayles, K., Tomoeda, C. K., Wood, J. A., Cruz, R. F., Azuma, T., & Montgomery, E. B. (1997). The effect of Parkinson's disease on language. *Journal of Medical Speech-Language Pathology, 5*, 157–166.

Berg, E., Björnram, C., Hartelius, L., Laakso, K., & Johnels, B. (2003). High-level language difficulties in Parkinson's disease. *Clinical Linguistics and Phonetics, 17*, 63–80.

Bertrand, J. A., Bedetti, C., Postuma, R. B., Monchi, O., Genier, M. D., Jubault, T., & Gagnon, J. F. (2012). Color discrimination deficits in Parkinson's disease are related to cognitive impairment and white-matter alterations. *Movement Disorders, 27*, 1781–1789.

Biundo, R., Weis, L., & Antonini, A. (2016). Cognitive decline in Parkinson's disease: The complex picture. *NPJ Parkinson's disease, 2*, 1–7.

Bodis-Wollner, I. (2002). Visualizing the next steps in Parkinson disease. *Archives of Neurology, 59*, 1233–1234.

Bom de Araujo, N., Barca, M. L., Engedal, K., Coutinho, E. S. F., Deslandes, A. C., & Laks, J. (2011). Verbal fluency in Alzheimer's disease, Parkinson's disease, and major depression. *Clinics, 66*, 623–627.

Bondi, M. W., Kaszniak, A. W., Bayles, K. A., & Vance, K. T. (1993). Contributions of frontal system dysfunction to memory and perceptual abilities in Parkinson's disease. *Neuropsychology, 7*, 89–102.

Boot, B. P., Boeve, B. F., Roberts, R. O., Ferman, T. J., Geda, Y. E., & Pankratz, V. S. (2012). Probable rapid eye movement sleep behavior disorder increases risk for mild cognitive impairment and Parkinson disease: A population-based study. *Annals of Neurology, 71,* 49–56.

Braak, H., & Braak, E. (2000). Pathoanatomy of Parkinson's disease. *Journal of Neurology, 247*(Suppl. 2), II3–II10.

Brainard, M. S., & Doupe, A. J. (2000). Interruption of a basal ganglia-forebrain circuit prevents the plasticity of learned vocalizations. *Nature, 404,* 762–766.

Brose, N., O'Connor, V., & Skehel, P. (2010). Synaptopathy: Dysfunction of synaptic function? *Biochemical Society Transactions, 38,* 443–444.

Bruna, O., Roig, C., Junque, C., & Vendrell, P. (2000). Relationship between visuospatial impairment and oculomotor parameters in Parkinson's disease. *Psicothema, 12,* 187–191.

Bulens, C., Meerwaldt, J. D., & van der Wildt, G. J. (1988). Effect of stimulus orientation on contrast sensitivity in Parkinson's disease. *Neurology, 38,* 76–81.

Büttner, T., Kuhn, W., Klotz, P., Steinberg, R., Voss, L., Bulgaru, D., & Przuntek, H. (1993). Disturbance of color perception in Parkinson's disease. *Journal of Neural Transmission Parkinson's Disease and Dementia Section, 6,* 11–15.

Büttner, T., Kuhn, W., Muller, T., Patzold, T., Heidbrink, K., & Przuntek, H. (1995). Distorted color discrimination in "de novo" parkinsonian patients. *Neurology, 45,* 386–387.

Cahn-Weiner, D. A., Grace, J., Ott, B. R., Fernandez, H. H., & Friedman, J. H. (2002). Cognitive and behavioral features discriminate between Alzheimer's and Parkinson's disease. *Neuropsychiatry, Neuropsychology, and Behavioral Neurology, 15,* 29–87.

Camicioli, R. M., Wieler, M., de Frias, C. M., & Martin, W. R. W. (2008). Early, untreated Parkinson's disease patients show reaction time variability. *Neuroscience Letters, 441,* 77-80.

Campdelacreu, J. (2014) Parkinson disease and Alzheimer disease: environmental risk factors. *Neurologia, 9,* 541–549.

Caplan, D., & Waters, G. S. (1999). Verbal working memory and sentence comprehension. *Behavioral and Brain Sciences, 22,* 77–126.

Chaudhuri, K. R., & Schapira, A. H. (2009). Nonmotor symptoms of Parkinson's disease: Dopaminergic pathophysiology and treatment. *Lancet Neurology, 8,* 464–474.

Chaudhury, S. (2010). Hallucinations: Clinical aspects and management. *Industrial Psychiatry Journal, 19,* 5–12.

Chenery, H. J., Angwin, A. J., & Copland, D. A. (2008). The basal ganglia circuits, dopamine and ambiguous word processing: A neurobiological account of priming studies in Parkinson's disease. *Journal of the International Neuropsychological Society, 14,* 351–364.

Colosimo, C., Hughes, A. J., Kilford, L., & Lees, A. J. (2003). Lewy body cortical involvement may not always predict dementia in Parkinson's disease. *Journal of Neurology, Neurosurgery and Psychiatry, 74,* 852–856.

Compta, Y., Parkkinen, L., O'Sullivan, S. S., Vandrovcova, J., Holton, J. L., Collins, . . . Revesz, T. (2011). Lewy- and Alzheimer-type pathologies in Parkinson's disease dementia: Which is more important? *Brain, 134,* 1493–1505.

Cools, R., Barker R. A., Sahakian, B. J., & Robbins, T. W. (2001). Enhanced or impaired cognitive function in Parkinson's disease as a function of dopaminergic medication and task demands. *Cerebral Cortex, 11,* 1136–1143.

Cooper, J. A., Sagar, H. J., Jordan, N., Harvey, N. S., Sullivan, E. V. (1991). Cognitive Impairment in early, untreated Parkinson's disease and its relationship to motor disability. *Brain, 114,* 2095–2122.

Copland, D. (2003). The basal ganglia and semantic engagement: Potential insights from semantic priming in individuals with subcortical vascular lesions, Parkinson's disease, and cortical lesions. *Journal of the International Neuropsychological Society, 9,* 1041–1052.

Copland, D. A., Chenery, H. J., & Murdock, B. E. (2000). Understanding ambiguous words in biased sentences: Evidence of transient contextual effects in individuals with nonthalamic subcortical lesions and Parkinson's disease. *Cortex, 36,* 601–622.

Dadgar, H., Khatoonabadi, A. R., & Bakhtiyari, J. (2013). Verbal fluency performance in patients with nondemented Parkinson's disease. *Iranian Journal of Psychiatry, 8,* 55–58.

Davidsdottir, S., Cronin-Golomb, A., & Lee, A. (2005). Visual and spatial symptoms in Parkinson's disease. *Vision Research, 45,* 1285–1296.

de Frias, C. M., Dixon, R. A., Fisher, N., & Camicioli, R. (2007). Intraindividual variability in neurocognitive speech: A comparison of Parkinson disease and normal older adults. *Neuropsychologia, 45,* 2499–2507.

de Rijk, M. C., Breteler, M. M., Graveland, G. A., Ott, A., Grobbee, D. E., van der Meché, F.G., & Hofman, A. (1995). Prevalence of Parkinson's disease in the elderly: The Rotterdam study. *Neurology, 45,* 2143–2146.

Dubois, B., Burn, D., Goetz, C., Aarsland, D., Brown, R. G., Broc, G. A., . . . Emre, M. (2007). Diagnostic procedures for Parkinson's disease dementia: Recommendations from the movement disorder society task force. *Movement Disorders, 22,* 2314–2224.

Dubois, B., & Pillon, B. (1997). Cognitive deficits in Parkinson's disease. *Journal of Neurology, 244,* 2–8.

Emre, M. (2003). What causes mental dysfunction in Parkinson's disease? *Movement Disorders, 18,* 63–71.

Esiri, M. M., & Morris, J. H. (2004). Practical approach to pathological diagnosis. In M. M. Esiri, V. M.-Y. Lee, & J. Q. Trojanowski (Eds.), *The neuropathology of dementia* (2nd ed., pp. 48–74). Cambridge, UK: Cambridge University Press.

Fall, P., Axelson, O., Fredriksson, M., Hansson, G., Lindvall, B., Olsson, J., . . . Granérus, A. K. (1996). Age-standardized incidence and prevalence of Parkinson's disease in a Swedish community. *Journal of Clinical Epidemiology, 49,* 637–641.

Fitzmaurice, A. G., Rhodes, S. L., Lulla, A., Murphy, N. P., Lam, H. A., O'Donnell, K. C., ... Bronstein, J. M. (2013). Aldehyde dehydrogenase inhibition as a pathogenic mechanism in Parkinson disease. *Proceedings of the National Academy of Sciences of the United States of America*, *110*, 636–641.

Folstein, M. F., Folstein, S. E., & McHugh, P. R. (1975). Mini-mental state. A practical method for grading the cognitive state of patients for the clinician. *Journal of Psychiatric Research*, *12*, 189–198.

Foltynie, T., Brayne, C. E. G., Robbins, T. W., & Barker, R. A. (2004). Cognitive ability of an incident cohort of Parkinson's patients in the UK. The Campaign study. *Brain*, *127*, 550–560.

Friederici, A. D., Kotz, S. A., Werheid, K., Hein, G., & von Cramon, D. Y. (2003). Syntactic comprehension in Parkinson's disease: Investigating early automatic and late integrational processes using event-related brain potentials. *Neuropsychology*, *17*, 133–142.

Galtier, I., Nieto, A., & Barroso, J. (2016). Cognitive impairment in Parkinson's disease: Historical review, past, and present. In J. Dorszewska (Ed.), *Mental and behavioural disorders and diseases of the nervous system: Challenges in Parkinson's disease* (pp. 155–180). London, UK: InTechOpen.

Galtier, I., Nieto, A., Barroso, J., & Lorenzo, N. (2009). Visuospatial learning impairment in Parkinson disease. *Psicothema*, *21*, 21–16

Garcia-Diaz, A. I., Segura, B., Baggio, H. C., Marti, M. J., Valldeoriola, F., Compta, Y., . . . Junque, C. (2014). Structural MRI correlates of the MMSE and pentagon copying test in Parkinson's disease. *Parkinsonism and Related Disorders*, *20*, 1405–1410.

Girotti, F., Soliveri, P., Carella, F., Piccolo, I., Caffarra, P., Musicco, M., & Caraceni, T. (1988). Dementia and cognitive impairment in Parkinson's disease. *Journal of Neurology, Neurosurgery, and Psychiatry*, *51*, 1498–1502.

Gorell, J. M., Johnson, C. C., Rybicki, B. A., Peterson, E. L., Kortsha, G. X., Brown, G. G., . . . Richardson, R. J. (1997). Occupational exposures to metals as risk factors for Parkinson's disease. *Neurology*, *48*, 650–658.

Grossman, M. (1999). Sentence processing in Parkinson's disease. *Brain and Cognition*, *40*, 387–413.

Grossman, M., Glosser, G., Kalmanson, J., Morris, J., Stern, M. B., & Hurtig, H. I. (2001). Dopamine supports sentence comprehension in Parkinson's disease. *Journal of the Neurological Sciences*, *184*, 123–130.

Hansen, L. A., Masliah, E., Galask, D., & Terry, R.D. (1993). Plaque-only Alzheimer's disease is usually the Lewy body variant, and vice versa. *Journal of Neuropathology and Experimental Neurology*, *6*, 648–654.

Harrington, D. L., Haaland, K. Y., Yeo, R. A., & Marder, E. (1990). Procedural memory in Parkinson's disease: Impaired motor but not visuoperceptual learning. *Journal of Clinical and Experimental Neuropsychology*, *12*, 323–339.

Helkala, E. L., Laulumaa, V., Soininen, H., & Riekkinen, P. J. (1989). Different error pattern of episodic and semantic memory in Alzheimer's disease and Parkinson's disease with dementia. *Neuropsychologia*, *27*, 1241–1248.

Henry, J. D., & Crawford, J. R. (2004). Verbal fluency deficits in Parkinson's disease: A metaanalysis. *Journal of the International Neuropsychological Society*, *10*, 608–622.

Hepp, D. H., Foncke, E. M. J., Olde Dubbelink, K. T. E., van de Berg, W. D. J., Berendse, H. W., & Schoonheim, M. M. (2017). Loss of functional connectivity in patients with Parkinson disease and visual hallucinations. *Radiology*, *285*, 896–903.

Hipp, G., Diederich, N. J., Pieria, V., & Vaillant, M. (2014). Primary vision and facial emotion recognition in early Parkinson's disease. *Journal of Neurological Sciences*, *338*, 178–182.

Hirsh, E. C. (2000). Glial cells and Parkinson's disease. *Journal of Neurology*, *247*(Suppl. 2), II58–II62.

Hirsch, L., Jette, N., Frolkis, A., Steeves, T., & Pringsheim, T. (2016). The incidence of Parkinson's disease: A systematic review and meta-analysis. *Neuroepidemiology*, *46*, 292–300.

Hobson, P., & Meara, J. (2015). Mild cognitive impairment in Parkinson's disease and its progression onto dementia: A 16-year outcome evaluation of the Denbighshire cohort. *International Journal of Geriatric Psychiatry*, *30*, 1048–1055.

Hochstadt, J., Nakano, H., Lieberman, P., & Friedman, J. (2006). The roles of sequencing and verbal working memory in sentence comprehension deficits in Parkinson's disease. *Brain and Language*, *97*, 243–257.

Imamura, K., Wada-Isoe, K., Kitayama, M., & Nakashima, K. (2008). Executive dysfunctions in non-demented Parkinson's disease patients with hallucinations. *Acta Neurologica Scandinavica*, *117*, 255–259.

Janvin, C. C., Aarsland, D., & Larsen, J. P. (2005). Cognitive predictors of dementia in Parkinson's disease: A community-based, 4-year longitudinal study. *Journal of Geriatric Psychiatry and Neurology*, *18*, 149–154.

Janvin, C. C., Larsen, J. P., Aarsland, D., & Hugdahl, K. (2006). Subtypes of mild cognitive impairment in Parkinson's disease: Progression to dementia. *Movement Disorders*, *21*, 1343–1349.

Johnson, D. K., & Galvin, J. E. (2011). Longitudinal changes in cognition in Parkinson disease with and without dementia. *Dementia and Geriatric Cognitive Disorders*, *31*, 98–108.

Kemps, E., Szmalec, A., Vandierendonck, A., & Crevits, L. (2005). Visuo-spatial processing in Parkinson's disease: Evidence for diminished visuo-spatial sketch pad and central executive resources. *Parkinsonism and Related Disorders*, *11*, 181–186.

Kempster, P. A., O'Sullivan, S. S., Holton, J. L., Revesz, T., & Lees, A. J. (2010). Relationships between age and late progression of Parkinson's disease: A clinico-pathological study. *Brain*, *133*, 1755–1762.

Koch, G., Costa, A., Brusa, L., Peppe, A, Gatto, I., Torriero, S., . . . Caltagirone, C. (2008). Impaired reproduction of second but not millisecond time intervals in Parkinson's disease. *Neuropsychologica, 46,* 1305–1313.

Koller, W., Vetere-Overfield, B., Gray, C., Alexander, C., Chin, T., Dolezal, J., . . . Tanner, C. (1990). Environmental risk factors in Parkinson's disease. *Neurology, 40,* 1218–1221.

Kotzbauer, P. T., Cairns, N. J., Campbell, M. C., Willis, A. W., Racette, B. A., Tabbal, S. D., & Perlmutter, J. S. (2012). Pathologic accumulation of alpha-synuclein and Abeta in Parkinson disease patients with dementia. *Archives of Neurology, 69,* 1326–1331.

Krysiak, A. P. (2011). Language, speech, and communication disorders in Parkinson's disease. *Neuropsychologia, 6,* 36–42.

Kuopio, A. M., Marttila, R. J., Helenius, H., & Rinne, U. (1999). Changing epidemiology of Parkinson's disease in southwest Finland. *Neurology, 52,* 302–308.

Kwakye, G. F., Paoliello, M. M. B., Mukhopadhyay, S., Bowman, A. B., & Aschner, M. (2015). Manganese-induced parkinsonism and Parkinson's disease: Shared and distinguishable features. *Internal Journal of Environmental Research and Public Health, 12,* 7519–7540.

Lees, A. J., & Smith, E. (1983). Cognitive deficits in the early stages of Parkinson's disease. *Brain, 106,* 257–270.

Lepeta, K., Lourenco, M. V., Schweitzer, B. C., Martino Adami, P. V., Banerjee, P., Catuara-Solarz, S., . . . Suska, A. (2016). Synaptopathies: Synaptic dysfunction in neurological disorders—A review from students to students. *Journal of Neurochemistry, 138,* 785–805.

Levin, B. E., Llabre, M. M., Resiman, S., Weiner, W. J., Sanchez-Ramos, J., Singer, C., . . . Brown, M. C. (1991). Visuospatial impairment in Parkinson's disease. *Neurology, 41,* 365–369.

Levy, G., Schupf, N., Tang, M. X., Cote, L. J., Louis, E. D., Mejia, H., ... Marder, K. (2002). Combined effect of age and severity on the risk of dementia in Parkinson's disease. *Annals of Neurology, 51,* 722–729.

Lieberman, P. (2000). *Human language and our reptilian brain: The subcortical bases of speech, syntax, and thought.* Cambridge, MA: Harvard University.

Lieberman, P. (2002). On the nature and evolution of the neural bases of human language. *Yearbook of Physical Anthropology, 45,* 36–62.

Litvan, I., Aarsland, D., Adler, C. H., Goldman, J. G., Kulisevsky, J., Mollenhauer, B., . . . Weintraub, D. (2011). MDS task force on mild cognitive impairment in Parkinson's disease: Critical review of PD-MCI. *Movement Disorders, 26,* 1814–1824.

Litvan, I., Goldman, J. G., Tröster, A. L., Schmand, B. A., Weintraub, D., Petersen, R. C., . . . Emre, M. (2012). Diagnostic criteria for mild cognitive impairment in Parkinson's disease. Movement disorder Society task Force guidelines. *Movement Disorders, 27,* 349–356.

Litvan, I., Mohr, E., Williams, J., Gomez, C., & Chase, T. N. (1991). Differential memory and executive functions in demented patients with Parkinson's and Alzheimer's disease. *Journal of Neurology, Neurosurgery, and Psychiatry, 54,* 25–29.

Liu, L., Luo, X-G., Dy, C-L., Ren, Y., Feng, Y., Yu, H-M., . . . He, Z-Y. (2015). Characteristics of language impairment in Parkinson's disease and its influencing factors. *Translational Neurodegeneration, 4,* 1–8.

Longhena, F., Faustini, G., Missale, C., Pizzi, M., Spano, P., & Bellucci, A. (2017). The contribution of a-synuclein spreading to Parkinson's disease synaptopathy. *Neural Plasticity, 2017,* 1–15.

Lozano, A. M., & Kalia, S. K. (2005). New movement in Parkinson's. *Scientific American, 293,* 68–75.

Mamikonyan, E., Moberg, P. J., Siderowf, A., Duda, J. E., Have, T. T., Hurtig, H. I., . . . Weintraub, D. (2009). Mild cognitive impairment is common in Parkinson's disease patients with normal Mini-Mental State Examination (MMSE) scores. *Parkinsonism and Related Disorders, 15,* 226–231.

Matilla, P. M., Rinne, J. O., Helenius, H., Dickson, D. W., & Roytta, M. (2000). Alpha-synucleinimmunoreactive cortical Lewy bodies are associated with cognitive impairment in Parkinson's disease. *Acta Neuropathologica* (Berlin), *100,* 285–290.

Matilla, R. J., & Rinne, U. K. (1976). Dementia in Parkinson's disease. *Acta Neurologica Scandinavia, 54,* 431–441.

Mayeux, R., Denaro, J., Hemenegildo, N., Marder, K., Tang, M.-X., Cote, L. J., . . . Stern, Y. (1992). A population-based investigation of Parkinson's disease with and without dementia: Relationship to age and gender. *Archives of Neurology, 49,* 492–497.

Mayeux, R., Marder, K., Cote, L. J., Denaro, J., Hemenegildo, N., Mejia, H., . . . Hauser, A. (1995). The frequency of idiopathic Parkinson's disease by age, ethnic group, and sex in northern Manhattan: 1988–1993. *American Journal of Epidemiology, 142,* 820–827.

Menza, M., Dobkin, R. D., Marin, H., Mark, M. H., Gara, M., Buyske, S., . . . Dicke, A. (2009). The impact of treatment of depression on quality of life, disability and relapse in patients with Parkinson's disease. *Movement Disorders, 24,* 1325–1332.

Mesulam, M. M. (1990). Large-scale neurocognitive networks and distributed processing for attention, language, and memory. *Annals of Neurology, 28,* 597–613.

Monchi, O., Petrides, M., Petre, V., Worsley, K., & Dagher, A. (2001). Wisconsin card Sorting revisited: Distinct neural circuits participating in different stages of the task identified by event-related functional magnetic resonance imaging. *Journal of Neuroscience, 21,* 7733–7741.

Monetta, L., Cheang, H. S., & Pell, M. D. (2008). Understanding speaker attitudes from prosody by adults with Parkinson's disease. *Journal of Neurophysiology, 2,* 415–430.

Monetta, L., Grindrod, C. M., & Pell, M. (2009). Irony comprehension and theory of mind deficits in patients with Parkinson's disease. *Cortex, 45,* 972–981.

Monetta, L., & Pell, M. D. (2007). Effects of verbal working memory deficits on metaphor comprehension in patients with Parkinson's disease. *Brain and Language*, *101*, 80–89.

Morens, D. M., Davis, J. W., Grandinetti, A., Ross, G. W., Popper, J. S., & White, L. R. (1996). Epidemiologic observations on Parkinson's disease: Incidence and mortality in a prospective study of middle-aged men. *Neurology*, *46*, 1044–1050.

Mrak, R. E., & Griffin, W. S. (2007). Dementia with Lewy bodies: Definition, diagnosis, and pathogenic relationship to Alzheimer's disease. *Neuropsychiatric Disease and Treatment*, *3*, 619–625.

Muslimovic, D., Post, B., Speelman, J. D., & Schmand, B. (2005). Cognitive profile of patients with newly diagnosed Parkinson disease. *Neurology*, *65*, 1239–1245.

Owen, A. M., James, M., Leigh, P. N., Summers, B. A., Marsden, C. D., Quinn, N. P., . . . Robbins, T. W. (1992). Fronto-striatal cognitive deficits at different stages of Parkinson's disease. *Brain*, *115*, 1727–1751.

Parkinson's Disease Foundation. (2017). *About PDF*. Retrieved December 4, 2017, from http://parkinson.org/understanding-parkinsons

Pedersen, K. F., Larsen, J. P., Tysnes, O. B., & Alves, G. (2013). Prognosis of mild cognitive impairment in early Parkinson disease: The Norwegian ParkWest study. *Journal of the American Medical Association Neurology*, *70*, 580–586.

Pillon, B., Deweer, B., Agid, Y., & Dubois, B. (1993). Explicit memory in Alzheimer's, Huntington's, and Parkinson's diseases. *Archives of Neurology*, *50*, 374–379.

Qureshi, G. A., Qureshi, A. A., Memon, S. A., & Parvez, S. H. (2006). Impact of selenium, iron, copper and zinc in on/off Parkinson's patients on L-dopa therapy. *Journal of Neural Transmission Supplementum*, *71*, 229–236.

Ramirez-Ruiz, B., Junque, C., Marti, M. J., Valledeoriola, F., & Tolosa, E. (2007). Cognitive changes in Parkinson's disease patients with visual hallucinations. *Dementia and Geriatric Cognitive Disorders*, *23*, 281–288.

Regan, D., & Maxner, C. (1987). Orientation-selective visual loss in patients with Parkinson's disease. *Brain*, *110*, 415–432.

Reeve, A., Simcox, E., & Turnbull, D. (2016). Ageing and Parkinson's disease: Why is advancing age the biggest risk factor? *Ageing Research Reviews*, *14*, 19–30.

Reid, W. G. (1992). The evolution of dementia in idiopathic Parkinson's disease: Neuropsychological and clinical evidence in support of subtypes. *International Psychogeriatrics*, *4*, 147–160.

Reid, W. G. J., Hely, M. A., Morris, J. G. L., Loy, C., & Halliday, G. M. (2011). Dementia in Parkinson disease: A 20-year neuropsychological study (Sydney Multicentre Study). *Journal of Neurology, Neurosurgery, and Psychiatry*, *82*, 1033–1037.

Repka, M. X., Claro, M. C., Loupe, D. N, & Reich, S. G. (1996). Ocular motility in Parkinson's disease. *Journal of Pediatric Ophthalmology and Strabismus*, *33*, 144–147.

Rippon, G. A., & Marder, K. S. (2005). Dementia in Parkinson's disease. *Advances in Neurology*, *96*, 95–113.

Rodnitzky, R. L. (1998). Visual dysfunction in Parkinson's disease. *Clinical Neuroscience*, *5*, 102–106.

Rodnitzky, R. L. (2017, February 5). Cognitive impairment and dementia in Parkinson disease. In S. T. DeKosky & A. F. Eichler (Eds.), *UpToDate*. Retrieved from http://www.uptodate.com/contents/cognitive-impairment-and-dementia-in-parkinson-disease

Rondeau, V., Jacqmin-Gadda, H., Commenges, D., Helmer, C., & Dartigues, J. F. (2009). Aluminum and silica in drinking water and the risk of Alzheimer's disease or cognitive decline: Findings from 15-year follow-up of the PAQUID cohort. *American Journal of Epidemiology*, *169*, 489–496.

Sabbagh, M. N., Adler, C. H., Lahti, T. J., Connor, D. J., Vedders, L., Peterson, L. K., . . . Beach, T. G. (2009). Parkinson disease with dementia: Comparing patients with and without Alzheimer pathology. *Alzheimer Disease and Associated Disorders*, *23*, 295–297.

Siegert R. J., Weatherall, M., Taylor, K. D., & Abernethy, D. A. (2008) A meta-analysis of performance on simple span and more complex working memory tasks in Parkinson's disease. *Neuropsychology. 22*, 450–461.

Silva, M. F., Faria, P., Regateiro, F. S., Forjaz, V., Januario, C., Freire, A., & Castelo-Branco, M. (2005). Independent patterns of damage within magno-parvo and koniocellular pathways in Parkinson's disease. *Brain*, *128*, 2260–2271.

Smith, S. J., Souchay, C., & Moulin, C. J. A. (2011). Metamemory and prospective memory in Parkinson's disease. *Neuropsychology*, *25*, 734–740.

Stefanova, E. D., Kostic, V. S., Ziropadja, L., Markovic, M., & Ocic, G. G. (2000). Visuomotor skill learning on serial reaction time task in patients with early Parkinson's disease. *Movement Disorders*, *15*, 1095–1103.

Stern, Y., Mayeux, R., Rosen, J., & Ilson, J. (1983). Perceptual motor dysfunction in Parkinson's disease: A deficit in sequential and predictive voluntary movement. *Journal of Neurology, Neurosurgery, and Psychiatry*, *46*, 145–151.

Stern, Y., Richards, M., Sano, M., & Mayeux, R. (1993). Comparison of cognitive changes in patients with Alzheimer's and Parkinson's disease. *Archives of Neurology*, *50*, 1040–1045.

Stowe, L. A., Paans, A. M. J., Wijers, A. A., & Zwarts, F. (2004). Activations of "motor" and other non-language structures during sentence comprehension. *Brain and Language*, *89*, 290–299.

Struck, L. K., Rodnitzky, R. L., & Dobson, J. K. (1990). Circadian fluctuations of contrast sensitivity in Parkinson's disease. *Neurology*, *40*, 467–470.

Takahashi, H., & Wakabayashi, K. (2005). Controversy: Is Parkinson's disease a single disease entity? Yes. *Parkinsonism and Related Disorders*, *11*, 31–37.

Taylor, A. E., Saint-Cyr, J. A., & Lang, A. E. (1986). Frontal lobe dysfunction in Parkinson's disease: The cortical focus of neostriatal outflow. *Brain*, *109*, 845–883.

Tremblay, C., Monchi, O., Hudon, C., Macoir, J., & Monetta, L. (2012). Are verbal fluency and nonliteral language comprehensiuon deficits related to depressive symptoms in Parkinson's disease. *Parkinson's Disease, 2012,* Article 308501.

Urwyler, P., Nef, T., Killen, A., Collerton, D., Thomas, A., Burn, D., . . . Mosimann, U. P. (2014). Visual complaints and visual hallucinations in Parkinson's disease. *Parkinsonism and Related Disorders, 20,* 313–322.

van den Eeden, S. K., Tanner, C. M., Bernstein, A. L., Fross, R. D., Leimpeter, A., Bloch, D. A., & Nelson, L. M. (2003). Incidence of Parkinson's disease: Variation by age, gender, and race/ethnicity. *American Journal of Epidemiology, 157,* 1015–1022.

van der Mark, M., Brouwer, M., Kromhout, H., Nijssen, P., Huss, A., & Vermeulen, R. (2012). Is pesticide use related to Parkinson disease? Some clues to heterogeneity in study results. *Environmental Health Perspectives, 120,* 340–347.

Watson, G. S., & Leverenz, J. B. (2010). Profile of cognitive impairment in Parkinson disease. *Brain Pathology, 20,* 640–645.

Wearden, J. H., Smith-Spark, J. H., Cousins, R., Edelstyn, N. M. J., Cody, F. W. J., & O'Boyle, D. J. (2008). Effect of click trains on duration estimates by people with Parkinson's disease. *Quarterly Journal of Experimental Psychology, 62,* 33–40.

Wengel, S. P., Bohac, D., & Burke, W. J. (2005). Depression in Parkinson's disease. In M. Ebadi & R. F. Pfeiffer (Eds.), *Parkinson's disease* (pp. 329–338). Boca Raton, FL: CRC Press.

Wirdefedlt, K., Adami, H. O., Cole, P., Trichopoulos, D., & Mandel, J. (2011). Epidemiology and etiology of Parkinson's disease: A review of the evidence. *European Journal of Epidemiology, 26*(Suppl. 1), S51–S58.

Wong, G. F., Gray, C. S., Hassanein, R. S., & Koller, W. C. (1991). Environmental risk factors in siblings with Parkinson's disease. *Archives of Neurology, 48,* 287–289.

Yang, Y., Tang, B-S., & Guo, J-F. (2016). Parkinson's disease and cognitive impairment. *Parkinson's Disease, 2016,* 1–8.

8

Dementia and Lewy Body Disease

Lewy Body Disease

In 1923, Fredrich Heinrich Lewy, a neurologist and contemporary of Alois Alzheimer, observed the round lumps of protein in the cell processes of neurons that characterize Lewy body disease (LBD; Figure 8–1) (Holdorff, 2002). However, it was not until 1961 that much attention was paid to the neuropathology and behavioral changes associated with the disease that today bears Lewy's name. In 1961, two individuals with progressive dementia and widespread cortical Lewy bodies were described by Okazaki, Lipton, and Aronson (1961) and their description rekindled interest in the disease. Subsequently, Kosaka (1978) detailed the characteristics and distribution of cortical Lewy bodies. Today, LBD is recognized as a major cause of dementia, perhaps even the second-most common cause (Aarsland et al., 2008; Donaghy & McKeith, 2014; Tsuboi & Dickson, 2005).

The protein in the brains of individuals with LBD that abnormally aggregates and forms clumps is alpha-synuclein (McKeith et al., 2004), a presynaptic neuronal protein that can also be found in the heart and other body tissues. One of the roles of alpha-synuclein is believed to be the compartmentalization, storage, and recycling of neurotransmitters (Reish & Standaert, 2015), among them dopamine. It is also associated with the regulation of certain enzymes (Lee, Lee, Lee, Chang, & Paik, 2002). In LBD, the brain areas most affected include the anterior frontal and temporal cortices, the cingulate area, insula, substantia nigra, nucleus basalis of Meynert, locus ceruleus, nucleus raphe dorsalis, and amygdala (Simard, van Reekum, & Cohen, 2000).

Lewy bodies also occur in the brains of patients with Parkinson's disease (PD) and those with Alzheimer's disease (AD) (Alzheimer's Association, 2017; Cummings & Mega, 2003; Reichman & Cummings, 1999), as well as in many individuals who appear healthy and cognitively normal. In fact, 8% to 16% of people 60 years or older have Lewy body pathology according to results of autopsy studies (Frigerio et al., 2011; Gibb & Lees, 1988). Because Lewy bodies are present in many diseases, Lewy body disease is considered a spectrum of disorders (Goldman, Williams-Gray, Barker, Duda, & Galvin, 2014).

With the fifth edition of the *Diagnostic and Statistical Manual of Mental Disorders* (DSM-5; American Psychiatric Association, 2013), dementia with Lewy bodies (DLB) was recognized as a diagnostic category equivalent to others such as AD and vascular disease, which will increase awareness of the disorder. The term "Lewy body dementias" refers to two clinical diagnoses: dementia with Lewy bodies (DLB) and Parkinson's disease dementia (PDD). The terms LBD and DLB can be confusing. LBD is an abbreviation for Lewy body disease; the term DLB refers to the condition of dementia *due to* Lewy body pathology.

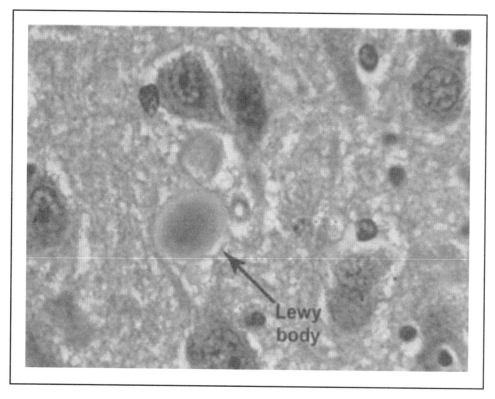

Figure 8–1. Brain cells containing a Lewy body, an abnormal aggregation of protein. (Courtesy of Kondi Wong, Armed forces Institute of Pathology, http://www.genome.gov)

Although LBD appears to affect individuals at a younger age than PD, it nonetheless increases substantially with age. The incidence and prevalence of LBD have not been definitively established, in part, because of the challenge of making an accurate diagnosis given that Lewy bodies are associated with several diseases (Huang & Halliday, 2013). People with the disease are often misdiagnosed with AD or PD (McKeith et al., 2017). The age at onset of LBD ranges from 50 to 83 years (Papka, Rubio, & Schiffer, 1998), and the mean disease duration is 6.4 years (Sreenath & Barber, 2009).

Diagnostic Criteria and Symptomatology

Individuals with LBD experience movement, cognitive, and affective disorders. Their parkinsonism is thought to result from a loss of dopamine-producing neurons in the substantia nigra, as is the case in PD; the dementia is thought to result from a loss of acetylcholine-producing neurons in the nucleus basalis of Meynert, as is the case in AD. The affective disorders are thought to be the result of widespread distribution of Lewy Bodies throughout the brain including the neocortex as well as neurochemical deficiencies. The three core symptoms of LBD are prominent and recurrent visual hallucinations or delusions, Parkinson's-like motor symptoms, and fluctuating awareness and concentration. If no mention is made of fluctuating attention/alertness and visual hallucinations, the clinician may fail to recognize LBD and the patient may be mistakenly diagnosed with PD (Auning et al., 2011). Unfortunately, not differentiating LBD from PD is serious because of the extreme sensitivity of LBD patients to treatment with neuroleptic medications that are tolerated by individuals with PD.

Other symptoms of LBD include depression, rapid eye movement (REM) sleep behavior disorder (RBD), decreased sense of smell, constipation, postural dizziness, problem solving difficulty, and memory impairment (57% of the time) (Auning et al., 2011; Donaghy & McKeith, 2014; McKeith et al., 2004; Mosimann & McKeith, 2003; Sreenath & Barber, 2009; Walker et al., 2000). The clinical features of LBD and PD are compared in Table 8–1 (Sulkava, 2003). Notice that the best differentiator of the disorder is visual hallucinations. Whereas they are often present in LBD, they are less common in PD. Similarly, fluctuating attention/alertness occurs in the majority of LBD patients but is uncommon in those with PD. Response to levodopa is another differentiator; LBD patients do not respond to levodopa, whereas most PD patients do (Louis, Klatka, Liu, & Fahn, 1997). When the clinical profiles of individuals with LBD were compared to those of individuals with PD, who were matched for score on the Unified Parkinson's Disease Motor Scale (that covers motor function, mentation, and mood), those with LBD had more axial motor, gait, and balance impairment and more daytime sleepiness, cognitive/behavioral fluctuations, hallucinations, and sleep apnea (Scharre et al., 2016).

The timing of the appearance of cognitive and motor symptoms is also typically different in the two conditions. In LBD, cognitive symptoms precede motor symptoms. When motor symptoms precede cognitive symptoms by a year, PDD is the likely diagnosis (Lee et al., 2010). In reality, clinicians often lack information about symptom onset and rely instead on lesion density data and immunohistochemistry. Neuropathologic and functional imaging data have shown that DLB is associated with greater density of Lewy bodies than PDD (Harding, Broe, & Halliday, 2002; Maetzler et al., 2008; Rowe et al., 2007).

Table 8–1. Clinical Features Helpful in the Differential Diagnosis of Early Parkinson's Disease (*PD*) and Dementia with Lewy Bodies (*DLB*) (Sulkava, 2003)

	PD	DLB
Impairment of psychomotor	Mild	More Marked
Executive dysfunction	Often	Often
Visuospatial impairment	Seldom	Often
Visual hallucinations	No	Often
Other hallucinations (e.g., auditory)	No	Sometimes
Extrapyramidal symptoms	Always	Often
Effect of levodopa	Good	Variable
Fluctuations of symptoms	Not Marked	Marked
Symptoms of depression	Often	Often
Delusions	No	Often
Absence of rest tremor	Sometimes	Often
Syncopal attacks	No	Sometimes
Episodes of unresponsiveness	No	Sometimes
Balance disorders	Sometimes	Seldom

Consortium Consensus Criteria for Diagnosis of Dementia

To facilitate diagnosis, the Dementia with Lewy Bodies Consortium created revised consensus criteria for diagnosis of "probable" and "possible" dementia with Lewy bodies (McKeith et al., 2017). A diagnosis of either "probable" or "possible" DLB requires a diagnosis of dementia plus one or more core clinical features. The core clinical features of DLB are fluctuating cognition, recurrent visual hallucinations, REM sleep behavior disorder, and at least one feature of parkinsonism. Probable DLB requires the presence of at least two of the core clinical features or one core clinical feature but with one or more biomarkers. Possible DLB requires one core clinical feature or one or more biomarkers without a core clinical feature.

The revision distinguishes more clearly between clinical features and biomarkers, and clinical signs and symptoms are weighted as core or supportive. Supportive clinical features include: frequent falls, negative response to antipsychotic agents, postural instability, syncope, autonomic dysfunction, apathy, anxiety, depression, and delusions. Biomarkers include chemical and structural abnormalities.

DLB fluctuations in cognition and behavior are described as occurring spontaneously. They are characterized as delirium-like with incoherent speech, staring or zoning out, and variable attention. The visual hallucinations occur in approximately 80% of patients and typically involve people and animals. The parkinsonism is spontaneous and not the result of antidopaminergic medications. Whereas PD is defined as bradykinesia (slowness of movement) as well as rigidity and rest tremor, individuals with possible DLB may have only one of these features. RBD is characterized as "vivid and often frightening dreams during REM sleep" (McKeith et al., 2005, p. 1866) in which patients vocalize, flail their limbs, and move around violently. Patients often have limited recollection of these episodes, though they are very memorable to their bed partners.

RBD may begin long before other symptoms, but the results of longitudinal investigations reveal that approximately 93% of individuals who experience them go on to develop a synucleinopthy; that is, PD, PDD, DLB, or multiple system atrophy (Iranzo et al., 2013; Postuma et al., 2009; Schenck, Boeve, & Mahowald, 2013).

The noted severe neuroleptic sensitivity of LBD patients refers to an adverse reaction to antipsychotic drugs that can manifest as exacerbation of parkinsonism and impaired consciousness. Low striatal dopamine transporter activity in functional imaging studies can help differentiate DLB from AD, in which striatal dopamine transporter activity is normal. Three other features have been associated with prodromal DLB: delirium, transient disturbances of consciousness (Vardy et al., 2014), and excessive daytime drowsiness.

Caregiver Report of Early Symptoms

Caregivers of LBD patients were interviewed by Auning and colleagues about the presenting symptoms (Auning et al., 2011). Caregivers were given a list of symptoms by the interviews and asked to designate those they had observed. The most commonly reported symptoms (with the percentage of caregivers who reported each) were

- Memory impairment (57%)
- Visual hallucinations (44%)
- Depression (34%)
- Specified difficulties in problem solving (33%)
- Gait problems (28%)
- Tremor/stiffness (25%)

LBD Risk Factors

Age is the primary risk factor for LBD. With age, the likelihood of LBD increases. Most individuals who develop the disease are at least 50 years of age. Apolipoprotein (APOE) carrier status is another risk factor. Of the gene variants that have been linked to DLB, it increases risk the most (Tsuang et al., 2012). The presence of the APOE e4 variant is also a risk factor for other dementias. It produces a 10-fold increase in the risk of pure AD; a 13-fold increase in the risk of AD with Lewy bodies; a 6-fold increase in the risk of pure DLB; and a 3-fold increase in the risk of PDD.

Given that many individuals with LBD have been found to have a diagnosis of Attention Deficit Hyperactive Disorder (ADHD), the APOE e4 gene is being investigated as a possible risk factor. Attention deficits are related in part to a frontal cholinergic deficit (Connor et al., 1998) and individuals with DLB also have cholinergic denervation; thus, researchers speculate that there may be a link between the two conditions (Bentley, Husain, & Dolan, 2004; Golimstok et al., 2011).

Effects of LBD on Cognition

A percentage of individuals diagnosed with MCI (a.k.a., mild neurocognitive disorder) will develop DLB and evolve to dementia. Rates vary from 5% to 25% (Bombois et al., 2008; Ferman et al., 2013; Fischer et al., 2007; Palmqvist et al., 2012). Memory deficits were the presenting disorder in 94% of individuals with DLB in the study by Noe et al. (2004). Other frequently reported effects of LBD on cognition are deficits in attention, executive functions, and visuoperceptual and spatial functions.

DLB may also present with noncognitive symptoms including depression, which can impact cognition. Results of a study of the psychiatric features of LBD (Klatka, Louis, & Schiffer, 1996) revealed that a history of depression was reported in 50% of patients with DLB who came to autopsy.

Executive Function and Attention

Executive dysfunction is an umbrella term referring to a host of abilities including initiating,

inhibiting, planning, organizing, self-monitoring, set shifting, and decision-making (Alvarez & Emory, 2006; Kobayakawa, Tsuruya, & Kawamura, 2010; Miyake et al., 2000; Royall et al., 2002; Spreen & Strauss, 1998; Stuss & Levine, 2002). Deficits in executive function occur early and throughout the disease course as a result of disrupted circuitry between the frontal cortex and subcortex (Dubois, Pillon, & McKeith, 2007; Goldman et al., 2014; Johns et al., 2009). As previously noted, fluctuations in cognitive ability, particularly the ability to direct and sustain attention are common. On some days, the individual with LBD is more disoriented and inattentive than on others. Delirium and transient disturbances of consciousness are reported to occur in the prodromal phase of LBD and thus may be the earliest symptoms of the disease (Vardy et al., 2014).

Visuoperceptual and Spatial Functions

Numerous reports exist of prominent impairment on a variety of visuospatial and visuoconstructional abilities (Oda, Yamamoto, & Maeda, 2009; Ota et al., 2015), among them deficits in the ability to draw a pentagon (Ala, Hughes, Kyrouac, Ghobrial, & Elble, 2001), do visual perception tasks (Mori et al., 2000), copy a cube (Palmqvist, Hansson, Minthon, & Londos, 2009), and arrange blocks or objects to match a target (Oda et al., 2009). Occipital dysfunction appears to account for functional disorders, and evidence exists of decreased regional glucose metabolism in the occipital association cortex and the primary visual area in individuals with autopsy-confirmed DLB (Albin et al., 1996). The same finding has been obtained in individuals with probable DLB who were compared with healthy control subjects (Ishii et al., 1998). Moreover, data from single photon emission computed tomography (SPECT) imaging reveal significantly lower occipital blood flow.

Visuopercental and visuoconstruction impairments can help distinguish DBL from normal aging and AD (Ota et al., 2015; Vann

Jones & O'Brien, 2014). Compared to individuals with AD, those with DLB perform worse on tasks of visuoperception, visuoconstruction, and spatial working memory, whereas those with AD are poorer in performance on memory and orientation tasks.

Memory

Working memory is impaired in DLB patients and is apparent in performance accuracy on digit vigilance, letter cancellation tasks, and slower reaction times. Deficits are particularly pronounced in those with Mini-Mental State Examination (MMSE) scores of 10 or less (Ballard et al., 2001). Episodic memory is affected, though less so than in individuals with AD, especially for verbal information (McLaughlin, Chang, & Malloy, 2012). Although few investigators have reported the effects of LBD pathology on procedural memory and learning, it is likely that affected individuals are compromised similarly to those with PD because of their pathology in the basal ganglia.

Language and Communicative Function

Whereas grammatical aspects of language are relatively preserved in LBD (Grossman et al., 2012), as they are in individuals with PD (Bayles, 1990), the process of communication and content of language are affected by disease-related cognitive deficits (Ash et al., 2011; Bastiaanse & Leenders, 2009; Chenery, Angwin, & Copland, 2008; Colman et al., 2009; Grossman, 1999; Hochstadt, 2009; Pereira et al., 2009). In a series of studies on sentence-processing skills in relation to integrity of executive function skills, Gross and colleagues (2012) demonstrated that individuals with DLB are significantly impaired relative to healthy elders in processing sentences when grammatical complexity and length are increased and when they are asked to do a secondary task. Similarly, DLB patients were impaired in understanding sentences lengthened by the addition of a prepositional phrase between sentence elements that must be linked to be comprehended. They were also impaired when the sentences contained additional prepositional phrases. Addition of these elements were interpreted by Gross and colleagues to stress working memory, thereby reducing the needed cognitive resources.

More recently, Grossman and colleagues (2012) extended their research on the effect of executive dysfunction on sentence processing in individuals with LBD by assessing their ability to process temporary structural ambiguities ("the tired passenger claimed the luggage was unidentified at the airport."). An online word detection procedure was used in which subjects heard sentences with a syntactic structure that had high or low compatibility with the main verb's statistically preferred syntactic structure. Half the sentences were strategically lengthened between the onset of the ambiguity and its resolution. Subjects were told to press a button when they heard a target word that was placed either right after the resolution of the ambiguity or preceding the verb by two words. Individuals with LBD were significantly impaired in processing the ambiguities and regression analyses related poor performance to significant cortical thinning in parietal and frontal brain areas.

Ash and colleagues (2011) studied the relation of executive function to the development of narrative discourse and reasoned that LBD pathology in basal ganglia and frontal lobes might compromise the planning and organization skills needed to produce coherent, logical narratives (Calderon et al., 2001; Kraybill et al., 2005; Lambon Ralph et al., 2001; Libon et al., 2001). Thirty-two individuals with LBD, 14 of whom had evidence of dementia, participated. Subjects were instructed to communicate an effective narrative from a series of drawings that portrayed a simple story. The narratives were evaluated in terms of local and global connectedness and theme maintenance. Results showed that all the LBD subjects had difficulty with the task, but those with dementia were significantly inferior to normal control subjects on all three narrative measures. Additionally, the degree of impairment was related to level of impairment on measures of executive functioning and speech fluency.

Future investigations of the effects of LBD on language and communication will likely reveal that communication is affected more than linguistic knowledge and affected individuals have performance profiles similar to those of individuals with AD and PDD. The form of language may include more sentence fragments, simplified grammar, less cohesion, and be less concise. Language content will likely be increasingly vague, tangential, and nonsensical. Ultimately, language use may diminish, become perseverative, or in some patients become echolalic.

A Case of Pure LBD

Few descriptions exist of the effects on communication of "pure" LBD, that is, LBD without coexistent Alzheimer's pathology. However, Gurd, Herzberg, Joachim, and Marshall (2000) described a 68-year-old man who was examined neuropsychologically and neuroradiologically several times in life and had autopsy confirmation of pure LBD. This contribution to the literature is valuable because it confirms reports of earlier investigations and adds new information about communicative functioning.

Early in the disease, Gurd et al.'s patient experienced periods of forgetfulness and described himself as having trouble putting thoughts into words. He sought advice from a general practitioner who referred him to specialists who followed him for 2 years. Gurd and colleagues reported that the patient was unable to shop with a list, sometimes forgot the beginning of a sentence by the end, and occasionally made comments that were out of context. At the first neuropsychological evaluation, cognitive impairment was obvious and he scored 15 of 30 on the MMSE. His attention was poor and he was disoriented for time and space. Furthermore, he was anosognosic for his

cognitive deficits. Over the disease course, the patient complained of visual hallucinations, confusion upon waking, and nightmares. He became depressed, irritable, stubborn, and preoccupied with death, which occurred 2.5 years after diagnosis.

In conversation, Gurd et al.'s patient made several tangential departures from topic and was extremely poor on semantic and letter category naming. Gurd et al. described the patient as having difficulty remembering and maintaining the semantic category as evident from several out-of-category errors. He could write his name and address and draw a house, man, and flower. One year after his initial examination, his spontaneous speech was grammatically sound but he was described as aphasic, although he did not display obvious language comprehension problems. His descriptions of a picture were plausible, though he confabulated at the end of picture description. Stress and intonation patterns were normal, but he was mildly deficient in word retrieval, articulation, and phrase completion. Word retrieval was often labored with long, frequent pauses. Some articulatory errors were noted and occasionally he mumbled his words. Although he named 18 of 21 pictured objects at his first test session, his object naming score diminished to 10 of 21 1.5 years later.

Definitions

Anosognosia: Unawareness of cognitive, linguistic, sensory, and/or motor deficits after brain disease or injury.

Neuroleptic drugs: Tranquilizers used to treat psychotic conditions.

Syncope: Fainting or temporary loss of consciousness due to inadequate blood flow to the brain.

Hallucination: A false perception; sensory experience of stimuli that are not actually present.

Neuroimaging (CT and SPECT) in life revealed progressive medial temporal lobe atrophy. Postmortem pathologic analysis documented Lewy bodies as well as degeneration in the substantia nigra, nucleus basalis of Meynert, and locus ceruleus, but none of the neuritic plaques and neurofibrillary tangles that characterize AD.

Summary of Changes in Communicative Functioning

The following are the early- and late-occurring changes in communicative functioning of the patient described by Gurd and colleagues (2000):

Early Features

- Grammatically sound speech
- Mild anomia on confrontation naming
- Forgot what he intended to say
- Some tangential comments
- Could write name and address
- Severe impairment in semantic and letter category naming

Later Features

- Grammatically sound speech
- Normal stress and intonation
- Occasional articulation error
- Occasional confabulation
- Slow in word retrieval
- Deficit in phrase completion
- Long, frequent pauses
- No obvious comprehension problems

Cognitive Profile of LBD Compared with AD

Whereas individuals with LBD experience cognitive deterioration, they are less susceptible to the hallmark early symptom of AD: episodic memory loss. However, many early symptoms mimic those associated with AD, among them attention deficits, constructional dyspraxia, and executive dysfunction (Byrne, Lennox, Lowe, &

Godwin-Austen, 1989; Gibb, Esiri, & Lees, 1985; Mondon et al., 2007; Salmon & Hamilton, 2005). Nonetheless, careful neuropsychological testing reveals significant differences (Scharre et al., 2016). Results of comparisons of individuals with DLB and those with AD—who were similar in age, mental status, and use of medications—revealed that DLB patients have more severe deficits in executive and visuospatial domains (Scharre et al., 2016), but are better on verbal episodic memory. The visuoperceptual and processing deficits are so prominent in DLB that Oda and colleagues (2009) consider neuropsychological assessment of visual perceptual and constructional functions to be critical in evaluating individuals suspected of having DLB or AD. The absence of visuospatial impairment may be the best negative predictor of DLB at autopsy (Tiraboschi et al., 2006).

In terms of performance on language tasks, individuals with LBD tend to have relative preservation of confrontation naming and better verbal recall and recognition memory than those with AD; however, greater impairment in verbal fluency (Connor et al., 1998; McKeith et al., 2005; Mormont, Grymonprez, Baisset-Mouly, & Pasquier, 2003; Walker, Allen, Shergill, Katona, 1997), particularly in the naming of action verbs (action fluency naming) (Delbeuck, Debachy, Pasquier, Moroni, 2013).

Finally, the key feature of DLB, fluctuation in attention, is unusual in individuals with AD. When family or patients report that on some days they are really confused and others more lucid, consider the possibility of LBD. Ballard and colleagues (2001) documented significant variability in reaction time (RT) in DLB patients when compared with AD patients, a finding that substantiates the commonly held belief that fluctuation in attention is a critical feature of DLB.

Cognitive Profile of LBD Compared with PDD

Twenty-one ambulatory LBD patients with mild dementia were individually matched by score on the Unified Parkinson's Disease Rating Scale motor score and MMSE score with 21 individuals with PD (Scharre et al., 2016). The LBD group had more cognitive/behavioral fluctuations, hallucinations, sleepiness, and sleep apnea than members of the PD group. Visual hallucinations occurred in 62% of the LBD group but in only 9.5% of the PD subjects.

Overall, the LBD subjects had significantly poorer gait and balance compared to PD subjects who had more resting tremor. Additionally, axial motor, gait, and balance disturbances correlated with executive, visuospatial, and global cognition function.

Summary of Important Points

- Lewy body disease (LBD) is considered a spectrum of disorders because Lewy bodies are common in individuals with PD, AD, and Down syndrome.
- DLB is an abbreviation for "dementia with Lewy bodies"; LBD is an abbreviation for Lewy body disease that is associated with dementia. Both terms are used in the literature.
- Lewy bodies are round lumps of the protein alpha-synuclein that are found in the cell processes of neurons. Between 15% and 25% of dementia patients have diffuse cortical Lewy bodies.
- Little attention was paid to LBD until 1961. Since then it has gained recognition as the second-most common cause of dementia.
- Individuals with LBD exhibit movement and cognitive disorders. The movement disorders are like those in PD and the cognitive disorders are similar to those associated with AD.
- The core features of the disease are prominent and recurrent visual hallucinations, Parkinson's-like motor symptoms, fluctuating awareness and concentration, and REM sleep disorder.
- Two core features are sufficient for a diagnosis of probable DLB, one for possible DLB.
- Because individuals with LBD often have extrapyramidal symptoms, they may be misdiagnosed as having PD.

- The timing of cognitive and motor symptoms helps clinicians differentiate PD and LBD. When cognitive symptoms precede motor symptoms, DLB is likely the diagnosis; when motor symptoms precede cognitive symptoms by a year, PDD is likely the diagnosis.
- Risk factors for LBD include age, APOE carrier status, and possibly ADHD.
- The most frequently reported effects of LBD on cognition are deficits in memory, executive functions, attention, and visuoperceptual and visuoconstruction functions.
- Many early symptoms of DLB mimic those associated with AD; namely, memory loss, attention deficits, constructional dyspraxia, and executive dysfunction. The visuospatial and visuoconstruction deficits of DLB are helpful in distinguishing it from AD.
- DLB can present with depression, which can impact cognition.
- With disease progression, severe behavioral problems and dementia develop.
- Whereas grammatical aspects of language are relatively preserved in LBD, as they are in individuals with PD, the process of communication and content of language are affected by disease-related cognitive deficits. An example is a deficient performance on category naming (verbal fluency) tests.
- Future investigations of the effects of LBD on language and communication will likely reveal that communication is affected more than linguistic knowledge and affected individuals have performance profiles similar to those of individuals with AD and PDD.

References

Aarsland, D., Rongve, A., Nore, S. P., Skogseth, R., Skulstad, S., Ehrt, U., . . . Ballard, C. (2008). Frequency and case identification of dementia with Lewy bodies using the revised consensus criteria. *Dementia and Geriatric Cognitive Disorders, 26*, 445–452.

Ala, T. A., Hughes, L. F., Kyrouac, G. A., Ghobrial, M. W., & Elble, R. J. (2001). Pentagon copying is more impaired in dementia with Lewy bodies than in Alzheimer's disease. *Journal of Neurology, Neurosurgery, and Psychiatry, 70,* 483–488.

Albin, R. L., Minoshima, S., d'Amato, C. J., Frey, K. A., Kuhl, D. A., & Sima, A. A. (1996). Flurodeoxyglucose positron emission tomography in diffuse Lewy body disease. *Neurology, 47,* 462–466.

Alvarez, J. A., & Emory, E. (2006). Executive function and the frontal lobes: A meta-analytic review. *Neuropsychology Review, 16,* 17–42.

Alzheimer's Association. (2017, November 6). Dementia with Lewy body: Symptoms, signs and diagnosis. Retrieved from https://www.alz.org/dementia/dementia-with-lewy-bodies-symptoms.asp

American Psychiatric Association. (2013). *Diagnostic and statistical manual of mental disorders* (5th ed.). Arlington, VA: American Psychiatric Publishing.

Ash, S., McMillan, C., Gross, R., Cook, P., Gunawardena, D., Morgan, B., . . . Grossman, M. (2012). Impairments of speech fluency in Lewy body spectrum disorder. *Brain and Language, 120,* 290–302.

Ash, S., McMillan, C., Gross, R. G., Cook, P., Morgan, B., Boller, A., . . . Grossman, M. (2011). The organization of narrative discourse in Lewy body spectrum disorder. *Brain and Language, 119,* 30–41.

Auning, E., Rongve, A., Fladby, T., Booij, J., Hortobágyi, T., Siepel, F. J., . . . Aarsland, D. (2011). Early and presenting symptoms of dementia with Lewy bodies. *Dementia and Geriatric Cognitive Disorders, 32,* 202–208.

Ballard, C., O'Brien, J., Gray, A., Cormack, F., Ayre, G., Rowan, E., . . . Tovee, M. (2001). Attention and fluctuating attention in patients with dementia with Lewy bodies and Alzheimer disease. *Archives of Neurology, 58,* 977–982.

Bastiaanse, R., & Leenders, K. L. (2009). Language and Parkinson's disease. *Cortex, 45,* 912–914.

Bayles, K. A. (1990). Language and Parkinson disease. *Alzheimer Disease and Associated Disorders, 4,* 171–180.

Bentley, P., Husain, M., & Dolan, R. J. (2004). Effects of cholinergic enhancement on visual stimulation, spatial attention, and spatial working memory. *Neuron, 41,* 969–982.

Bombois, S., Debette, S., Bruandet, A., Delbeuck, X., Delmaire, C., Leys, D., & Pasquier, F. (2008). Vascular subcortical hyperintensities predict conversion to vascular and mixed dementia in MCI patients. *Stroke, 39,* 2046–2051.

Byrne, E. J., Lennox, G., Lowe, J., & Godwin-Austen, R. B. (1989). Diffuse Lewy body disease: Clinical features in 15 cases. *Journal of Neurology. Neurosurgery, and Psychiatry, 52,* 709–717.

Calderon, J., Perry, R. J., Erzinclioglu, S. W., Berrios, G. E., Dening, T. R., & Hodges, J. R. (2001). Perception, attention, and working memory are disproportionately impaired in dementia with Lewy bodies compared with Alzheimer's disease. *Journal of Neurology, Neurosurgery, and Psychiatry, 70,* 157–164.

Chenery, H. J., Angwin, A. J., & Copland, D. A. (2008). The basal ganglia circuits, dopamine, and ambiguous word processing: A neurobiological account of priming studies in Parkinson's disease. *Journal of the International Neuropsychological Society, 14,* 351–364.

Colman, K. S., Koerts, J., Van Beilen, M., Leenders, K. L., Post, W. J., & Bastiaanse, R. (2009). The impact of executive functions on verb production in patients with Parkinson's disease. *Cortex, 45,* 930–942.

Connor, D. J., Salmon, D. P., Sandy, T. J., Galasko, D., Hansen, L. A., & Thal, L. J. (1998). Cognitive profiles of autopsy-confirmed Lewy body variant vs. pure Alzheimer disease. *Archives of Neurology, 55,* 994–1000.

Cummings, J. L., & Mega, M. S. (2003). *Neuropsychiatry and behavioral neuroscience.* New York, NY: Oxford University Press.

Delbeuck, X., Debachy, B., Pasquier, F., & Moroni, C. (2013). Action and noun fluency testing to distinguish between Alzheimer's disease and dementia with Lewy bodies. *Journal of Clinical and Experimental Neuropsychology, 35,* 259–268.

Donaghy, P. C., & McKeith, I. G. (2014). The clinical characteristics of dementia with Lewy bodies and a consideration of prodromal diagnosis. *Alzheimer's Research and Therapy, 6,* 46.

Dubois, B., Pillon, B., & McKeith, I. G. (2007). Parkinson's disease with and without dementia and Lewy body dementia. In B. Miller & J. L. Cummings (Eds.), *The human frontal lobes: Functions and disorders* (pp. 472–504). New York, NY: Guilford Press.

Ferman, T. J., Smith, G. E., Kantarci, K., Boeve, B. F., Pankratz, V. S., Dickson, D. W., Graff-Radford, N. R., Wszolek, Z., ... Petersen, R. C. (2013). Nonamnestic mild cognitive impairment progresses to dementia with Lewy bodies. *Neurology, 81,* 2032–2038.

Fischer, P., Jungwirth, S., Zehetmayer, S., Weissgram, S., Hoenigschnabl, S., Gelpi, E., ... Tragl, K. H. (2007). Conversion from subtypes of mild cognitive impairment to Alzheimer dementia. *Neurology, 68,* 288–291.

Frigerio, R., Fujishiro, H., Ahn, T.-B., Josephs, K. A., Maraganore, D. M., DelleDonne, A., ... Ahskog, E. J. (2011). Incidental Lewy body disease: Do some cases represent a preclinical stage of dementia with Lewy bodies? *Neurobiology of Aging, 32,* 857–863.

Gibb, W. R. G., Esiri, M. M., & Lees, A. J. (1985). Clinical and pathological features of diffuse cortical Lewy body disease (Lewy body dementia). *Brain, 110,* 1131–1153.

Gibb, W. R., & Lees, A. J. (1988). The relevance of the Lewy body to the pathogenesis of idiopathic Parkinson's disease. *Journal of Neurology, Neurosurgery, and Psychiatry, 51,* 745–752.

Goldman, J. G., Williams-Gray, C., Barker, R., Duda, J. E., & Galvin, J. E. (2014). The spectrum of cognitive impairment in Lewy body disease. *Movement Disorders, 29,* 608–621.

Golimstok, A., Rojas, J. I., Romano, M., Zurru, M. C., Doctorovich, D., & Cristiano, E. (2011). Previous adult attention-deficit and hyperactivity disorder symptoms and risk of dementia with Lewy bodies: A case-control study. *European Journal of Neurology, 18*, 78–84.

Gross, R. G., McMillan, C. T., Chandrasekaran, K., Dreyfuss, M., Ash, S., Avants, B., . . . Grossman, M. (2012). Sentence processing in Lewy body spectrum disorder: The role of working memory. *Brain and Cognition, 78*, 85–93.

Grossman, M. (1999). Sentence processing in Parkinson's disease. *Brain and Cognition, 40*, 387–413.

Grossman, M., Gross, R. G., Moore, P., Dreyfuss, M., McMillan, C. T., Cook, P. A., . . . Siderowf, A. (2012). Difficulty processing temporary syntactic ambiguities in Lewy body spectrum disorder. *Brain and Language, 120*, 52–60.

Gurd, J. M., Herzberg, L., Joachim, C., & Marshall, J. C. (2000). Dementia with Lewy bodies: A pure case. *Brain and Cognition, 44*, 307–323.

Harding, A. J., Broe, G. A., & Halliday, G. M. (2002). Visual hallucinations in Lewy body disease relate to Lewy bodies in the temporal lobe. *Brain, 125*, 391–403.

Hochstadt, J. (2009). Set-shifting and the on-line processing of relative clauses in Parkinson's disease: Results from a novel eye-tracking method. *Cortex, 45*, 991–1011.

Holdorff, B. (2002). Friedrich Heinrich Lewy (1885–1950) and his work. *Journal of the History of Neuroscience, 11*, 19–28.

Huang, Y., & Halliday, G. (2013). Can we clinically diagnose dementia with Lewy bodies yet? *Translational Neurodegeneration, 2*, 4.

Iranzo, A., Tolosa, E., Gelpi, E., Molinuevo, J. L., Valldeoriola, F., Serradell, M., ... Santamaria, J. (2013). Neurodegenerative disease status and post-mortem pathology in idiopathic rapid-eye-movement sleep behaviour disorder: An observational cohort study. *Lancet Neurology, 12*, 443–453.

Ishii, K., Imamura, T., Sasaki, M., Yamaji, S., Sakamoto, S., Kitagaki, H., . . . Mori, E. (1998). Regional cerebral glucose metabolism in dementia with Lewy bodies and Alzheimer's disease. *Neurology, 51*, 125–130.

Johns, E. K., Phillips, N. A., Belleville, S., Goupil, D., Babins, L., Kelner, N., . . . Chertkow, H. (2009). Executive functions in frontotemporal dementia and Lewy body dementia. *Neuropsychology, 23*, 765–777.

Klatka, L. A., Louis, E., & Schiffer, R. B. (1996). Psychiatric features in diffuse Lewy body disease: A clinicopathologic study using Alzheimer's disease and Parkinson's disease comparison groups. *Neurology, 47*, 1148–1152.

Kobayakawa, M., Tsuruya, N., & Kawamura, M. (2010). Sensitivity to reward and punishment in Parkinson's disease: An analysis of behavioral patterns using a modified version of the Iowa gambling task. *Parkinsonism and Related Disorders, 16*, 453–457.

Kosaka, K. (1978). Lewy bodies in cerebral cortex: Report of three cases. *Acta Neuropathologica, 42*, 127–134.

Kraybill, M. L., Larson, E. B., Tsuang, D. W., Teri, L., McCormick, W. C., Bowen, J. D., . . . Cherrier, M. M. (2005). Cognitive differences in dementia patients with autopsy-verified AD, Lewy body pathology, or both. *Neurology, 64*, 2069–2073.

Lambon Ralph, M. A., Powell, J., Howard, D., Whitworth, A. B., Garrard, P., & Hodges, J. R. (2001). Semantic memory is impaired in both dementia with Lewy bodies and dementia of Alzheimer's type: A comparative neuropsychological study and literature review. *Journal of Neurology, Neurosurgery, and Psychiatry, 70*, 149–156.

Lee, D. Lee, S.-Y., Lee, E.-N., Change, C.-S., & Paik, S. R. (2002). α-Synuclein exhibits competitive interaction between calmodulin and synthetic membranes. *Journal of Neurochemistry, 82*, 1007–1017.

Lee, J. E., Park, H.-J., Park, B., Song, S. K., Sohn, Y.H., Lee, J. D., & Lee, P. H. (2010). A comparative analysis of cognitive profiles and white matter alterations using voxel-based diffusion tensor imaging between patients with Parkinson's disease dementia and dementia with Lewy Bodies. *Journal of Neurology, Neurosurgery, and Psychiatry, 81*, 320–326.

Libon, D. J., Bogdanoff, B., Leopold, N., Hurka, R., Bonavita, J., Skalina, S., . . . Ball, S. K. (2001). Neuropsychological profiles associated with subcortical white matter alterations and Parkinson's disease: implications for the diagnosis of dementia. *Archives of Clinical Neuropsychology, 16*, 19–32.

Louis, E. D., Klatka, L. A., Liu, Y., & Fahn, S. (1997). Comparison of extrapyramidal features in 31 pathologically confirmed cases of diffuse Lewy body disease and 34 pathologically confirmed cases of Parkinson's disease. *Neurology, 48*, 376–380.

Maetzler, W., Reimold, M., Liepelt, I., Solbach, C., Leyhe, T., Schweitzer, K., . . . Berg, D. (2008). [11C] PIB binding in Parkinson's disease dementia. *Neuroimage, 39*, 1027–1033.

McKeith, I., Mintzer, J., Aarsland, D., Burn, D., Chiu, H., Cohen-Mansfield, J., . . . Reid, W. (2004). Dementia with Lewy bodies. *Lancet Neurology, 3*, 19–28.

McKeith, I. G. (2005). Dementia with Lewy bodies: A clinical overview. In A. Burns, J., O'Brien, & D. Ames (Eds.), *Dementia* (pp. 603–614). London, UK: Hodder Arnold.

McKeith, I. G., Boeve, B. F., Dickson, D. W., Halliday, G., Taylor, J-P. Weintraub, D., ... Kosaka, K. (2017). Diagnosis and management of dementia with Lewy bodies. *Neurology, 89*, 88–100.

McKeith, I. G., Dickson, D. W., Lowe, J., Emre, M., O'Brien, J. T., Feldman, H., . . . Yamada, M. (2005). Diagnosis and management of dementia with Lewy bodies: Third report of the DLB consortium. *Neurology, 65*, 1863–1872.

McLaughlin, N. C. R., Change, A. C., & Malloy, P. (2012). Verbal and nonverbal learning and recall in dementia with Lewy bodies and Alzheimer's disease. *Applied Neuropsychology, 19*, 86–89.

Miyake, A., Friedman, N. P., Emerson, M. J., Witzki, A. H., Howerter, A., & Wager, T. D. (2000). The unity and diversity of executive functions and their contributions to complex "Frontal Lobe" tasks: A latent variable analysis. *Cognitive Psychology, 41*, 49–100.

Mondon, K., Gochard, A., Marque, A., Armand, A., Beauchamp, D., Prunier, C., . . . Hommet, C. (2007). Visual recognition memory differentiates dementia with Lewy bodies and Parkinson's disease dementia. *Journal of Neurology, Neurosurgery, and Psychiatry, 78*, 738–741.

Mori, E., Shimomura, T., Fujimori, M., Hirono, N., Imamura, T., Hashimoto, M., . . . Hanihara, T. (2000). Visuoperceptual impairment in dementia with Lewy bodies. *Archives of Neurology, 57*, 489–493.

Mormont, E., Grymonprez, L. L., Baisset-Mouly, C., & Pasquier, F. (2003). The profile of memory disturbance in early Lewy body dementia differs from that in Alzheimer's disease. *Review Neurologique, 159*, 762–766.

Mosimann, U. P., & McKeith, I. G. (2003). Dementia with Lewy bodies: Diagnosis and treatment. *Swiss Medical Weekly, 133*, 131–142.

Noe, E., Marder, K., Bell, K. L., Jacobs, D. M., Manly, J. J., & Stern, Y. (2004). Comparison of dementia with Lewy bodies to Alzheimer's disease and Parkinson's disease with dementia. *Movement Disorders, 19*, 60–67.

Oda, H., Yamamoto, Y., & Maeda, K. (2009). Neuropsychological profile of dementia with Lewy bodies. *Psychogeriatrics, 9*, 85–90.

Okazaki, H., Lipton, L. S., & Aronson, S. M. (1961). Diffuse intracytoplasmic ganglionic inclusions (Lewy type) associated with progressive dementia and quadriparesis in flexion. *Journal of Neurology, Neurosurgery, and Psychiatry, 20*, 237–244.

Ota, K., Murayama, N., Kasanuki, K., Kondo, D., Fujishiro, H., Sato, K., & Iseki, E. (2015). Visuoperceptual assessments for differentiating dementia with Lewy bodies and Alzheimer disease: Illusory contours and other neuropsychological examinations. *Archives of Clinical Neuropsychology, 30*, 256–263.

Palmqvist, S., Hansson, O., Minthon, L., & Londos, E. (2009). Practical suggestions on how to differentiate dementia with Lewy bodies from Alzheimer's disease with common cognitive tests. *International Journal of Geriatric Psychiatry, 24*, 1405–1412.

Palmqvist, S., Hertze, J., Minthon, L., Wattmo, C., Zetterberg, H., Blennow, K., ... Hansson, O. (2012). Comparison of brief cognitive tests and CSF biomarkers in predicting Alzheimer's disease in mild cognitive impairment: 5-year follow-up study. *Plos ONE, 7*, 1–7.

Papka, M., Rubio, A., & Schiffer, R. B. (1998). A review of Lewy body disease: An emerging concept of cortical dementia. *Journal of Neuropsychiatry and Clinical Neuroscience, 10*, 267–279.

Pereira, J. B., Junque, C., Marti, M. J., Ramirezruiz, B., Bartres-Faz, D., & Tolosa, E. (2009). Structural brain correlates of verbal fluency in Parkinson's disease. *NeuroReport, 20*, 741–744.

Postuma, R. B., Gagnon, J. F., Vendette, M., Fantini, M. L., Massicotte-Marquez, J., & Montplaisir, J. (2009). Quantifying the risk of neurodegenerative disease in idiopathic REM sleep behavior disorder. *Neurology, 72*, 1296–1300.

Reichman, W. E., & Cummings, J. L. (1999). Dementia. In E. H. Duthie & P. R. Katz (Eds.), *Practice of geriatrics* (pp. 295–304). Philadelphia, PA: W. B. Saunders.

Reish, H. E. A., & Standaert, D. G. (2015). Role of α-synuclein in inducing innate and adaptive immunity in Parkinson disease. *Journal of Parkinson's Disease, 5*, 1–19.

Rowe, C. C., Ng, S., Ackermann, U., Gong, S.J., Pike, K., Savage, G., . . . Villemagne, V. L. (2007). Imaging beta-amyloid burden in aging and dementia. *NeuroImage, 68*, 1718–1725.

Royall, D. R., Lauterbach, E. C., Cummings, J. L., Reeve, A., Rummans, T. A., Kaufer, D. I., . . . Coffey, C. E. (2002). Executive control function: A review of its promise and challenges for clinical research. A report from the Committee on Research of the American Neuropsychiatric Association. *Journal of Neuropsychiatry and Clinical Neurosciences, 14*, 377–405.

Salmon, D. P., & Hamilton, J. M. (2005). Neuropsychological changes in dementia with Lewy bodies. In A. Burns, J. O'Brien, & D. Ames (Eds.), *Dementia* (pp. 634–647). London, UK: Hodder Arnold.

Scharre, D. W., Change, S-I., Nagaraja, H. N., Park, A., Adeli, A., Agrawal, P., ... Kataki, M. (2016). Paired studies comparing clinical profiles of Lewy body dementia with Alzheimer's and Parkinson's diseases. *Journal of Alzheimer's Disease, 54*, 995–1004.

Schenck, C. H., Boeve, B. F., & Mahowald, M. W. (2013). Delayed emergence of a parkinsonian disorder or dementia in 81% of older males initially diagnosed with idiopathic REM sleep behavior disorder (RBD): 16-year update on a previously reported series. *Sleep Medicine, 14*, 744–748.

Simard, M., Van Reekum, R., & Cohen, T. (2000). A review of the cognitive and behavioral symptoms in dementia with Lewy bodies. *Journal of Neuropsychiatry and Clinical Neurosciences, 12*, 425–450.

Spreen, O., & Strauss, E. (1998). *A compendium of neuropsychological tests: Administration, norms, and commentary.* New York, NY: Oxford University Press.

Sreenath, S., & Barber, R. (2009). Dementia with Lewy bodies. *The AvMA Medical and Legal Journal, 15*, 115–119.

Stuss, D. T., & Levine, B. (2002). Adult clinical neuropsychology: Lessons from studies of the frontal lobes. *Annual Review of Psychology, 53*, 401–433.

Sulkava, R. (2003). Differential diagnosis between early Parkinson's disease and dementia with Lewy bodies. In A. Gordin, S. Kaakkola, & H. Teravainen (Eds.), *Parkinson's disease: Advances in neurology* (pp. 411–413). Philadelphia, PA: Lippincott Williams & Wilkins.

Tiraboschi, P., Salmon, D. P., Hansen, L. A., Hofstetter, R. C., Thal, L. J., & Corey-Bloom, J. (2006). What best differentiates Lewy body from Alzheimer's disease in early-stage dementia? *Brain, 129,* 729–735.

Tsuang, D., Leverenz, J. B., Lopez, O., Hamilton, R. L., Bennett, D. A., Schneider, J. A., . . . Zabetian, C. P. (2012). GBA mutations increase risk for Lewy body disease with and without Alzheimer pathology. *Neurology, 79,* 1944–1950.

Tsuboi, Y., & Dickson, D. W. (2005). Dementia with Lewy bodies Parkinson's disease with dementia: Are they different? *Parkinsonism and Related Disorders, 11*(Suppl. 1), 47–51.

Vann Jones, S. A., & O'Brien, J. T. (2014). The prevalence and incidence of dementia with Lewy bodies: A systematic review of population and clinical studies. *Psychological Medicine, 44,* 673–683.

Vardy, E., Holt, R., Gerhard, A., Richardson, A., Snowden, J., & Neary, D. (2014). History of a suspected delirium is more common in dementia with Lewy bodies than Alzheimer's disease: A retrospective study. *International Journal of Geriatric Psychiatry, 29,* 178–181.

Walker, A., Allen, R. L., Shergill, S., & Katona, C. L. E. (1997). Neuropsychological performance in Lewy body dementia and Alzheimer's disease. *British Journal of Psychiatry, 170,* 156–158.

Walker, M. P., Ayre, G. A., Perry, E. K., Wesnes, J., Mckeith, I. G., Tovee, M., . . . Ballard, C. G. (2000). Quantification and characterization of fluctuating cognition in dementia with Lewy bodies and Alzheimer's disease. *Dementia and Geriatric Cognitive Disorders, 11,* 327–335.

9

Dementia and Huntington's Disease

Overview and Genetics of Huntington's Disease

Huntington's disease (HD), also known as Huntington's chorea, is an inherited degenerative disease of the nervous system characterized by dementia and uncontrollable dancelike movements known as chorea. George Huntington, the physician for whom the disease was named, described the uncoordinated movements as "chorea" from the Greek word *choros* for "dance."

The mutant gene that causes HD is called huntingtin and is autosomal dominant (Chua & Chiu, 2005; Kordasiewicz et al., 2012). "Autosomal" means that the gene is located on a chromosome other than the sex chromosome and therefore the disease is not sex-linked; males and females are equally likely to be affected. "Dominant" means that the defective gene dominates its normal partner gene from the unaffected parent. Each child of an affected parent has a 50% chance of inheritance. If a child has not received the Huntington's gene from a parent, the child and his or her children will be free of the disease, but children who inherit the gene will develop the disease if they live long enough. HD affects roughly 1 in every 10,000 persons.

In 1983, the gene causing HD was identified by a team of scientists from around the world (Gusella et al., 1983). It lies at one end of chromosome 4 and makes a mutant form of huntingtin protein in which the same amino acid, glutamine, repeats dozens of times (Cattaneo, Rigamonti, & Zuccato, 2002; Nopoulos, 2016). Mutant huntingtin appears to be toxic to certain nerve cells and lacks the ability to trigger the production of a necessary growth factor. There is no known cure for HD; however, soon after the discovery of huntingtin, genetic tests were developed enabling individuals with a family member with HD to determine whether they carry the HD gene. Many individuals at risk for developing HD have taken advantage of genetic testing. Yet, with this advantage is the possibility of significant stress at the prospect of symptom onset (Barema, 2005; Wexler, 1995).

The median age at onset of HD is late 40s or early 50s (Kremer, 2003); however, in 5% to 10% of cases, symptoms occur in persons under 20 years of age (Freckelton, 2012). Young et al. (1986) reported that 94% of individuals with HD developed it as adults and only 6% developed it as juveniles. In the large majority of individuals with juvenile onset (90%), the gene was inherited from the father (Harper, 1996). Once symptoms appear, death usually occurs within 15 to 20 years (Saldert & Hartelius, 2011), most commonly from pneumonia, but suicide is the second most-common cause (Roos, 2010).

Neuropathology of HD

The signs and symptoms of HD result from brain atrophy and neurochemical deficiencies. Atrophy is most prominent in the head of the caudate nucleus but exists to a lesser extent in the putamen and globus pallidus (Bamford, Caine, Kido, Cox, & Shoulson, 1995; Bamford, Caine, Kido, Plassche, & Shoulson, 1989; Roth et al., 2005; Zakzanis, 1998), the cortex, and the substantia nigra. The atrophy of the caudate nucleus and putamen is the most striking neuropathologic feature. Atrophy of the frontal lobes is also apparent in 80% of HD brains (Aylward et al., 1998; Vonsattel et al., 1985). Other regions of the brain often show atrophy that varies in severity. Typically, the brains of individuals who have suffered with HD weigh 10% to 20% less than the brains of age-matched controls (Lange, Thorner, Hofp, & Schroder, 1976; MacMillan & Quarrell, 1996). To understand the movement disorder of HD, it is necessary to appreciate that components of the basal nuclei are part of reverberating neuronal networks that control body movements. These networks rely on specific neurotransmitters and a particular balance between them. In HD, an imbalance occurs within the caudate nucleus in which dopamine becomes excessive in relation to acetylcholine and gamma-aminobutyric acid (GABA). When the balance between these three neurotransmitters is restored, choreiform movements are reduced (Stipe, White, & Van Arsdale, 1979).

Definitions

Hypokinesia: Abnormally decreased motor function.
Dystonia: Impairment of voluntary movement.

Symptomatology

Affect and Motor Symptoms

Most individuals who carry the HD gene develop and function normally into early adulthood before experiencing a change in affect, motor, or cognitive function that signals disease onset. Changes in affect often present before motor symptoms (Roos, 2010). For example, sadness, irritability, depression, and occasionally an episode of verbal or physical abuse is the first evidence of the disease (Kirkwood, Su, Conneally, & Foroud, 2001).

Early motor symptoms include facial grimaces, abnormal eye movements, impaired finger tapping, excessive movements of the fingers or hands, and sometimes a mild dysarthria (Penney et al., 1990). These abnormalities usually precede the more obvious signs of extrapyramidal dysfunction by several years (Penney et al., 1990). When clear extrapyramidal signs appear, such as chorea (Figure 9–1), hypokinesia, rigidity, or dystonia, the diagnosis of HD becomes definitive. Other less known but debilitating symptoms of Huntington's include autonomic nervous system dysfunction, sleep and circadian rhythm disturbances, and unintended weight loss (Roos, 2010).

Effects of HD on Speech

Over the disease course, the jerky, involuntary, dancelike movements of chorea increase in severity and eventually become disabling. Speech is affected and hyperkinetic dysarthria develops. In late-stage disease, natural speech may be unintelligible (Hamilton et al., 2012). The chorea affects all the muscle groups that support respiration, phonation, and articulation, and unpredictable involuntary movements disrupt breath support, voicing, and articulation. As a result, speech rate varies unpredictably as does loudness, prosody, and the accuracy of vowel and consonant production

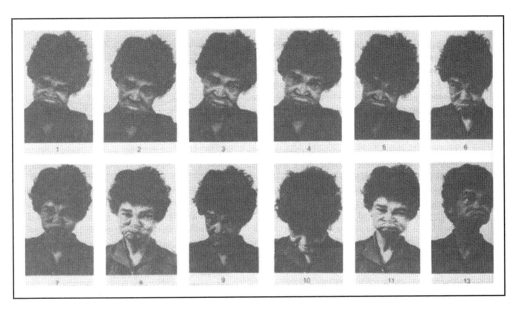

Figure 9–1. Sequential photographs taken at 1-s intervals show choreiform movements of the face and neck. (From Hayden, 1981.)

(Skodda, Schlegel, Hoffman, & Saft, 2014). Voice quality can be distorted and harsh.

Hartelius, Carlstedt, Ytterberg, Malin, and Laakso (2003) characterized the dysarthric speech signs of 19 individuals with mild and moderate HD. The most severe deviations were observed in phonation, oral motor performance, and prosody; all resulted from the excessive and involuntary choreatic movements. Other signs included shortened phrase length and prolongation of interword and intersyllable intervals, increased pitch, harsh phonation, and consonant distortions. Severity of dysarthria was highly correlated with disease severity.

Effects on Cognition

The neurodegenerative effects of HD occur insidiously over years until victims develop multiple cognitive deficits and dementia (Paulsen et al., 2011). Cognitive impairments are evident many years prior to a motor diagnosis. Duff, Beglinger, Theriault, Allison, and Paulsen

(2011) used standardized measures to evaluate cognitive function in a large sample of individuals with prodromal HD and reported that the performance of 38% of the sample met the criteria for mild cognitive impairment. In the early stage, subtle changes occur in memory (Brouwers, Cox, Martin, Chase, & Fedio, 1984; Butters, Salmon, & Heindel, 1994; Butters, Sax, Montgomery, & Tarlow, 1978; Josiassen, Curry, & Mancall, 1983; Kirkwood et al., 2001; Lemiere, Decruyenaere, Evers-Kiebooms, Vandenbussche, & Dom, 2004; Shirbin et al., 2013), attention (Beatty, Salmon, Butters, Heindel, & Granholm, 1988; Butters, Wolfe, Granholm, & Martone, 1986; Montoya, Pelletier, et al., 2006), and executive function (Brandt, Bylsma, Aylward, Rothlind, & Gow, 1995; Hart, Middelkoop, Jurgens Witjes-Ané, Roos, 2011; Watkins et al., 2000). Several investigators report that persons with HD are impaired in their ability to estimate time (Hinton et al., 2007; Rowe et al., 2010; Zimbelman et al., 2007). Moreover, the ability to self-pace timing has been shown to track changes in HD individuals in the early phase of the disease.

Visual and Verbal Memory and Attention

Visual and verbal memory and psychomotor speed are affected because of disruption of the circuitry connecting the basal ganglia to the frontal lobe (Kirkwood et al., 2001). Focusing and maintaining attention, searching long-term memory, and self-monitoring diminish. Recall of factual and episodic information becomes harder. Recognition is better than recall, though evidence exists that it is impaired (Montoya, Pelletier, et al., 2006). Because factual and episodic information are generally intact for much of the disease course, HD patients benefit from cueing (Hart et al., 2011; Montoya, Pelletier, et al., 2006).

Montoya, Pelletier, et al. (2006) conducted a meta-analysis of the data from 544 symptomatic HD patients, 224 presymptomatic gene carriers, and 963 control subjects to evaluate the magnitude of deficits in memory recall and recognition. Both mild and moderately demented HD patients showed significant deficits in recall and recognition, although recall was more impaired in the mild group. Lemiere et al. (2004) also found that memory tasks differentiated *asymptomatic carriers* of the mutated HD gene from those with clinically verified HD.

Motor Procedural Memory

Motor memory and motor learning are diminished because of subcortical pathology in the basal ganglia. HD patients have trouble learning new motor skills, especially those requiring a sequence of movements (Gabrieli, Stebbins, Singh, Willingham, & Goetz, 1997; Heindel, Butters, & Salmon, 1988). Willingham, Koroshetz, and Peterson (1996) observed that HD subjects had no difficulty learning to track a moving target with a joystick on a computer screen, provided the target moved randomly; however, when the target moved in a repeated sequence, they were impaired. Mickes and colleagues (2013) documented motor slowing prior to diagnosis of HD. Previously acquired motor skills deteriorate and actions that could be done premorbidly without thinking take conscious attention to complete.

Executive Function

The early deficits in executive function (Ho et al., 2003; Lawrence et al., 1996) result from striatal and extrastriatal atrophy (Peinemann et al., 2005). They are apparent on numerous executive function tests such as the Stroop, Trail Making, Symbol Digit Modalities Test, and WAIS-R arithmetic (Hart et al., 2011; Lemiere et al., 2004; Smith, 1982). The Symbol Digit Modalities Test (a simple 90-s task in which examinees use a reference key to pair specific numbers with given geometric figures) was the best of those in a large neuropsychological battery used by Lemiere and colleagues (2004) for detecting the onset of cognitive problems and tracking disease progression.

Language

Individuals with early HD do not typically exhibit impairment of everyday language (Brandt, 1991; Paulsen, 2011); however, if given linguistically based neuropsychological tests, deficits can be demonstrated that are proportional to task difficulty. In fact, the literature on HD and language contains reports of impaired confrontation naming, repetition, decreased conversational initiative, syntactic deficits in spontaneous speech, and decreased language output in written narratives in individuals with early HD (Bayles & Tomoeda, 1983; Caine, Bamford, Schiffer, Shoulson, & Levy, 1986; Podoll, Caspary, Lange, & Noth, 1988; Wallesch & Fehrenbach, 1988). Paulsen (2011) characterized the communicative function of HD individuals as difficulty speaking clearly, starting conversation, and organizing and understanding what's coming in and going out. According to Hartelius, Jonsson, Rickeberg, and Laakso (2010), HD patients report that the primary barriers to conversing are mustering the increased effort and concentration needed.

Bayles and Kaszniak (1987) observed impairment of object recognition and semantic processing in 11 individuals with HD, and mild or moderate dementia as can be seen from the following language sample of an HD subject with moderate dementia.

Sample of Language from Individual with HD and Moderately Severe Dementia

The examiner asked the HD patient to describe a button and define two words.

Examiner: What is this? [button]
Subject: Oh, that's a needle. But . . . button hole scissors. And they go ahead they put buttons or they put, ss, that's how they put buttons your coat with it, I guess.
Examiner: What does it mean to describe?
Subject: Well like you're a buttoning your blouse would be an example.
Examiner: What does it mean to guarantee?
Subject: Guarantee you're gonna get it. I guess we're gonna have company. Something. That would be a guarantee, wouldn't it?

Common Communication Difficulties

The most common communication difficulties are (Hamilton et al., 2012; Liou, 2010):

- Initiating conversation
- Word finding
- Speaking clearly
- Organizing what is to be said
- Understanding what is said
- Difficulty making inferences
- Perseveration
- Maintaining topic
- Decrease in length of utterances

With disease progression, expression and comprehension are increasingly affected (Chenery, Copland, & Murdoch, 2002; Saldert, Fors, Stroberg, Hartelius, 2010; Saldert & Hartelius, 2011); ultimately, advanced-stage individuals may no longer initiate conversation (Saldert & Hartelius, 2011; Yorkston, Miller, & Klasner, 2004). However, language comprehension is generally better than language production (Paulsen, 2011).

Striatal Degeneration and Language

Numerous investigators have considered the question of whether the striatum supports language-specific processes such as syntax (Sambin et al., 2012). Although it is beyond the scope of this book to review the extensive literature on this subject, it is worth pointing out that many researchers have observed deficits in the production and comprehension of words and sentences in individuals with caudate pathology or damage (Cambier, Elghozi, & Strube, 1979; Damasio, Damasio, Rizzo, Varney, & Gersh, 1982; Hochstadt, 2009; Kumral, Evyapan, & Balkir, 1999; Lieberman et al., 1992; Teichmann et al., 2005; Ullman et al., 1997). Gronholm, Roll, Horne, Sundgren, and Lindgren (2016) reported that the left caudate nucleus and adjacent corona radiata were the brain areas most frequently affected in 34 individuals with first-ever ischemic strokes who had language and speech problems. Less than one-fourth of the patients had damage in Broca's and Wernicke's areas. Their findings are evidence that the basal ganglia have a critical role in control over language and speech processing.

Teichmann and colleagues (2005) tested the hypothesis that the left caudate is involved in the application of grammatical rules as theorized by Ullman (2001). In the Teichmann et al. study, 30 HD patients and 20 control subjects were administered a verb-conjugation task, a sentence-picture matching task, and arithmetic tasks. HD patients were found to be impaired in rule application in both the linguistic and nonlinguistic domains (morphology, syntax, and subtraction).

Sambin and colleagues (2012) concluded that the striatum does have a genuine role in complex syntactic processing because HD patients in their study had difficulty processing certain syntactic rules. Fifteen individuals with

HD-related striatal damage and 15 matched healthy controls participated. Whereas the HD patients could correctly establish noun-pronoun coreference, they failed to block it in certain rule-governed conditions. The fact that they performed well with both center-embedded and right-branching relatives indicated that their sentence comprehension difficulties did not arise from the memory load.

Also interested in the role of the caudate in language processing, Nemeth and colleagues (2012) examined language production in Hungarian patients with presymptomatic HD and found them to be impaired in the production of morphologically complex nouns. They concluded that the caudate is involved in rule-processing, particularly for nonautomatic behavior.

Dysphagia Is Also a Concern

In addition to the cognitive, speech, and communication deficits that victims of HD endure, they also have swallowing problems (de Tommaso et al., 2015). Aspiration pneumonia is the number one cause of death. Although the focus of this book is on the cognitive-communication disorders, clinicians should be alert to the possibility of dysphagia. The American Speech-Language Hearing Association provides a list of swallowing problems and their signs. Clinicians who observe one or more of these signs should refer HD patients for a swallowing evaluation.

Swallowing problems associated with HD include the following:

- Impulsivity while eating
- Difficulty controlling rate of food or liquid intake
- Difficulty chewing food
- Delayed swallow reflex (does not kick in even when food moves to the back of the throat)
- Holding food/liquid in the mouth
- Difficulty initiating a swallow
- Inability to swallow

- Incomplete swallows in which food or liquid is left in the mouth and/or throat
- Lack of coordination between swallowing process and breathing or speaking
- Need to swallow repeatedly for each bite/sip
- Chorea of the oral or pharyngeal muscles (tongue, lips, throat, esophagus)
- Drooling and/or spillage of food or liquid from the mouth.

The following signs at mealtime may indicate swallowing problems:

- Coughing
- Choking
- Gurgly voice quality
- Wet sounding breathing
- Spillage of food and liquid from the mouth
- Frequent throat clearing
- Progressively slower rate of food intake
- Regurgitation of food after it has been swallowed
- Food or liquid left in the mouth after swallowing
- Difficulty manipulating food or liquid in the mouth
- Frequent congestion
- Frequent fever
- Consistent or significant weight loss

Cognition and Communication

Individuals with HD have cognitive-communication impairments that are proportional to the severity of their nonlinguistic cognitive deficits and neuropathology. Results of structural neuroimaging studies support a relation between degree of striatal and cortical atrophy and performance on tests of attention, working memory, and executive functions. Striatal hypoperfusion and decreased glucose uptake correlate with degree of executive dysfunction. Degree of cortical hypometabolism correlates with impairment on recognition memory, language, and perceptual tests (see Montoya, Price, Menear, & Lepage, 2006 for a review of brain imaging and cognitive dysfunction in HD); thus, early in the disease when neuropathology is less extensive and cognitive deficits are mild, everyday language functioning is good, but as pathology increases and deficits in executive function, attention, memory, and perceptual processing worsen, expressive and receptive language are markedly affected.

The cognitive-communication disorders of individuals with HD combined with the dysarthria that commonly develops and the not uncommon occurrence of dysphagia, provide the speech-language pathologist with a prominent role in patient management. Not only should assessment include a thorough evaluation of speech and language strengths and weaknesses, but it should also include evaluation of the impact of the disease on everyday social communicative interactions. Augmentative communication is an option for individuals with HD that may improve their ability to communicate and participate socially (Hamilton et al., 2012).

Summary of Important Points

- HD is an inherited degenerative disease of the nervous system characterized by dementia and uncontrollable dancelike movements known as chorea.
- The mutant gene that causes HD is called huntingtin and is autosomal dominant.
- Most individuals with HD develop and function normally until mid-life. The mean age at onset is 40 years.
- The gene that causes HD was identified in 1983 and genetic tests were developed that enable at-risk individuals to determine if they are carriers.
- The signs and symptoms of HD result from brain atrophy and neurochemical deficiencies. Atrophy is most pronounced in the head of the caudate nucleus but exists to a lesser extent in the putamen and globus pallidus. In HD, an imbalance occurs between the neurochemicals needed to control movement.
- As HD progresses, cognitive deficits become increasingly pronounced and dementia always develops.

- Executive functions are those most vulnerable to the effects of HD.
- Episodic memory deficits are apparent in HD but not to the extent that they exist in individuals with AD.
- HD patients have trouble learning new motor skills involving a repeated sequence of movements.
- Many reports exist of diminished performance of individuals with HD on linguistic tasks such as naming, sentence comprehension, and discourse production; however, at issue is whether diminished performance reflects nonlinguistic cognitive deficits or deficits in linguistic knowledge.
- It may be that individuals with HD have a "signature language" impairment of disrupted lexical-semantic processing and the application of grammatical rules that are the consequences of striatal pathology.
- Overall, communicative functioning reflects the degree of dementia severity.
- Swallowing problems are common in individuals with HD and clinicians should be alert to the possibility of dysphagia.

References

Aylward, E., Anderson, N., Bylsma, F., Wagster, M., Barta, P., Sherr, M., . . . Ross, C. (1998) Frontal lobe volume in patients with Huntington's disease. *Neurology, 50,* 252–258.

Bamford, K. A., Caine, E. D., Kido, D. K., Cox, C., & Shoulson, I. (1995). A prospective evaluation of cognitive decline in early Huntington's disease: Functional and radiographic correlates. *Neurology, 45,* 1867–1873.

Bamford, K. A., Caine, E. D., Kido, D. K., Plassche, W. M., & Shoulson, I. (1989). Clinical-pathologic correlation in Huntington's disease: A neuropsychological and computer tomography study. *Neurology, 39,* 796–801.

Barema, J. (2005). *The test: Living in the shadow of Huntington's disease.* New York, NY: Franklin Square Press.

Bayles, K. A., & Kaszniak, A. W. (1987). *Communication and cognition in normal aging and dementia.* Austin, TX: Pro-Ed.

Bayles, K. A., & Tomoeda, C. K. (1983). Confrontation naming impairment in dementia. *Brain and Language, 19,* 98–114.

Beatty, W. W., Salmon, D. P., Butters, N., Heindel, W. C., & Granholm, E. L. (1988). Retrograde amnesia in patients with Alzheimer's disease or Huntington's disease. *Neurobiology of Aging, 9,* 181–186.

Brandt, J. (1991). Cognitive impairments in Huntington's disease: Insights into the neuropsychology of the striatum. In F. Boller & J. Grafman (Eds.), *Handbook of neuropsychology* (Vol. 5, pp. 241–264). New York, NY: Elsevier Science.

Brandt, J., Bylsma, F. W., Aylward, E. H., Rothlind, J., & Gow, C. A. (1995). Impaired source memory in Huntington's disease gene carriers: A comparison with gene negative at-risk subjects. *Acta Psychiatrica Scandinavica, 105*, 224–230.

Brouwers, P., Cox, C., Martin, A., Chase, T., & Fedio, P. (1984). Differential perceptual-spatial impairment in Huntington's and Alzheimer's dementias. *Archives of Neurology, 41*, 1073–1076.

Butters, N., Salmon, D., & Heindel, W. C. (1994). Specificity of the memory deficits associated with basal ganglia dysfunction. *Revue Neurologique (Paris), 150*, 580–587.

Butters, N., Sax, D., Montgomery, K., & Tarlow, S. (1978). Comparison of the neuropsycholoical deficits associated with early and advanced Huntington's disease. *Archives of Neurology, 35*, 585–589.

Butters, N., Wolfe, J., Granholm, E., & Martone, M. (1986). An assessment of verbal recall, recognition and fluency abilities in patients with Huntington's disease. *Cortex, 22*, 11–32.

Caine, E. D., Bamford, K. A., Schiffer, R. B., Shoulson, I., & Levy, S. (1986). A controlled neuropsychological comparison of Huntington's disease and multiple sclerosis. *Archives of Neurology, 43*, 249–254.

Cambier, J., Elghozi, D., & Strube, E. (1979). Hemorrhage of the head of the left caudate nucleus: Disorganization of speech and graphic expression, and disturbances in gestures [Author's translation]. *Revue Neurologique (Paris), 135*, 763–774.

Cattaneo E., Rigamonti, D., & Zuccato, D. (2002). Huntington's disease. *Scientific American, 287*, 93–97.

Chenery, H. J., Copland, D. A., & Murdoch, B. E. (2002). Complex language functions and subcortical mechanisms: Evidence from Huntington's disease and patients with non-thalamic subcortical lesions. *International Journal of Language and Communication Disorders, 37*, 459–474.

Chua P., & Chiu, E. (2005). Huntington's disease. In A. Burns, J. O'Brien, & D. Ames (Eds.), *Dementia* (3rd ed., pp. 754–762). London, UK: Hodder Arnold.

Damasio, A. R., Damasio, H., Rizzo, M., Varney, N., & Gersh, F. (1982). Aphasia with nonhemorrhagic lesions in the basal ganglia and internal capsule. *Archives of Neurology, 39*, 15–24.

de Tommaso, M., Nuzzi, A., Dellomonaco, A. R., Sciruicchio, V., Serpino, C., Cormio, C., . . . Megna, M. (2015). Dysphagia in Huntington's disease: Correlation with clinical features. *European Neurology, 74*, 49–53.

Duff, K., Beglinger, L. J., Theriault, D., Allison, J., & Paulsen, J. S. (2011). Cognitive deficits in Huntington's disease on the Repeatable Battery for the Assessment of Neuropsychological Status. *Journal of Clinical and Experimental Neuropsychology, 32*, 231–238.

Freckelton, I. (2012). Expert evidence by mental health professionals: The communication challenge posed by evidence about autism spectrum disorder, brain injuries, and Huntington's disease. *International Journal of Law and Psychiatry, 35*, 372–379.

Gabrieli, J. D. E., Stebbins, G. T., Singh, J., Willingham, D. B., & Goetz, C. G. (1997). Intact mirror-tracing and impaired rotary-pursuit skill learning in patients with Huntington's disease: Evidence for dissociable memory systems in skill learning. *Neuropsychology, 11*, 272–281.

Gronholm, E. O., Roll, M. C., Horne, M. A., Sundgren, P. C., & Lindgren, A. G. (2016). Predominance of caudate nucleus lesions in acute ischaemic stroke patients with impairment in language and speech. *European Journal of Neurology, 23*, 148–153.

Gusella J., Wexler, N. S., Conneally, P. M., Naylor, S. L., Anderson, M. A., Tanzi, R. E., . . . Martin, J. B. (1983). A polymorphic DNA marker genetically linked to Huntington's disease. *Nature, 306*, 234–238.

Hamilton, A., Ferm, U., Heemskerk, A. W., Twiston-Davies, R., Matheson, K. Y., Simpson, S. A., & Rae, D. (2012). Management of speech, language, and communication difficulties in Huntington's disease. *Neurodegenerative Disease Management, 2*, 67–77.

Harper, P. S. (1996). *Huntington's disease. Major problems in neurology* (2nd ed.). London, UK: W. B. Saunders.

Hart, E., Middelkoop, H., Jurgens, C. K., Witjes-Ané, M. N., & Roos, R. A. (2011). Seven-year clinical follow-up of premanifest carriers of Huntington's disease. *PLoS Currents, 3*, RRn1288.

Hartelius, L., Carlstedt, A., Ytterberg, M., Malin, L., & Laakso, K. (2003). Speech disorders in mild and moderate Huntington disease: Results of dysarthria assessments of 19 individuals. *Journal of Medical Speech-Language Pathology, 11*, 1–14.

Hartelius, L., Jonsson, M., Rickeberg, A., & Laakso, K. (2010). Communication and Huntington's disease: Qualitative interviews and focus groups with persons with Huntington's disease, family members, and carers. *International Journal of Language and Communication Disorders, 45*, 381–393.

Hayden, M. R. (1981). *Huntington's chorea*. New York, NY: Springer-Verlag.

Heindel, W. C., Butters, N., & Salmon, D. P. (1988). Impaired learning of a motor skill in patients with Huntington's disease. *Behavioural Neuroscience, 102*, 141–147.

Hinton, S. C., Paulsen, J. S., Hoffman, R. G., Reynolds, N. C., Zimbelman, J. L., & Rao, S. M. (2007). Motor timing variability increases in preclinical Huntington's disease patients as estimated onset of motor symptoms approaches. *Journal of International Neuropsychological Society, 13*, 539–543.

Ho, A. K., Sahakian, B. J., Brown, R. G., Barker, R. A., Hodges, J. R., Ané, M.N., . . . NEST-HD Consortium. (2003). Profile of cognitive progression in early Huntington's disease. *Neurology, 61,* 1702–1706.

Hochstadt, J. (2009). Set-shifting and the on-line processing of relative clauses in Parkinson's disease: Results from a novel eye-tracking method. *Cortex, 45,* 991–1011.

Josiassen, R. C., Curry, L. M., & Mancall, E. L. (1983). Development of neuropsychological deficits in Huntington's disease. *Archives of Neurology, 40,* 791–796.

Kirkwood, S. C., Su, J. L., Conneally, P., & Foroud, T. (2001). Progression of symptoms in the early and middle stages of Huntington disease. *Archives of Neurology, 58,* 273–278.

Kordasiewicz, H., Stanek, L., Wancewicz, E., Mazur, C., MCAlonis, M., Pytel, K., . . . Cleveland, D. (2012). Sustained therapeutic reversal of Huntington's disease by transient repression of Huntington synthesis. *Neuron, 74,* 1031–1044.

Kremer, B. (2003). Clinical neurology of Huntington's disease. In G. Bates, P. Harper, & L. Jones (Eds.), *Huntington's disease* (3rd ed., pp. 28–61). Oxford, UK: Oxford University Press.

Kumral, E., Evyapan, D., & Balkir, K. (1999). Acute caudate vascular lesions. *Stroke, 30,* 100–108.

Lange, H., Thorner, G., Hofp, A., & Schroder, K. F. (1976). Morphometric studies of the neuropathological changes in choreatic diseases. *Journal of Neurological Science, 28,* 401–425.

Lawrence, A. D., Sahakian, B. J., Hodges, J. R., Rosser, A. E., Lange, K. W., & Robbins, T. W. (1996). Executive and mnemonic functions in early Huntington's disease. *Brain, 119,* 1633–1645.

Lemiere, J., Decruyenaere, M., Evers-Kiebooms, G., Vandenbussche, E., & Dom R. (2004). Cognitive changes in patients with Huntington's disease (HD) and asymptomatic carriers of the HD mutation: A longitudinal follow-up study. *Journal of Neurology, 251,* 935–942.

Lieberman, P., Kako, E., Friedman, J., Tajchman, G., Feldman, L. S., & Jimenez, E. B. (1992). Speech production, syntax comprehension, and cognitive deficits in Parkinson's disease. *Brain and Language, 43,* 169–189.

Liou, S. (2010). The cognitive symptoms of Huntington's disease. *HOPES: Huntington Outreach Project Education, at Stanford.* Retrieved from http://web.stanford.edu/group/hopes/cgi-bin/hopes_test/the-cognitive-symptoms-of-huntingtons-disease/

MacMillan, J., & Quarrell, O. (1996). The neurobiology of Huntington's disease. In P. S. Harper (Ed.), *Huntington's disease* (2nd ed., pp. 317– 357). London, UK: W. B. Saunders.

Mickes, L., Wixted, J. T., Peavy, G. M., Jacobson, M. W., Goldstein, J. L., & Corey-Bloom, J. (2013). Difficulty modifying a sustained motor response in prodromal Huntington's disease. *Journal of Clinical and Experimental Neuropsychology, 35,* 35–40.

Montoya, A., Pelletier, M., Menear, M., Duplessis, E., Richer, F., & Lepage, M. (2006). Episodic memory impairment in Huntington's disease: A meta-analysis. *Neuropsychologia, 44,* 1984–1994.

Montoya, A. L., Price, B. H., Menear, M., & Lepage, M. (2006). Brain imaging and cognitive dysfunctions in Huntington's disease. *Journal of Psychiatry and Neuroscience, 31,* 21–29.

Nemeth, D., Dye, C. D., Sefcsik, T., Janacsek, K., Turi, Z., Londe, Z., . . . Ullman, M. T. (2012). Language deficits in pre-symptomatic Huntington's disease: Evidence from Hungarian. *Brain and Language, 121,* 248–253.

Nopoulos, P. C. (2016). Huntington disease: A single-gene degenerative disorders of the striatum. *Dialogues in Clinical Neuroscience, 18,* 91–98.

Paulsen, J. (2011). Cognitive impairment in Huntington's disease: Diagnosis and treatment. *Current Neurology and Neuroscience Reports, 11,* 474–483.

Peinemann, A., Schuller, S., Pohl, C., Jahn, T., Weindl, A., & Kassubek, J. (2005). Executive dysfunction in early stages of Huntington's disease is associated with striatal and insular atrophy: A neuropsychological and voxelbased morphometric study. *Journal of the Neurological Sciences, 239,* 11–19.

Penney, J. B., Jr., Young, A. D., Shoulson, I., Starosta-Rubenstein, S., Snodgrass, S. R., Sanchez-Ramos, J., . . . Wexler, N. S. (1990). Huntington's disease in Venezuela: 7 years of follow-up on symptomatic and asymptomatic individuals. *Movement Disorders, 5,* 93–99.

Podoll, K., Caspary, P., Lange, H. S., & Noth, J. (1988). Language functions in Huntington's disease. *Brain, 111,* 1475–1503.

Roos, R. (2010). Huntington's disease: A clinical review. *Orphanet Journal of Rare Diseases, 5,* 40.

Roth, J., Klempir, J., Jech, R., Zidovska, J., Uhrova, T., Doubek, P., & Ruzicka, E. (2005). Caudate nucleus atrophy in Huntington's disease and its relationship with clinical and genetic parameters. *Functional Neurology, 20,* 127–130.

Rowe, K. C., Paulsen, J. S., Langbehn, D. R., Wang, C., O'Rourke, J. J., Stout, J. C., . . . Moser, D. J. (2010). Self-paced timing detects and tracks change in prodromal Huntington disease. *Neuropsychology, 24,* 435–442.

Saldert, C., Fors, A., Stroberg, S., & Hartelius, L. (2010). Comprehension of complex discourse in different stages of Huntington's disease. *International Journal of Language and Communication Disorders, 45,* 656–669.

Saldert, C., & Hartelius, L. (2011). Echlalia or functional repetition in conversation—a case study of an individual with Huntington's disease. *Disability and Rehabilitation, 33,* 253–260.

Sambin, S., Teichmann, M., Balaguer, de Diego Balaguer, R., Giavazzi, M., Sportiche, D., . . . Bacoud-Lévi, A.-C. (2012). The role of the striatum in sentence processing: Disentangling syntax from working memory in Huntington's disease. *Neuropsychologia, 50,* 2625–2635.

Shirbin, A., Chua, P., Churchyard, A., Hannan, A., Lowndes, G., & Stout, J. (2013). The relationship between cortisol and verbal memory in the early stages of Huntington's disease. *Journal of Neurology, 260,* 891–902.

Skodda, S., Schlegel, U., Hoffman, R., & Saft, C. (2014). Impaired motor speech performance in Huntington's disease. *Journal of Neural Transmission, 121,* 399–407.

Smith, A. (1982). *Symbol Digit Modalities Test (SDMT) manual–revised.* Los Angeles, CA: Western Psychological Services.

Stipe, J., White, D., & Van Arsdale, E. (1979). Huntington's disease. *American Journal of Nursing, 79,* 1428–1433.

Teichmann, M., Dupoux, E., Kouider, S., Brugiéres, P., Boissé, M. F., Baudic, S., . . . Bachoud-Lévi, A.C. (2005). The role of the striatum in rule application: the model of Huntington's disease at early stage. *Brain, 128,* 1155–1167.

Ullman, M. T. (2001). The declarative/procedural model of lexicon and grammar. *Journal of Psychololinguistic Research, 30,* 37–69.

Ullman, M. T., Corkin, S., Coppola, M., Hickok, G., Growdon, J. H., Koroshetz, W. J., . . . Pinker, S. (1997). A neural dissociation within language: Evidence that the mental dictionary is part of declarative memory, and that grammatical rules are processed by the procedural system. *Journal of Cognitive Neuroscience, 9,* 266–276.

Vonsattel, J. P. G., Myers, R. H., Stevens, T. J., Ferrante, R. J., Bird, E. D., & Richardson, E. P., Jr. (1985). Neuropathological classification of Huntington's disease. *Journal of Neuropathology and Experimental Neurology, 44,* 559–577.

Wallesch, C. W., & Fehrenbach, R. A. (1988). On the neurolinguistic nature of language abnormalities in Huntington's disease. *Journal of Neurology, Neurosurgery, and Psychiatry, 51,* 367–373.

Watkins, L. H., Rogers, R. D., Lawrence, A. D., Sahakian, B. J., Rosser, A. E., & Robbins, T. W. (2000). Impaired planning but intact decision making in early Huntington's disease: Implications for specific frontostriatal pathology. *Neuropsychologia, 38,* 1112–1125.

Wexler, A. (1995). *Mapping fate: A memoir of family, risk, and genetic research.* Berkeley, CA: University of California Press.

Willingham, D. B., Koroshetz, W. J., & Peterson, E. W. (1996). Motor skills have diverse neural bases: Spared and impaired skill acquisition in Huntington's disease. *Neuropsychology, 10,* 315–321.

Yorkston, K. M., Miller, R. M., & Klasner, E. R. (2004). Huntington's disease. In K. M. Yorkston, R. M. Miller, & E. A. Strand (Eds.), *Management of speech and swallowing in degenerative disease* (pp. 139–154). Austin, TX: Pro-Ed.

Young, A. B., Shoulson, I., Penney, J. B., Starosta-Rubinstein, S., Gomez, F., Travers, H., . . . Wexler, N. S. (1986). Huntington's disease in Venezuela: Neurologic features and functional decline. *Neurology, 36,* 244–249.

Zakzanis, K. K. (1998). The subcortical dementia of Huntington's disease. *Journal of Clinical and Experimental Neuropsychology, 20,* 565–578.

Zimbelman, J. L., Paulsen, J. S., Mikos, A., Reynolds, N. C., Hoffman, R. G., & Rao, S. M. (2007). *Journal of International Neuropsychology Society, 13,* 758–769.

10

Frontotemporal Dementia

Introduction

Frontotemporal dementia (FTD) is a syndrome of cognitive impairment associated with a variety of heterogeneous neurodegenerative disorders and characterized by frontotemporal lobar degeneration (FTLD) (McKhann et al., 2001). Three types are now recognized (National Institute on Aging, 2017): a behavioral type in which abnormal behavior is the presenting symptom; a language type in which the presenting symptom is one of three types of progressive aphasia; and a type in which movement disorders are the presenting symptom. For many years, FTD was thought to be rare, but is now acknowledged as a common form of dementia, accounting for 20% of adults who visit memory-disorder clinics (Grossman, 2002). Of people with early-onset dementia, FTD is the most common cause (Brunnström, Gustafson, Passant, & Englund, 2009).

Mean age at onset varies across FTD subtypes; however, the prevalence of FTD across subtypes is similar, approximately 10.8/100,000 person/years. The age-adjusted prevalence peaks in the 60s at 42.6/100,000. According to Coyle-Gilchrist et al. (2016), the age-adjusted prevalence for persons older than 65 years is double the prevalence for those between 40 and 64 years. The lifetime risk is 1 in 742.

The first paper describing an individual with FTD was written by Arnold Pick in 1892. The individual was a 71-year-old man with a history of progressive mental deterioration and severe aphasia whose postmortem examination revealed atrophy of the left temporal cortex. In subsequent years, Pick described several other patients with similar symptoms who had temporal or frontotemporal atrophy (Pick, 1901, 1904, 1906). In 1911, Alois Alzheimer identified the microscopic brain changes that caused the clinical profile described earlier by Pick. Alzheimer found intraneuronal inclusions (later called Pick bodies), circumscribed atrophy, and ballooned cortical neurons. In 1922, Gans used the name Pick's disease to refer to individuals with the morphologic changes first noted by Pick and later described by Alzheimer, and usage of the term became widespread.

Subsequently, many clinicians reported individuals with dementia and prominent language and personality changes but whose neuropathology *did not match* that described by Pick. Confusion developed over whether to label them as having Pick's disease and the question arose as to whether Pick's disease was a spectrum of disorders. Over the years, various terms were used to refer to these patients, as can be seen in Table 10–1, and the need developed for consensus terminology. The National Institutes of Health responded to the need and an international consortium of clinicians and scientists formulated diagnostic criteria that are still undergoing modest revisions as more is known about the myriad conditions associated with the syndrome (Chare et al., 2014; Rascovsky et al., 2011).

Table 10–1. Terms Used to Refer to Individuals with Frontotemporal Dementia *(FTD)*

Pick complex

Frontal lobe degeneration frontal lobe dementia

Frontal lobe degeneration of the non-Alzheimer type

Frontotemporal lobar degeneration

Dementia lacking distinct histopathologic features

Semantic dementia

Primary progressive aphasia

Progressive nonfluent aphasia

Source: Kertesz (2004).

Diagnosis of Frontotemporal Dementia (FTD)

As previously noted, the primary types of frontotemporal degeneration are *distinguished by the symptoms that present first* (Hall, Shapira, Gallagher & Denny, 2013): progressive behavioral and personality decline; progressive language decline; or progressive motor decline (Figure 10–1). Most individuals presenting with progressive behavioral symptoms have Pick's disease and are now commonly referred to as having the behavioral variant of FTD (bvFTD). Patients presenting with progressive language impairment are said to have primary progressive aphasia (PPA) that takes one of three forms (Gorno-Tempini et al., 2011): a logopenic form (PPA-L), a nonfluent-agrammatic form (PPA-G), and a semantic-variant form (PPA-S). Patients presenting with progressive motor impairment are less common and often have corticobasal syndrome, progressive supranuclear palsy, or motor neuron disease (Rohrer et al., 2011).

The word "presents" is emphasized because a behavioral presentation does not mean that language and communicative function are necessarily spared throughout the disease course, but rather that the *early* symptoms are notable changes in behavior and personality. A language presentation does not mean that cognitive, behavioral, and personality changes will not be part of the syndrome but that the *early* symptoms are notable changes in language. Similarly, a movement disorder presentation does not mean that cognitive, behavioral, personality and language changes will not be part of the syndrome.

Behavioral Presentation

Behavioral Variant Frontotemporal Dementia (bvFTD)

The bvFTD is the result of neurodegeneration of the anterior temporal and/or frontal lobes. Average age of onset is approximately 58 years, yet the literature contains reports of onset as early as the 20s and as late as the 80s (Warren, Rohrer, & Rossor, 2013; Westbury & Bub, 1997; Woodward et al., 2010; Yener & Didem, 2016). It is equally common in men and women. While mean life expectancy for individuals with the behavioral variant is around three years from diagnosis (Yener & Didem, 2016), disease duration can vary from three to 17 years. The median survival for bvFTD is estimated to be 10.5 years (Nunnemann et al., 2011). Principal causes of death are pneumonia, choking, cardiovascular failure, excessive loss of weight, and cancer.

Because of frontal pathology, bvFTD patients exhibit changes in personality, character, social skills (Rascovsky et al., 2011), and comportment (Mendez, Shapira, Woods, Licht, & Saul, 2008). These changes often appear before brain abnormalities can be detected with neuroimaging (Gregory, Serra-Mestres, & Hodges, 1999) and many patients first seek advice from psychiatrists. It is common for symptoms to overlap with those associated with primary psychiatric disorders; for example, schizophrenia, obsessive-compulsive disorder, borderline personality disorder, and bipolar disorder (Pressman & Miller, 2014). Lack of concern about the disease process is common in bvFTD patients as are poor judgment, emotional blunting, compulsive exploration of environmental stimuli, hyperorality, altered die-

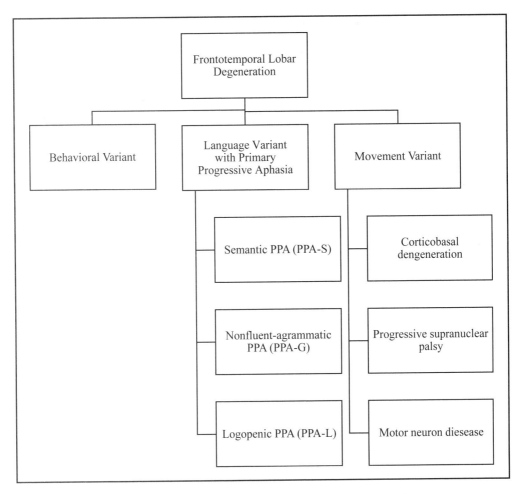

Figure 10–1. Categorization of types of frontotemporal dementia.

tary preferences, changes in sexual behavior, and visual and auditory agnosia (Cummings & Benson, 1983). Repetitive behaviors are also common and occur in approximately 78% of bvFTD (Banks & Weintraub, 2008.) Unsurprisingly, many bvFTD patients are misdiagnosed because of the lack of biomarkers for primary psychiatric disorders and the limited use of bvFTD biomarkers by psychiatrists (Lanata & Miller, 2016).

Cognitive Changes in bvFTD Patients

The cognitive deficits of bvFTD patients reflect the previously noted frontal lobe pathology and include executive dysfunction, deficits in attention, difficulty shifting mental set, and poor performance on frontal/executive tests such as category fluency (Elfgren, Passant, & Risberg, 1993; Hodges et al., 1999; Neary, Snowdon & Mann, 2005; Rosen et al., 2004; Warren, Rohrer, & Rossor, 2013). Although memory disturbance is demonstrable with neuropsychological testing (Elfgren et al., 1993; Gregory et al., 1999; Hodges et al., 1999; Hornberger & Piguet, 2012; Rahman, Sahakian, Hodges, Rogers, & Robbins, 1999), bvFTD patients do not have a true amnestic syndrome and can track day-to-day events until late in the disease (Hodges et al., 1999; McKhann et al., 2001;

Rascovsky et al., 2002; Warren, Rohrer, & Rossor, 2013). Another striking feature of these patients is preservation of visuospatial abilities (Hodges, 2001; Pressman & Miller, 2014).

Language and Communication in bvFTD Patients

Although language disturbance is common in individuals with bvFTD, frank aphasia early in the disease course is not (Blair, Marczinski, Davis-Faroque, & Kertesz, 2007; Hodges et al., 1999; Karbe, Kertesz, & Polk, 1993; Mesulam, 2001; Siri, Benaglio, Frigerio, Binetti, & Cappa, 2001; Snowden & Neary, 1993; Weintraub & Mesulam, 1993). When language symptoms develop, they often take the form of nonfluent aphasia with phonologic and articulatory impairment and agrammatism.

Blair and colleagues (2007) administered the Western Aphasia Battery to 54 individuals with bvFTD and 105 with Alzheimer's disease (AD) two times one year apart and reported that decline in language was faster in those with bvFTD than in individuals with AD. Holland, McBurney, Moossy, and Reinmuth (1985) published a comprehensive account of the deterioration of language in an individual with Pick's disease, a man known as Mr. E, who today would be classified as having bvFTD. They conducted a retrospective study of his communicative functioning from the time of his first speaking difficulty in 1967 until his death 12 years later. Upon postmortem examination, Mr. E was found to have the neuropathologic features typical of Pick's disease and neurofibrillary tangles but no neuritic plaques. Recall that in Alzheimer's disease (AD), both neurofibrillary tangles and neuritic plaques are present. In the earlier stages, Mr. E's speech slowed, became more deliberate, and was interspersed with inordinately long pauses. Thereafter, he began to substitute lower frequency words for words of higher frequency, a tendency that continued throughout the language-dissolution process. In a speech-language evaluation in 1971, Mr. E

was observed to have language formulation and word-finding problems, although his responses were clear and concise. Particularly troublesome was what appeared to be a progressive auditory agnosia. After 1971, he became more and more reluctant to talk, preferring to communicate in writing. From letters written in his last years of life, it is apparent that Mr. E retained memory for names of people and environments. In his final 24 months, marked personality changes occurred and Mr. E became increasingly passive, impulsive, and exhibited poor judgment. Thus, unlike individuals with AD, Mr. E first lost the formal syntactic elements of language but retained access to semantic memory throughout the disease course, a fact clearly revealed in letters he wrote.

Differentiating bvFTD from AD

Before routine use of neuroimaging, individuals with bvFTD were often misdiagnosed as having AD. Today, evidence of focal atrophy in younger persons (individuals in their 50s), who have relatively preserved memory, makes bvFTD easier to diagnose. A comparison of AD and bvFTD was carried out by Mendez, Selwood, Mastri, and Frey (1993) who compared 21 pathologically confirmed cases of Pick's disease/bvFTD to 42 pathologically confirmed cases of AD. The two groups of patients were matched by sex and duration of dementia. All the Pick/bvFTD patients, but none of the AD patients, had onset before age 65 years. The Pick/bvFTD patients had early change in personality (roaming, disinhibition, and hyperorality) and a tendency toward reiterative and other speech disturbances, such as decreased verbal output, poor articulation, verbal stereotypies, and echolalia. These characteristics contrasted with the fluent speech and impaired memory of AD patients. Lobar atrophy of temporal and frontal lobes, or both, was apparent on CT scans in 44% of the Pick/bvFTD patients, but not on the scans of AD patients. Whereas patients with bvFTD have severe frontal and anterior temporal lobe atrophy primarily in the left hemisphere, individuals with AD show atrophy in medial posterior cortex and hippocampus (Harciarek & Jodzio, 2005; Warren, Rohrer, & Rossor, 2013).

Although the various subtypes of FTD are associated with distinct pathology and cognitive-linguistic characteristics, a proportion of individuals in each FTD subtype have been found to also have AD pathology (Mesulam et al., 2008; Padovani et al., 2013). As a result, differentiation of AD and FTD remains challenging (Chare et al., 2014).

Language Presentation of FTD: Primary Progressive Aphasia

A diagnosis of primary progressive aphasia (PPA) is made when individuals present with progressive aphasia in the absence of other cognitive or behavioral problems. Progressive aphasia typically predates other behavioral changes by at least two years (Banks & Weintraub, 2008; Mesulam, 1987, 2001), and although the aphasia may interfere with performance on memory and reasoning tests, PPA patients generally have no difficulty recalling day-to-day events or problem solving.

Variants of PPA

Three variants of PPA were characterized by an international group of PPA investigators with the support of the National Institutes of Health (Gorno-Tempini et al., 2011): logopenic PPA (PPA-L), nonfluent-agrammatic PPA (PPA-G), and semantic PPA (PPA-S). Tables 10–2, 10–3, and 10–4 describe the characteristics of PPA variants.

PPA-L: Primary Progressive Aphasia Logopenic Variant (PPA-L)

From recent research, we now know that most individuals with the PPA-L have AD pathology (Lanata & Miller, 2016; Spinelli et al., 2017); in fact, approximately 77%. They also have left perisylvian atrophy in the temporal–parietal junction region (Abe, Ukita, & Yanagihara, 1997; Hodges, 2001). Many cases also have the histologic features of neuronal loss, gliosis, and spongiosis in layers ii and iii of the cortex (Kirshner, Tanridag, Thurman, & Whetsell, 1987; Turner, Kenyon, Trojanowski, Gonatas, & Grossman, 1996).

The cardinal features of PPA-L are impaired short-term memory and trouble repeating and retrieving names. Spontaneous speech is often slow, interspersed with pauses related to word-retrieval failures and phonologic errors. There is no agrammatism and single-word comprehension is typically good. With disease progression, comprehension worsens, reading and spelling often deteriorate, paraphasias are more evident, and language becomes increasingly empty (Ballard et al., 2014; Mesulam, 2001).

PPA-G: Primary Progressive Aphasia Nonfluent-Agrammatic Variant (PPA-G)

Brain imaging of individuals with PPA-G reveals predominant left hemisphere pathology in the posterior frontoinsular region, the inferior frontal gyrus, insula, premotor and supplementary motor areas, as well as hypoperfusion and hypometabolism (Gorno-Tempini et al., 2011). As the name indicates, nonfluency and agrammatism are the cardinal features of PPA-G patients who exhibit effortful speech and often apraxia (Ballard et al., 2014; Clark, Charuvastra, Miller, Shapira, & Mendez, 2005; Gorno-Tempini et al., 2004; Josephs et al., 2006; Mesulam, 2001; Warren, Rohrer, & Rossor, 2013). The narratives of these patients contain many speech sound errors and prosody is disrupted. Patients have difficulty maintaining grammatical constructs and frequently use the improper tense of verbs. Comprehension is good except for grammatically complicated sentences (Mesulam, 2001). Some affected individuals have impaired repetition, stuttering,

Table 10–2. Diagnostic Criteria for Logopenic Variant of Primary Progressive Aphasia *(PPA-L)*

Clinical Diagnosis of PPA-L

Both of the following core features must be present:

1. Impaired single-word retrieval in spontaneous speech and naming
2. Impaired repetition of sentences and phrases

At least three of the following other features must be present:

1. Speech (phonologic) errors in spontaneous speech and naming
2. Spared single-word comprehension and object knowledge
3. Spared motor speech
4. Absence of frank agrammatism

Imaging-Supported PPA-L Diagnosis

Both criteria must be present:

1. Clinical diagnosis of logopenic-variant PPA
2. Imaging must show at least one of the following results:
   a. Predominant left posterior perisylvian or parietal atrophy on magnetic resonance imaging
   b. Predominant left posterior perisylvian or parietal hypoperfusion or hypometabolism on single photon emission computed tomography or positron emission tomography

PPA-L with Definite Pathology

Clinical diagnosis (criterion 1 below) and either criterion 2 or 3 must be present:

1. Clinical diagnosis of logopenic-variant PPA
2. Histopathologic evidence of a specific neurodegenerative pathology (e.g., Alzheimer's disease, FTLD-tau, FTLD-TDP, other)
3. Presence of a known pathogenic mutation

dyslexia, dysgraphia, and develop mutism late in the course of the disease (Neary et al., 1998). Grossman (2002) speculated that their difficulties constructing and decoding complex grammar result from the existence of an underlying grammatical disorder caused by frontal lobe pathology.

PPA-S: Primary Progressive Aphasia Semantic Dementia Variant (PPA-S)

PPA-S is an uncommon but distinctive syndrome in which affected individuals progressively lose their conceptual (semantic) knowledge. It presents most often in individuals who are between 50 and 65 years of age although some sources report that the most common age range is between 66 to 70 years (Hodges & Patterson, 2007). The median du-

ration of illness approximates eight years and ranges from three to 15 years (Snowden, 2005). Although Arnold Pick reported the syndrome much earlier, it was not until 1975 that the behavioral symptoms of PPA-S were characterized by Warrington as a loss of knowledge for objects and their names. Warrington reported on three individuals with progressive anomia without phonologic or syntactic deficits who had difficulty comprehending verbal and pictorial presentations of the same stimuli. Her patients had preserved episodic memory and intact perceptual and visuospatial abilities. In 1982, Mesulam published a description of six patients who experienced progressive deterioration of spoken language but who did not have frank dementia. This publication generated considerable interest in the dementias, and in the next decade,

Table 10–3. Diagnostic Criteria for the Nonfluent-Agrammatic Variant of Primary Progressive Aphasia *(PPA-G)*

Clinical Diagnosis of PPA-G

At least one of the following core features must be present:

1. Agrammatism in language production
2. Effortful, halting speech with inconsistent speech sound errors and distortions (apraxia of speech)

At least two of three of the following other features must be present:

1. Impaired comprehension of syntactically complex sentences
2. Spared single-word comprehension
3. Spared object knowledge

Imaging-Supported PPA-G Diagnosis

Both of the following criteria must be present:

1. Clinical diagnosis of nonfluent/agrammatic variant PPA
2. Imaging must show one or more of the following results:
   a. Predominant left posterior frontoinsular atrophy on magnetic resonance imaging
   b. Predominant left posterior frontoinsular hypoperfusion of hypometabolism on single photon emission computed tomography or positron emission tomography

PPA-G with Definite Pathology

Clinical diagnosis (criterion 1 below) and either criterion 2 or 3 must be present:

1. Clinical diagnosis of nonfluent/agrammatic variant PPA
2. Histopathologic evidence of a specific neurodegenerative pathology (e.g., FTLD-tau, FTLD-TDP, Alzheimer's disease, other)
3. Presence of a known pathogenic mutation

---

many papers appeared in the literature with descriptions of individuals who presented with similar problems. Snowden, Goulding, and Neary (1989) drew attention to the similarity between patients with a progressive fluent aphasia and Warrington's cases and introduced the term "semantic dementia" to define what Warrington believed to be the underlying deficit.

Neuropathology of PPA-S. Results of magnetic resonance imaging scans indicate that individuals with PPA-S have bilateral but asymmetric pathology of the anterior portion of the temporal lobes with the left more affected (Thompson, Patterson, & Hodges, 2003; Wittenberg et al., 2008); however, it is also common for the pathology to extend to the frontal lobes. Within the temporal lobes, the areas most involved are the middle and inferior

gyri, particularly in the polar and inferolateral regions (Hodges, Patterson, Oxbury, & Funnell, 1992). Medial temporal structures, such as the hippocampus and parahippocampal gyrus, typically are spared, at least in the early stage of the disease (Mummery, Hodges, Patterson, & Price, 1998). There is also a loss of the large pyramidal nerve cells in the temporal and frontal lobes.

Language Characteristics of PPA-S. Individuals with PPA-S typically complain of a loss of memory for words and objects. They are verbally fluent with intact grammar and syntax. Testing reveals that nouns are more problematic than verbs. When presented with an object—for example, a key—they are unable to provide its name or explain the object's use, nor can they provide appropriate associations for the object such as "a key is used

Table 10–4. Diagnostic Criteria for the Semantic Dementia Variant of Primary Progressive Aphasia *(PPA-S)*

Clinical Diagnosis of PPA-S

Both of the following core features must be present:

1. Impaired confrontation naming
2. Impaired single-word comprehension

At least three of the following other diagnostic features must be present:

1. Impaired object knowledge, particularly for low-frequency or low-familiarity items
2. Surface dyslexia or dysgraphia
3. Spared repetition
4. Spared speech production (grammar and motor speech)

Imaging-Supported PPA-S Diagnosis

Both of the following criteria must be present:

1. Clinical diagnosis of semantic-variant PPA
2. Imaging must show one or more of the following results:
   a. Predominant anterior temporal lobe atrophy
   b. Predominant anterior temporal hypoperfusion or hypometabolism on single photon emission computed tomography or positron emission tomography

PPA-S with Definite Pathology

Clinical diagnosis (criterion 1 below) and either criterion 2 or 3 must be present:

1. Clinical diagnosis of semantic-variant PPA
2. Histopathologic evidence of a specific neurodegenerative pathology (e.g., FTLD-tau, FTLD-TDP, Alzheimer's disease, other)
3. Presence of a known pathogenic mutation

---

to open doors" (Hodges & Patterson, 2007). They perform poorly when asked to identify the correct referent for a word when the target and foils are from the same semantic category. Also present are deficits in the comprehension of single words and the ability to provide definitions.

Occasionally, individuals with PPA-S have word-finding problems in conversation that are masked by circumlocution (Mahendra & Hopper, 2017). As might be expected, they struggle to perform category fluency tests in which they must think of as many examples as possible from the same semantic category (Rosser & Hodges, 1994). Often, they have difficulty with reading and spelling irregular words and make regularization errors (Graham, Patterson, & Hodges, 2000; Jeffries, Lambon Ralph, Jones, Bateman, & Patterson, 2004; Macoir & Bernier,

2002). Nonetheless, they typically perform relatively well on measures of grammar and phonology (Hodges & Patterson, 2007; Meteyard & Patterson, 2009). Also preserved are visuoperceptual and spatial abilities, nonverbal reasoning, executive functions, and episodic memory (Hodges et al., 1999; Hodges & Patterson, 2007).

A clue that deterioration of semantic memory is causing the communication problem is the fact that PPA-S patients also perform poorly on nonverbal tests of conceptual knowledge (Howard & Patterson, 1992). Their problem is not one of perception but of assigning meaning to perception. Garrard and Hodges (1999) published examples of the spontaneous speech of an individual with PPA-S and an individual with nonfluent aphasia (Table 10–5).

Table 10–5. Spontaneous Speech Sample of Individual with PPA-S

Individual with Semantic Dementia
[*On being shown a picture of a soldier*]: oh gosh, this seems to be, oh come on, try to remember the name; i know what they are 'cause there's three of these so it's not the two and three, it's the one which, er . . . Some of them will be in Britain because, er, you know with our stuff in Britain, some of them are also outside Britain, some of them are also in Britain as well. What d'you call them again because n.'s son, no not son, his brother, he's one of these as well.

Individual with Primary Progressive Aphasia
Examiner: *Could you tell me something about your holiday in Norway?*
Patient: Er (holding up nine fingers) nides (= nine days) and an aeropload (= aeroplane) have flow and a mawnd bandelez and er the (unintelligible). When we came out a coach and took us (= us) all round hoadle (= hotel) three days and er we a coach or two days and a splip ote and er ote five days it was all right. (Gives "thumbs up" sign)

Source: Garrard & Hodges (1999).

Differentiating the Behavioral Variant of FTD from the Primary Progressive Aphasia Variants

Kirshner (2014) published a review of the variants of FTD that provides clinicians a good sense of the key differences between them. The features that best discriminate the behavioral variants from the PPA variants is aberrant behavior and relative lack of language and motor deficits. In terms of language, individuals with early stage bvFTD are verbally fluent and able to name, repeat, and comprehend language. The features that best discriminate the PPA-S variant are impaired word and object comprehension but fluent speech, normal grammar, an ability to repeat, and normal behavior. Most discriminating of the PPA-G variant are nonfluent and agrammatic speech with normal behavior early in the disease course. Most discriminating of the PPA-L variant are word finding difficulty but preserved word comprehension for simple items, fluent repetition, and normal behavior early.

Amyotrophic Lateral Sclerosis and FTD

Amyotrophic lateral sclerosis (ALS) is a progressive, adult-onset motor neuron disease characterized by loss of motor function and ultimately death. The incidence rate is 1.8 to 2.8 in 100,000 and the average age of symptom onset is 64 years (Al-Chalabi, Calvo, Chio, Colville, Ellis, & Hardiman, 2014). Patients with ALS-FTD have a rapid disease course and typically die from respiratory failure within three years of symptom onset. Amyotrophic refers to muscle atrophy, lateral refers to affected areas of the spinal cord, and sclerosis refers to thickening and hardening of motor neurons (Palmieri, 2005). Affected individuals experience weakness and progressive wasting of muscles that ultimately produces paralysis and the inability to speak and swallow.

Although ALS has long been regarded as a motor disorder that spares cognitive function, it is now apparent that cognitive deficits are present in approximately 40% of ALS patients and a relation exists between ALS and FTD (Rabkin, Goetz, Murphy, Factor-Litvak, & Mitsumoto, 2016; Strong, 2008). Guedji and colleagues (2007) reported in their study that 58% of patients with ALS, who also had FTD, experienced the onset of FTD more than three years *before* they developed ALS symptoms. Then too, as many as 30% of FTD patients exhibit signs of motor system dysfunction (Burrell, Kiernan, Vucic, & Hodges, 2011). Frank dementia has been reported to develop in 3% to 5% of individuals with ALS (Kiernan, 2012).

Results of a study of the neuropsychological profiles of 20 individuals with bvFTD, 20 with ALS, and 20 healthy controls—who were given a neuropsychiatric and neuropsychological assessment that included cognitive screening, working memory, inhibitory control, decision making, and emotion recognition

(Lillo, Savage, Mioshi, Kiernan, & Hodges, 2012)—revealed that ALS subjects had a similar performance profile to bvFTD subjects on tests of working memory, inhibitory control, and behavioral measures. Nine of the ALS patients (45%) had cognitive impairment and five (25%) met criteria for bvFTD. Although ALS-FTD patients are reported to have memory impairment, hippocampal structures are relatively spared and memory impairment is thought to be secondary to executive function deficits (Neary, Snowden, & Mann, 2000). Today, substantial evidence exists of frontal lobe pathology in ALS victims from neuropathologic (Nagy, Kato, & Kushner, 1994), neuroimaging (Abe et al., 1993; Abrahams, Goldstein, Al-Chalabi, Pickering, & Passingham, 1997; Frank, Haas, Heinze, Stark, & Münte, 1997), and electrophysiologic studies (Münte, Tröger, Nusser, Wieringa, Johannes, et al., 1998; Münte, Tröger, Nusser, Wieringa, Matzke, et al., 1998).

Effects of ALS-FTD on Language

The most frequently reported language change in individuals with ALS-FTD is progressive reduction in verbal output progressing to mutism (van Bogaert, 1925; Ziegler, 1930). Other reported changes include difficulty with the use and understanding of grammar, sentence comprehension (Saxon et al., 2017; Taylor et al., 2013; Tsermentseli et al., 2016), syntactic comprehension deficits (Kamminga et al., 2016), perseveration, echolalia, and use of stereotypic expressions (Constantinidis, 1987; Meyer, 1929; Zago, Poletti, Morelli, Doretti, Silani, 2011). Several reports exist of aphasia (Caselli et al., 1993; Mitsuyama, 1984; Tsuchiya et al., 2000) that can present early. Caselli et al. described seven patients in whom progressive nonfluent aphasia was the first symptom. Five ALS patients reported by Doran, Xuereb, and Hodges (1995) had a similar clinical profile. Bak and Hodges (2001) documented language dysfunction in the seven ALS-FTD cases in the Cambridge series. In every case, language dysfunction preceded motor symptoms and both

production and comprehension were compromised. Several of the patients in the Cambridge series used nonverbal means of communicating, indicating that reduction in verbal output was not the result of apathy. Other interesting observations made by Bak and Hodges were that verbs were affected more than nouns in both language production and comprehension. This greater vulnerability of verbs has also been noted in individuals with nonfluent-agrammatic PPA (Cappa et al., 1998; Hillis, Tiffiash, & Caramazza, 2002) and those with progressive supranuclear palsy (Daniele, Giustolisi, Silveri, Colosimo, & Gainotti, 1994). The finding of selective vulnerability of action words in ALS-FTD patients, who have severe motor dysfunction, is intriguing given the finding of a relation between verb processing and motor function in healthy adults (Pülvermuller, Härle, & Hummel, 2000; Pülvermuller, Lutzenberger, & Preiss, 1999).

More recently Ichikawa and Kawamura (2010) reported that language impairment including progressive nonfluent aphasia and PPA-S are linked to bulbar-onset ALS. They suggest that the language problems in ALS victims may have gone unrecognized because the pseudobulbar palsy that produces dysarthria makes language evaluations challenging. Ichikawa and Kawamura report observing frequent omissions and paragraphias of kana letters and syntactic errors in writing.

Summary of Important Points

- Frontotemporal dementia is syndrome of cognitive impairment associated with a variety of heterogeneous neurodegenerative disorders and characterized by frontotemporal lobar degeneration.
- Three types have been distinguished: behavioral presentation, language presentation, and movement disorder presentation
- The variants are distinguished by their presenting symptoms. The behavioral variant presents with aberrant behavior, the language variant present with language deficits, and

the movement type presents with movement disorders.

- The behavioral variant, referred to as Pick's disease by some clinicians, is a rare disorder resulting primarily from lobar atrophy of the frontal and temporal lobes.
- Pick's disease typically manifests when individuals are in their 50s and lasts from three to 17 years.
- The cognitive and personality changes of individuals with bvFTD include disinhibition, apathy, decreased sympathy, perseverative and stereotypic behaviors, executive dysfunction, hyperorality, and sparing of visuospatial function.
- Individuals with the behavioral variant are often misdiagnosed because many symptoms of the variant are also associated with primary psychiatric disorders.
- The communication disorder associated with bvFTD is characterized by decreased verbal output, nonfluency, poor articulation, verbal stereotypies, and echolalia.
- Memory is better preserved in individuals with bvFTD than those with Alzheimer's disease.
- The diagnosis of primary progressive aphasia (PPA) is made when individuals present with progressive aphasia without other cognitive or behavioral problems (that, nonetheless, typically occur later).
- Three variants of primary progressive aphasia syndromes have been distinguished: nonfluent-agrammatic, logopenic, and semantic.
- The primary features of individuals with progressive nonfluent-agrammatic PPA are agrammatism and effortful, halting speech with speech sound errors and word finding difficulty.
- The primary features of individuals with logopenic PPA are impaired word finding and naming, difficulty with word and sentence repetition, and phonologic errors.
- The primary features of the semantic variant of PPA (a.k.a., semantic dementia) are impaired word comprehension and gradual loss of conceptual knowledge, surface dyslexia, object agnosia, prosopagnosia, and stereotyped behaviors.

- Movement disorder presentation is generally associated with corticobasal degeneration or progressive supranuclear palsy.
- Amyotrophic lateral sclerosis (ALS) is a progressive, adult-onset motor neuron disease that is characterized by loss of motor function and untimely death. Historically, ALS was thought to spare cognitive functions; however, research has shown that cognitive deficits are present in approximately 40% of patients and FTD dementia in 3% to 5% of cases.
- Several reports exist of aphasia presenting early before motor symptoms in individuals with ALS, with comprehension and production of language both affected.
- The most common change in language function in ALS is progressive reduction in verbal output often progressing to mutism. Other reported language changes include difficulty using and understanding grammar, perseveration, echolalia, and used of stereotypic expressions. Verbs appear to be affected more than nouns.

References

Abe, K., Fujimura, H., Toyooka, K., Hazama, T., Hirono, N., Yorifuji, S., & Yanagihara, T. (1993). Single-photon emission computed tomographic investigation of patients with motor neuron disease. *Neurology, 43*, 1569–1573.

Abe, K., Ukita, H., & Yanagihara, T. (1997). Imaging in primary progressive aphasia. *Neuroradiology, 39*, 556–559.

Abrahams, S., Goldstein, L. H., Al-Chalabi, A., Pickering, A., & Passingham, R. E. (1997). Relation between cognitive dysfunction and pseudo-bulbar palsy in amyotrophic lateral sclerosis. *Journal of Neurology, Neurosurgery, and Psychiatry, 62*, 464–472.

Al-Chalabi, A., Calvo, A., Chio, A., Colville, S., Ellis, C. M., & Hardiman, O. (2014). Analysis of amyotrophic lateral sclerosis as a multistep process: A population-based modelling study. *The Lancet Neurology, 13*(11), 1108–1113.

Alzheimer, A. (1911). Uber eigenartige Krankheits-falle des spateren Alters. *Zeitschrift fur die Gesamte Neurologie und Psychiatrie, 4*, 356–385.

Bak, T. H., & Hodges, J. R. (2001). Motor neurone disease, dementia and aphasia: Coincidence, co-occurrence or continuum? *Journal of Neurology, 248*, 260–270.

Ballard, K. J., Savage, S., Leyton, C. E., Vogel, A. P., Hornberger, M., & Hodges, J. R. (2014). Logopenic and nonfluent variants of primary progressive aphasia are differentiated by acoustic measures of speech production. *PLoS One, 9*(2), 1–14.

Banks, S. J., & Weintraub, S. (2008). Neuropsychiatric symptoms in behavioral variant frontotemporal dementia and primary progressive aphasia. *Journal of Geriatric Psychiatry and Neurology, 21*(2), 133–141.

Blair, M., Marczinski, C. A., Davis-Faroque, N., & Kertesz, A. (2007). A longitudinal study of language decline in Alzheimer's disease and frontotemporal dementia. *Journal of the International Neuropsychological Society, 13*, 237–245.

Brunnström, H., Gustafson, L., Passant, U., & Englund, E. (2009). Prevalence of dementia subtypes: A 30-year retrospective survey of neuropathological reports. *Archives of Gerontology and Geriatrics, 49*, 146–149.

Burrell, J. R., Kiernan, M. C., Vucic, S., & Hodges, J. R. (2011). Motor neuron dysfunction in frontotemporal dementia. *Brain, 9*, 2582–2594.

Cappa, S. F., Binetti, G., Pezzini, A., Padovani, A., Rozzini, L., & Trabucchi, M. (1998). Object and action naming in Alzheimer's disease and frontotemporal dementia. *Neurology, 50*, 351–355.

Caselli, R. J., Windebank, A. J., Petersen, R. C., Komori, T., Parisi, J. E., Okazaki, H., . . . Stein, S. D. (1993). Rapidly progressive aphasic dementia and motor neuron disease. *Annals of Neurology, 33*, 200–207.

Chare, L., Hodges, J. R., Leyton, C. E., McGinley, C., Tan, R. H., Kril, J. J., & Halliday, G. M. (2014). New criteria for frontotemporal dementia syndromes: Clinical and pathological diagnostic implications. *Journal of Neurology, Neurosurgery, and Psychiatry, 85*, 866–871.

Clark, D. G., Charuvastra, A., Miller, B. L., Shapira, J. S., & Mendez, M. F. (2005). Fluent versus nonfluent primary progressive aphasia: A comparison of clinical and functional neuroimaging features. *Brain and Language, 94*, 54–60.

Constantinidis, J. (1987). Syndrome familial: Association de Maladie de Pick at sclérose latérale amyotrophique. *Éncephale, 13*, 285–298.

Coyle-Gilchrist, I. T. S., Dick, K. M., Patterson, K., Rodriquez, P. V., Wehmann, E., Wilcox, A., . . . Rowe, J. B. (2016). Prevalence, characteristics, and survival of frontotemporal lobar degeneration syndromes. *Neurology, 86*(18), 1736–1743.

Cummings, J. L., & Benson, D. R. (1983). *Dementia: A clinical approach*. Boston, MA: Butterworth.

Daniele, A., Giustolisi, L., Silveri, M. C., Colosimo, C., & Gainotti, G. (1994). Evidence for a possible neuroanatomical basis for lexical processing of nouns and verbs. *Neuropsychologia, 32*, 1325–1341.

Doran, M., Xuereb, J., & Hodges, J. R. (1995). Rapidly progressive aphasia with bulbar motor neuron disease: A clinical and neuropsychological study. *Behavioural Neurology, 8*, 169–180.

Elfgren, C., Passant, U., & Risberg, J. (1993). Neuropsychological findings in frontal lobe dementia. *Dementia, 4*, 214–219.

Frank, B., Haas, J., Heinze, H. J., Stark, E., & Münte, T. F. (1997). Relation of neuropsychological and magnetic resonance findings in amyotrophic lateral sclerosis: Evidence for subgroups. *Clinical Neurology and Neurosurgery, 99*, 79–86.

Gans, A. (1922). Pick Betrachtungen über Art und Ausbreitung des krankhaften Prozesses in einem Fall von Pickscher Atrophie des Stirnhirns. *Zeitschrift für die Gesamte Neurologie und Psychiatrie, 80*, 10–28.

Garrard, P., & Hodges, J. R. (1999). Semantic dementia: Implications for the neural basis of language and meaning. *Aphasiology, 13*, 609–623.

Gorno-Tempini, M. L., Dronkers, N. F., Rankin, K. P., Ogar, J. M., Phengrasamy, L., Rosen, H. J., . . . Miller, B. L. (2004). Cognition and anatomy in three variants of primary progressive aphasia. *Annals of Neurology, 55*, 335–346.

Gorno-Tempini, M. L., Hillis, A. E., Weintraub, S., Kertesz, A., Mendez, M., Cappa, S. F., . . . Grossman, M. (2011). Classification of primary progressive aphasia and its variants. *Neurology, 76*, 1006–1014.

Graham, N. L., Patterson, K., & Hodges, J. R. (2000). The impact of semantic memory impairment on spelling: Evidence from semantic dementia. *Neuropsychologia, 38*, 143–163.

Gregory, C. A., Serra-Mestres, J., & Hodges, J. R. (1999). Early diagnosis of the frontal variant of frontotemporal dementia: How sensitive are standard neuroimaging and neuropsychologic tests? *Neuropsychiatry, Neuropsychology, and Behavioral Neurology, 12*, 128–135.

Grossman, M. (2002). Progressive aphasic syndromes: Clinical and theoretical advances. *Current Opinion in Neurology, 15*, 409–413.

Guedji, E., Le Ber, I., Lacomblez, L., Dubois, B., Verpillat, P., Didic, M., . . . Puel, M. (2007). Brain spect perfusion of frontotemporal dementia associated with motor neuron disease. *Neurology, 69*(5), 488–490.

Hall, G. R., Shapira, J., Gallagher, M., & Denny, S. S. (2013). Managing differences: Care of the person with frontotemporal degenerationg. *Journal of Gerontological Nursing, 39*(3), 10–14.

Harciarek, M., & Jodzio, K. (2005). Neuropsychological differences between frontotemporal dementia and Alzheimer's disease: A review. *Neuropsychology Review, 15*, 131–145.

Hillis, A. E., Tiffiash, E., & Caramazza, A. (2002). Modality-specific deterioration in naming verbs in nonfluent primary progressive aphasia. *Journal of Cognitive Neuroscience, 14*, 1099–1108.

Hodges, J. R. (2001). Frontotemporal dementia (Pick's disease): Clinical features and assessment. *Neurology, 56*(Suppl. 4), S6–S10.

Hodges, J. R., & Patterson, K. (2007). Semantic dementia: A unique clinicopathological syndrome. *Lancet Neurology, 6*, 1004–1014.

Hodges, J. R., Patterson, K., Oxbury, S., & Funnell, E. (1992). Semantic dementia. Progressive fluent aphasia with temporal lobe atrophy. *Brain, 115*, 1783–1806.

Hodges, J. R., Patterson, K., Ward, R., Garrard, P., Bak, T., Perry, R., & Gregory, C. (1999). The differentiation of semantic dementia and frontal lobe dementia (temporal and frontal variants of frontotemporal dementia) from early Alzheimer's disease: A comparative neuropsychological study. *Neuropsychology, 13*, 31–40.

Holland, A. L., McBurney, D. H., Moossy, J., & Reinmuth, O. M. (1985). The dissolution of language in Pick's disease with neurofibrillary tangles: A case study. *Brain and Language, 24*, 36–58.

Hornberger, M., & Piguet, O. (2012). Episodic memory in frontotemporal dementia: A critical review. *Brain, 135*, 678–692.

Howard, D., & Patterson, K. (1992). *Pyramids and palm trees: A test of semantic access from pictures and words.* Bury St. Edmunds, UK: Thames Valley.

Ichikawa, H., & Kawamura, M. (2010). Language impairment in amyotrophic lateral sclerosis. *Brain Nerve, 62*(4), 435–440.

Jeffries, E., Lambon Ralph, M. A., Jones, R., Bateman, D., & Patterson, K. (2004). Surface dyslexia in semantic dementia: A comparison of the influence of consistency and regularity. *Neurocase, 10*, 290–299.

Josephs, K. A., Duffy, J. R., Strand, E. A., Whitwell, J. L., Layton, K. F., Parisi, J. E., . . . Petersen, R. C. (2006). Clinicopathological and imaging correlates of progressive aphasia and apraxia of speech. *Brain, 129*, 1385–1398.

Kamminga, J., Leslie, F. V., Hsieh, S., Caga, J., Mioshi, E., Hornberger, M., . . . Burrell, J. R. (2016). Syntactic comprehension deficits across the FTD-ALS continuum. *Neurobiology of Aging, 41*, 11–18.

Karbe, H., Kertesz, A., & Polk, M. (1993). Profiles of language impairment in primary progressive aphasia. *Archives of Neurology, 50*, 193–201.

Kertesz., A. (2004). Frontotemporal dementia/Pick's disease. *Archives of Neurology, 61*, 969–971.

Kiernan, M. C. (2012). Amyotrophic lateral sclerosis and frontotemporal dementia. *Journal of Neurology, Neurosurgery, and Psychiatry, 83*, 355.

Kirshner, H. S. (2014). Frontotemporal dementia and primary progressive aphasia, a review. *Neuropsychiatric Disease and Treatment, 10*, 1045–1055.

Kirshner H. S., Tanridag, O., Thurman L., & Whetsell Jr., W. O. (1987). Progressive aphasia without dementia: Two cases with focal spongiform degeneration. *Annals of Neurology, 22*, 527–532.

Lanata, S. C., & Miller, B. L. (2016). The behavioural variant frontotemporal dementia (bvFTD) syndrome is psychiatry. *Journal of Neurology, Neurosurgery, and Psychiatry, 87*(5), 501–511.

Lillo, P., Savage, S., Mioshi, E., Kiernan, M. C., & Hodges, J. R. (2012). Amyotrophic lateral sclerosis and frontotemporal dementia: A behavioural and cognitive continuum. *Amyorophic Lateral Sclerosis, 13*, 102–109.

Macoir, J., & Bernier, J. (2002). Is surface dysgraphia tied to semantic impairment? Evidence from a case of semantic dementia. *Brain and Cognition, 48*, 452–457.

Mahendra, N., & Hopper, T. (2017). Dementia and related cognitive disorders. In I. Papathanasiou & P. Coppens (Eds.), *Aphasia and related neurogenic communication disorders* (2nd ed., pp. 455–491). Burlington: MA: Jones and Bartlett Learning.

McKhann, G. M., Albert, M. S., Grossman, M., Miller, B., Dickson, D., & Trojanowski, J. Q. (2001). Clinical and pathological diagnosis of frontotemporal dementia. *Archives of Neurology, 58*, 1803–1809.

Mendez, M. F., Selwood, A., Mastri, A. R., & Frey, W. H. (1993). Pick's disease versus Alzheimer's disease: A comparison of clinical characteristics. *Neurology, 43*, 280–292.

Mendez, M. F., Shapira, J. S., Woods, R. J., Licht, E. A., & Saul, R. E. (2008). Psychotic symptoms in frontotemporal dementia: Prevalence and review. *Dementia and Geriatric Cognitive Disorders, 25*(3), 206–211.

Mesulam, M. M. (1982). Slowly progressive aphasia without dementia. *Annals of Neurology, 11*, 592–598.

Mesulam, M. M. (1987). Primary progressive aphasia: differentiation from Alzheimer's disease. *Annals of Neurology, 22*, 522–524.

Mesulam, M. M. (2001). Primary progressive aphasia. *Annals of Neurology, 49*, 425–432.

Mesulam, M., Wicklund, A., Johnson, N., Rogalski, E., Leger, G. C., Rademaker, A., . . . Bigio, E. (2008). Alzheimer and frontotemporal pathology in subsets of primary progressive aphasia. *Annals of Neurology, 63*(6), 709–719.

Meteyard, L., & Patterson, K. (2009). The relation between content and structure in language production: An analysis of speech errors in semantic dementia. *Brain and Language, 110*, 121–134.

Meyer, A. (1929). Uber eine der amyotrophischen Lateralsklerose nahestehende erkrankung mit psychischen Storungen. Zugleich ein Beitrag zur Frage der spastischen pseudosklerose (A. Jakob, Ed.). *Zeitschrift für die Gesamte Neurologie und Psychiatrie, 121*, 107–128.

Mitsuyama, Y. (1984). Presenile dementia with motor neuron disease in Japan: Clinico-pathological review of 26 cases. *Journal of Neurology, Neurosurgery, and Psychiatry, 47*, 953–959.

Mummery, C. J., Hodges, J. R., Patterson, K., & Price, C. J. (1998). Functional neuroanatomy of the semantic system: Divisible by what? *Journal of Cognitive Neuroscience, 10*, 766–777.

Münte, T. F., Tröger, M., Nusser, I., Wieringa, B. M., Johannes, S., Matzke, M., & Dengler, R. (1998). Alterations of early components of the visual evoked potential in amyotrophic lateral sclerosis. *Journal of Neurology, 245*, 206–210.

Münte, T. F., Tröger, M., Nusser, I., Wieringa, B. M., Matzke, M., Johannes, S., & Dengler, R. (1998). Recognition memory deficits in amyotrophic lateral sclerosis assessed with eventrelated brain potentials. *Acta Neurologica Scandinavia, 98*, 110–115.

Nagy, D., Kato, T., & Kushner, P. D. (1994). Reactive astrocytes are widespread in the cortical gray matter of amyotrophic lateral sclerosis. *Journal of Neuroscience Research, 38*, 336–347.

National Institute on Aging. (2017).*What are frontotemporal dementias?* Retrieved from https://www.nia.nih.gov /health/what-are-frontotemporal-disorders.

Neary, D., Snowden, J. S., Gustafson, L., Passant, U., Stuss, D., Black, S., . . . Benson, D. F. (1998). Frontotemporal lobar degeneration: A consensus on clinical diagnostic criteria. *Neurology, 51*, 1546–1554.

Neary, D., Snowden, J., & Mann, D. (2005). Frontotemporal dementia. *Lancet Neurology, 4*(11), 771–780.

Neary, D., Snowden, J. S., & Mann, D. M. A. (2000). Cognitive change in motor neuron disease/amyotrophic lateral sclerosis. *Journal of the Neurological Sciences, 180*, 15–20.

Nunnemann, S., Last, D., Schuster, T., Förstl, H., Jurz, A., & Diehl-Schmid, J. (2011). Survival in a German population with frontotemporal lobal degeneration. *Neuroepidemiology, 37*, 160–165.

Padovani, A., Premi, E., Pilotto, A., Gazzina, S., Cosseddu, M., Archetti, S., . . . Borroni, B. (2013). Overlap between frontotemporal dementia and Alzheimer's disease: Cerebrospinal fluid pattern and neuroimaging study. *Journal of Alzheimer's Disease, 36*(1), 49–55.

Palmieri, R. L. (2005). Take aim at amyotrophic lateral sclerosis. *Nursing, 35*, 32hn1–32hn2.

Pick, A. (1901). Senile hirnatrophie als grundlage für hernderscheinungen. *Wiener Klinische Wochenschrift, 14*, 403–404.

Pick, A. (1904). Zur symptomatologie der linksseitigen. Schlafenlappenatrophie. *Monatschrift für Psychiatrie und Neurologie, 16*, 378–388.

Pick, A. (1906). Uber einen weiteren symptomenkomplex in rahmen der dementia senilis, bedingt durch umschriebene starkere hirnatrophie (gemischte apraxie). *Monatsschrift für Psychiatrie und Neurologie, 19*, 97–108.

Pressman, P. S., & Miller, B. L. (2014). Diagnosis and management of behavioral variant frontotemporal dementia. *Biological Psychiatry, 75*(7), 574–581.

Pülvermuller, F., Härle, M., & Hummel, F. (2000). Neurophysiological distinction of verb categories. *NeuroReport, 11*, 2789–2793.

Pülvermuller, F., Lutzenberger, W., & Preiss, H. (1999). Nouns and verbs in the intact brain: Evidence from event-related potentials and high-frequency cortical responses. *Cerebral Cortex, 9*, 497–506.

Rabkin, J., Goetz, R., Murphy, J. M., Factor-Litvak, P., & Mitsumoto, H. (2016). Cognitive impairment, behavioral impairment, depression, and wish to die in an ALS cohort. *Neurology, 87*(13), 1320–1328.

Rahman, S., Sahakian, B. J., Hodges, J. R., Rogers, R. D., & Robbins, T. W. (1999). Specific cognitive deficits in mild frontal variant frontotemporal dementia. *Brain, 122*, 1469–1493.

Rascovsky, K., Hodges, J. R., Knopman, d., Mendea, M. F., Kramer, J. H., Neuhaus, J., . . . Miller, B. L. (2011). Sensitivity of revised diagnostic criteria for the behavioral

variant of frontotemporal dementia. *Brain, 134*(Pt. 9), 2456–2477.

Rascovsky, K., Salmon, D. P., Ho, G. J., Galasko, D., Peavy, G. M., Hansen, L. A., & Thal, L. J. (2002). Cognitive profiles differ in autopsyconfirmed frontotemporal dementia and AD. *Neurology, 58*, 1801–1808.

Rohrer, J. D., Lashley, T., Schott, J. M., Warren, J. E., Mead, S. Isaacs, A. M., . . . Warren, J. D. (2011). Clinical and neuroanatomical signatures of tissue pathology in frontotemporal lobar degeneration. *Brain, 134*(9), 2565–2581.

Rosen, H. J., Narvaez, J. M., Hallam, B., Kramer, J. H., Wyss-Coray, C., Gearhart, R., . . . Miller, B. L. (2004). Neuropsychological and functional measures of severity in Alzheimer's disease, frontotemporal dementia, and semantic dementia. *Alzheimer Disease and Associated Disorders, 18*, 202–207.

Rosser, A., & Hodges, J. R. (1994). Initial letter and semantic category fluency in Alzheimer's disease, Huntington's disease, and progressive supranuclear palsy. *Journal of Neurology, Neurosurgery, and Psychiatry, 57*, 1389–1394.

Saxon, J. A., Thompson, J. C., Jones, M., Harris, J. M., Richardson, A. M., Langheinrich, T., . . . Snowden, J. S. (2017). Examining the language and behavioural profile in FTD and ALS-FTD. *Journal of Neurology, Neurosurgery, and Psychiatry*, pp. 1–6.

Siri, S., Benaglio, I., Frigerio, A., Binetti, G., & Cappa, S. F. (2001). A brief neuropsychological assessment for the differential diagnosis between frontotemporal dementia and Alzheimer's disease. *European Journal of Neurology, 8*, 125–132.

Snowden, J. S. (2005). Semantic dementia. In A. Burns, J. O'Brien, & D. Ames (Eds.), *Dementia* (3rd ed., pp. 702–712). London, UK: Hodder Arnold.

Snowden, J. S., Goulding, P. J., & Neary, D. (1989). Semantic dementia: A form of circumscribed cerebral atrophy. *Behavioural Neurology, 2*, 167–182.

Snowden, J. S., & Neary, D. (1993). Progressive language dysfunction and lobar atrophy. *Dementia, 4*, 226–231.

Spinelli, E. G., Mandelli, M. L., Miller, Z. A., Santos-Santos, M. A., Wilson, S. M., Agosta, F., . . . Henry, M. L. (2017). Typical and atypical pathology in primary progressive aphasia variants. *Annals of Neurology, 81*(3), 430–443.

Strong, M. J. (2008). The syndromes of frontotemporal dysfunction in amyotrophic lateral sclerosis. *Amyotrophic Lateral Sclerosis, 9*, 323–338.

Taylor, L. J., Brown, R. G., Tsermentseli, S., Al-Chalabi, A., Shaw, C. E., Ellis, C. M., . . . Goldstein, L. H. (2013). Is language impairment more common than executive dysfunction in amyotrophic lateral sclerosis? *Journal of Neurology, Neurosurgery, and Psychiatry, 84*(5), 494–498.

Thompson, S. A., Patterson, K., & Hodges, J. R. (2003). Left/right asymmetry of atrophy in semantic dementia: Behavioral-cognitive implications. *Neurology, 61*, 1196–1203.

Tsermentseli, S., Leigh, P. N., Taylor, L. J., Radunovic, A., Catani, M., & Goldstein, L. H. (2016). Syntactic processing as a marker for cognitive impairment in amyotrophic lateral sclerosis. *Amyotrophic Lateral Sclerosis and Frontotemporal Degeneration*, *17*(1–2), 69–76.

Tsuchiya, K., Ozawa, E., Fukushima, J., Yasui, H., Kondo, H., Nakano, I., & Ikeda, K. (2000). Rapidly progressive aphasia and motor neuron disease: A clinical, radiological and pathological study of an autopsy case with circumscribed lobar atrophy. *Acta Neuropathologica*, *99*, 81–87.

Turner, R. S., Kenyon, L. C., Trojanowski, J. Q., Gonatas, N., & Grossman, M. (1996). Clinical, neuroimaging, and pathologic features of progressive nonfluent aphasia. *Annals of Neurology*, *39*, 166–173.

van Bogaert, L. (1925). Les troubles mentaux dans la sclérose latérale amyotrophique. Éncephale, *20*, 27.

Warren, J. D., Rohrer, J. D., & Rossor, M. N. (2013). Frontotemporal dementia. *British Medical Journal*, *347*, 1–9.

Warrington, E. K. (1975). The selective impairment of semantic memory. *Quarterly Journal of Experimental Psychology*, *27*(4), 635–657.

Weintraub, S., & Mesulam, M. (1993). Four neuropsychological profiles in dementia. In F. Boller & J. Grafman (Eds.), *Handbook of neuropsychology* (Vol. 8, pp. 253–281). Amsterdam, The Netherlands: Elsevier.

Westbury, C., & Bub, D. (1997). Primary progressive aphasia: A review of 112 cases. *Brain and Language*, *60*(3), 381–406.

Wittenberg, D., Possin, K. L., Rascovsky, K., Rankin, K. P., Miller, B. L., & Kramer, J. H. (2008). The early neuropsychological and behavioral characteristics of frontotemporal dementia. *Neuropsychological Review*, *18*, 91–102.

Woodward, M., Jacova, C., Black, S. E., Kertesz, A., Mackenzie, I. R., & Feldman, H. (2010). Differentiating the frontal variant of Alzheimer's disease. *International Journal of Geriatric Psychiatry*, *25*(7), 732–738.

Yener, G., & Didem, O. Z. (2016). Behavioral variant frontotemporal dementia. *Journal of Neurological Sciences (Turkish)*, *33*(4), 526–544.

Zago, S., Poletti, B., Morelli, C., Doretti, A., & Silani, V. (2011). Amyotrophic lateral sclerosis and frontotemporal dementia (ALS-FTD). *Archives Italiennes de Biologie*, *149*(1), 39–56.

Ziegler, L. H. (1930). Psychotic and emotional phenomena associated with amyotrophic lateral sclerosis. *Archives of Neurology and Psychiatry*, *24*, 930–936.

CLINICAL MANAGEMENT GUIDE

Assessments and Interventions
for Cognitive-Communication
Disorders of Dementia

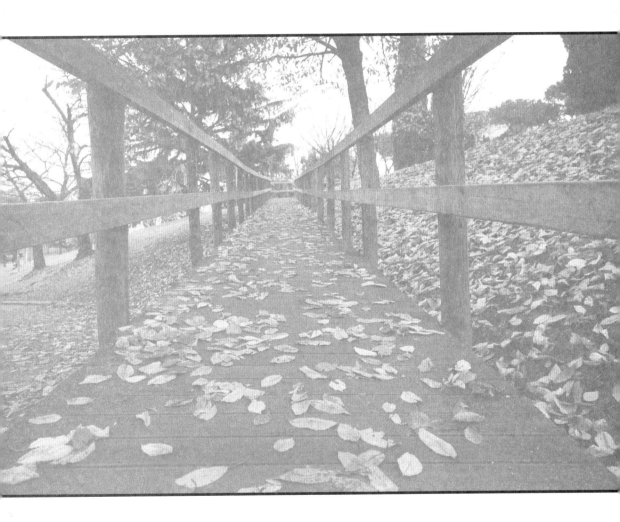

I

Assessment

Introduction

Assessment of cognitive function is critical to the early identification of individuals with mild cognitive impairment (MCI) or dementia. For individuals with MCI, early identification has profound benefits because lifestyle changes, cognitive stimulation, and drug therapy can prevent or slow evolution to dementia. Comprehensive evaluation of cognitive and linguistic functions is needed to correctly diagnose and treat those affected and for family counseling. In this section three major topics are addressed:

Assessment procedures that produce valid and reliable data

Tests for diagnosing MCI and dementia

Differentiating the types of dementia

Assessment Procedures that Produce Valid and Reliable Data

The diagnosis of MCI or dementia is made on the basis of history, performance on neuropsychological tests, perceptions of patients and families, and biomarker data from laboratory and imaging results. Currently, however, biomarker data are generally unavailable and results of cognitive-linguistic assessment are the primary basis primarily used for making a diagnosis. Therefore, clinicians should use assessments for which there are normative data on the performance of healthy individuals of a similar age and, if possible, individuals with MCI or dementia. Additionally, clinicians must control for sensory loss and other age-related conditions that can affect cognitive functioning and lead to inaccurate conclusions about mental status and functional abilities.

Prior to Testing

Take a Case History

- What were the presenting symptoms?
- When did they develop?
- Are the symptoms variable? Variability in mental status is characteristic of individuals with Lewy body dementia.
- Is there evidence of more than one neurologic problem? Individuals with Alzheimer's disease (AD) frequently have vascular disease and those with vascular disease often have AD.
- Does the client have other medical problems?
- Does the client have a history of depression?
- What, if any, drugs does the client take?
- What, if any, laboratory tests or neuroimaging has the client had? And, what are the results?
- If the client has a diagnosis of dementia, what is the presumptive cause?
- What is the severity of dementia? Clinicians should be familiar with the commonly used severity rating scales and the scores that correspond to mild, moderate, and severe dementia (Table I–1).

Table I–1. Three Commonly Used Measures of Dementia Severity and Scores/Ratings that Correspond to Mild, Moderate, and Severe Dementia

Measure	Mild Dementia	Moderate-Moderately Severe Dementia	Severe Dementia
Global Deterioration Scale (GDS; Reisberg, Ferris, de Leon, & Crook, 1982): The course of dementia is defined in seven stages that have specific observational criteria. GDS stage 1 represents "normal" aging without evidence of cognitive decline. GDS stage 7 represents "late dementia" with very severe cognitive decline.	3 or 4	5 or 6	7
Clinical Dementia Rating Scale (CDR; Hughes et al., 1982): The CDR provides a rating of global cognitive function based on clinical information about memory, orientation, judgment, problem solving, community affairs, home and hobbies, and personal care. Level of impairment is rated as none (0), questionable (0.5), mild (1), moderate (2), or severe (3).	CDR 1	CDR 2	CDR 3
Dementia Rating Scale (DRS; Mattis, 1976): The DRS contains items that evaluate five cognitive functions: attention, initiation and perseveration, construction, conceptualization, and memory. A maximum of 144 points can be awarded and normal elders obtain scores of 140 or more.	120–130	90–119	<90

- Review the patient's medical history for information about sensory impairment (i.e., macular degeneration, moderate to severe hearing loss) and other conditions that can alter cognitive function (i.e., depression, drug effects).

Arrange for a Good Test Environment

Testing should be conducted in a quiet room with adequate lighting. Illuminate test materials in a way that prevents shadows and remember that elders need two to three times more illumination than young adults. Glare can impair an elder's vision. Avoid sitting with your back to a bright light or window that makes your facial features hard to perceive. Test stimuli should be printed in a font size that is readily perceptible. Black print on a white background is the easiest for elders to see. Avoid putting words in all caps as they are harder to comprehend.

Check Vision

Visual acuity diminishes with age and many elders need glasses to read. If the patient's vision status is unknown, a standard eye chart can be used to screen for a visual deficit or the patient can be asked to read simple words in a print size *smaller* than the test stimuli. If the patient can read text in the smaller print, you can be assured that the patient has adequate visual acuity to see the printed test materials.

Check Hearing

Hearing loss is more common with age (Cruickshanks, 2009; NIDCD, 2017). Indeed, age is the strongest predictor of hearing loss and those with the greatest amount of loss are typically older than 60 years. Men are twice as likely as women to have hearing loss (Hoffman, Dobie, Losonczy, Themann, & Flamme, 2017). Nearly one-quarter of adults aged 65 to 74 and 50% of those who are 75 and older have disabling hearing loss.

If the patient has hearing aids, have the patient wear them during testing. If a full audiometric evaluation cannot be obtained, a simple speech discrimination test can be given to ensure that the examinee can hear the clinician's voice in the test environment. Have the client repeat words that sound similar (like "cake" and "take") to determine if they can discriminate subtle differences. Use the same intonation and loudness level when presenting the stimulus word pairs. An example of this type of speech discrimination task can be found in the Arizona Battery for Cognitive-Communication Disorders (ABCD-2) (Bayles & Tomoeda, 2019). An error rate of 30% or greater indicates that the patient's hearing will likely impact test performance.

Check Literacy

Check for literacy by having the examinee read two or three simple sentences. Generally, even individuals with moderately severe dementia are able to read aloud if they were literate prior to the onset of dementia.

Take Steps to Reduce Test-Taking Anxiety

Before testing, visit with the examinee and describe what will occur during the session. Position score sheets so the examinee cannot see you record responses. When examinees ask about their performance, tell them the testing is going well. During testing, do not tell examinees if their responses are correct.

Some individuals, particularly those with dementia, become anxious about where their spouse or family member is. Give assurance that the caregiver is nearby. If an examinee will not participate in the evaluation without the caregiver being present, allow the caregiver to be present but refrain from giving cues.

Be Alert to Depression

Depression is common in older adults and can negatively affect test performance. In fact, its effects can mimic dementia. Historically, the term "pseudodementia" was used to designate a dementia-like performance in a cognitively intact but depressed individual (Kiloh, 1961). However, in recent years, the term has fallen out of favor (Alexopoulos, 2003; Dobie, 2002; Emery & Oxman, 2003) because research has shown that depression is frequently an early sign of a dementing disease (Alexopoulos, Young, & Meyers, 1993; Kral & Emery, 1989; Saczynski et al., 2010).

Individuals who are depressed generally convey a sense of distress. Often, they make self-deprecatory comments. Some are uninterested in the testing and its outcome. A subsequent part of this section is devoted to differentiating mild AD from delirium and depression. Table I–2 contains brief descriptions of tests that can be used to screen for depression in adults.

Be Alert to Drug Effects on Performance

Most elders and many middle-aged individuals at risk for dementia take several medications to manage age-associated chronic disease (Lamy, 1986). The potential for adverse drug interactions rises with advancing age because of age-related physiologic change, greater occurrence of comorbid diseases, and an increase in the number of medications prescribed (Hines & Murphy, 2011; Seymour & Routledge, 1998). Sloan (1983) reported that the potential for drug interaction is 5.6% when patients take two drugs and increases to 100% when patients take eight or more drugs. Similarly, Larson, Kukull, Buchner, and Reifler (1987) found that drug reactions that impair cognitive function increase as the number of prescription drugs increases. In a review of 16 studies that included 1,551 patients, Weytingh, Bossuyt, and van Crevel (1995) found that drugs were a frequent cause of reversible dementia.

Table I–2. Screening Tests for Depression

Name of Measure	Reference	Description
Hamilton Rating Scale for Depression (HRS-D)	Hamilton (1967, 1970)	The HRS-D is one of the first-developed and best-known interview-based rating scales for depression. It is a 17-item inventory of symptoms that are rated for severity by an experienced clinician, based on an interview and other available data.
Beck Depression Inventory (BDI)	Beck, Ward, Mendelson, Mock, & Erbaugh (1961)	The BDI is a 21-item inventory of depressive symptoms and attitudes that are rated from 0 to 3 in terms of intensity. The BDI is commonly used as a self-administered measure, although it was designed for administration by trained interviewers.
Zung Self-rating Depression Scales (SDS)	Zung (1965)	The SDS comprises 20 items that evaluate four areas of disturbance: pervasive psychic, physiologic, psychomotor, and psychologic. The patient rates the applicability, within the past week, of each item according to the following terms: "none or a little of the time," "some of the time," "good part of the time," and "most or all of the time."
Zung Depression Status Inventory (DSI)	Zung (1972)	The 20 items of the DSI correspond to the SDS; however, the interviewer rates the severity of symptoms or signs on a four-point scale from none to severe based on the results of a clinical interview.
Dementia Mood Assessment Scale	Sunderland et al. (1988)	This two-part instrument is designed to measure the severity of mood disturbance of demented patients based on direct observation and a semistructured interview by health professionals. The first 17 items evaluate mood and are scaled from 0 (within normal limits) to 6 (most severe). The remaining seven items measure the patient's functional capacities.
Cornell Scale for Depression in Dementia	Alexopoulus, Abrams, Young, & Shamoian (1988)	The Cornell Scale is a 19-item clinician-administered instrument that uses information obtained from interviews with the patient and a member of the nursing staff. This instrument was specifically designed for measuring depression in demented patients.

Orange (2001) listed classes of drugs that commonly interfere with speech, language, and cognition in persons with dementia. They include:

Sedatives

Antidepressants

Anxiolytics (antianxiety drugs)

Antipsychotics

Anticoagulants

Antihypertensives

Narcotic-based analgesics

Massey (2005) cautioned that long-term use of benzodiazepines can interfere with the ability to learn, and long-term use of anticholinergic medications (Artane, Cogentin, Atropine) and antihistamines (Benadryl, Dimetapp, Chlortrimeton) can contribute to confusion. Mental status changes also occur with medications for incontinence (Detrol, Ditropan), motility (Levsin, Bentyl), and pain.

Know the Criteria for Diagnosing MCI and Dementia

The criteria for diagnosing MCI and dementia provide a guideline for the assessment.

Criteria for diagnosing MCI (Albert et al., 2011) are as follows:

1. **Concern regarding a change in cognition.** Concern can be expressed by the person

or an informant who knows the individual well or a skilled clinician.

2. **Impairment in one or more cognitive domains.** Evidence is needed of lower performance in one or more cognitive domains that is greater than would be expected for the patient's age and education. Remember that change can occur in a variety of cognitive domains, including language, attention, visuospatial skills, memory, and executive function. Scores on tests of those with MCI are typically 1 to 1.5 standard deviations (SD) below the mean for age and education.
3. **Preservation of independence in basic functional abilities.**
4. **No dementia.**

Take Into Account Degree of Intelligence and Education in Evaluating Test Performance

The challenge of identifying MCI or mild dementia is that intelligence and degree of education vary considerably in the healthy population. Without taking into account intelligence and education, you can mistakenly conclude that a low-average or average performance is normal in a highly intelligent and educated individual when, in fact, the individual has MCI. Similarly, you can mistakenly conclude that a below average performance of a person, who has below average intelligence, is evidence of impairment. To cope with these challenges, the authors of the diagnostic clinical criteria for MCI established the following performance cutoffs.

> **A performance of 1 to 2 SD below the mean of healthy elders with similar education is considered indicative of cognitive impairment** (Albert et al., 2011).

Clearly, to make this comparison, you need to administer tests for which there are normative data for healthy adults.

Criteria for diagnosing dementia (American Psychiatric Association, 2013) are as follows:

1. **Individual exhibits significant cognitive decline from a previous level of performance.**

2. **The cognitive deficits are sufficient to interfere with independence in everyday activities.** At a minimum, assistance should be required with complex instrumental activities of daily living, such as paying bills or managing medications.
3. **The cognitive deficits do not occur exclusively in the context of delirium.**
4. **The cognitive deficits are not better explained by another mental disorder.**

The National Institutes of Health–Alzheimer's Disease and Related Disorders Association (NIH-ADRDA) working group acknowledges that specifying the definitive points at which individuals transition from MCI to dementia and mild to moderate dementia is difficult. Efforts to refine the criteria for characterizing the various stages of dementing diseases (asymptomatic preclinical, symptomatic predementia, and clinically apparent dementia) are ongoing (Albert et al., 2011; McKhann et al., 2011; Sperling et al., 2011). Thus, some degree of clinical judgment is involved. However, to improve decision making, use tests for which there are normative data on the performance of healthy adults, and, if possible, measures that also have data on the performance of individuals with mild and moderate dementia (for whom etiology is specified).

Severity of Cognitive Impairment Affects Test Selection

We have found, and others have confirmed (Locascio, Growdon, & Corkin, 1995), that tests suitable for early detection of cognitive impairment are unsuitable for documenting abilities in severely demented individuals. If a test is sufficiently cognitively challenging for identifying individuals with MCI, it is usually too difficult for individuals with moderate dementia and *floor effects* emerge. Similarly, tests designed to characterize cognitive-communicative functioning in the later stages of dementia are generally too easy for individuals in the mild stage, and the result is a *ceiling effect*. It is the

Table I–3. Definitions of Terms Related to Testing

Ceiling Effect	The failure of a test to identify the highest performance of the most competent examinees because of a limited number of difficult test items.
Floor Effect	The failure of a test to identify the lowest possible performance because of a limited number of easy or simple test items.
Sensitivity	A statistical term that refers to the ability of a measure to correctly identify individuals who have a condition or disease.
Specificity	A statistical term that refers to the ability of a measure to correctly identify individuals who do not have a condition or disease.

clinician's responsibility to administer measures that have demonstrated sensitivity for detecting the condition and high specificity for distinguishing it from those without the condition. See Table I–3 for brief definitions of terms used in describing tests.

Tests for Diagnosing MCI and Dementia

When deciding what cognitive domains to assess, it is important to remember that certain cognitive deficits are red flags for a specific disease.

- The presence of impairment in episodic memory is a red flag for possible AD. Thus, an episodic memory test should always be included in the assessment.
- Prominent visual spatial impairments are a red flag for possible Lewy body disease (Aarsland et al., 2003; Collerton, Burn, McKeith, & O'Brien, 2003; Johnson, Morris, & Galvin, 2005). Thus, tests of visuospatial (construction and perception) should be included in the assessment.
- Prominent language disorders that occur early are a red flag for possible primary progressive aphasia. Thus, the clinical assessment should include tests of language functions.
- Aberrant behavior early is a red flag for the behavioral variant of frontotemporal dementia (FTD). Thus, if possible, clinicians need to interview informants about the client's behavior over the last year.

To adequately evaluate for either MCI or dementia, clinicians should conduct a *comprehensive evaluation* of cognitive-linguistic functions that includes measures to detect any of the noted "red flags." This is the gold standard for providing good patient care. The NIH-ADRDA working group recommendations include assessing the following cognitive domains: language, attention, memory, executive, and visuoconstructive/visuospatial skills.

Arizona Battery for Communication Disorders of Dementia (ABCD-1) aka Arizona Battery for Cognitive-Communicative Disorders (ABCD-2)

The original battery, ABCD-1 (Bayles & Tomoeda, 1993) was designed by speech-language pathologists and researchers to characterize the cognitive and communicative abilities of persons with early and mid-stage dementia and to differentiate them from healthy older adults. The battery evolved from NIH supported cross-sectional and longitudinal studies of adults with etiologically different neurodegenerative diseases that are associated with dementia. The original standardization sample included individuals with mild and moderate AD, Parkinson's disease (PD), and young and older nondemented community-dwelling individuals. Later, it was also given to individuals with multiple sclerosis (Wallace & Holmes, 1993) and to individuals with Down syndrome with and without dementia (Moss, Tomoeda, &

Table I–4. The Domains and Subtests of the Arizona Battery for Cognitive-Communicative Disorders-2

Domain 1	**Mental Status**
	Subtests: Mental Status
Domain 2	**Episodic Memory**
	Subtests: Story Retelling–Immediate Story Retelling–Delayed Word Learning
Domain 3	**Linguistic Expression**
	Subtests: Object Description Generative Naming Confrontation Naming Concept Definition
Domain 4	**Linguistic Comprehension**
	Subtests: Following Commands Comparative Questions Repetition Reading Comprehension
Domain 5	**Visuospatial Construction**
	Subtests: Generative Drawing Figure Copying

Source: Bayles and Tomoeda (2019).

Bayles, 2000). Also, it was modified for use with individuals in the United Kingdom (Armstrong, Borthwick, Bayles, & Tomoeda, 1996), Australia (Moorhouse, Douglas, Panaccio, & Steel, 1999), and The Netherlands.

A second edition of the ABCD was released in 2019, the ABCD-2 (Bayles & Tomoeda, 2019). This edition, that has a slightly different name, relies on the same underlying principles and theory as the first edition but has a larger and more geographically diverse standardization sample that includes individuals with MCI. Both editions contain the same tests that evaluate the same five cognitive domains and both produce 17 scores. However, in the second edition the three components of the original Word Learning subtest are considered to be separate subtests. The 17 subtests of the ABCD-2 and the domains evaluated are listed in Table I–4.

ABCD-2 subtests can be used alone or the full battery can be given. When all subtests are administered, four types of scores are obtainable: a raw score for each subtest, a severity score (the result of converting raw scores for the individual subtests to the same scale), a domain score, and a total overall score (Table I–5). The full ABCD-2 typically requires 60 to 90 min to complete.

Test-Retest Reliability of the ABCD-2

Reliability refers to the consistency with which repeated administrations of a test will produce the same results. To answer this question,

Table I–5. Four Types of Scores Available from the Arizona Battery for Communication Disorders of Dementia-2 and Their Uses

Raw	Scores on the individual subtests
Severity	Standardized scores that permit performance comparisons between subtests
Domain	Standardized scores that permit interdomain performance comparisons
Total	One score that represents performance on the entire test

19 individuals with dementia were given the ABCD-2 twice seven days apart. After the two administrations, the severity and domain scores for each testing were correlated. As can be seen in Table I–6, all subtest severity score correlations were impressive with one exception, reading comprehension of words which has few items and low variance. When a correlation is below .70, it does not necessarily mean that reliability is low and can indicate that a test was very easy or hard. Reading comprehension is a very easy test and most examinees scored at ceiling. The correlations for domain scores were uniformly solid, and the total score correlation was excellent.

Internal Consistency. Internal consistency, or the degree to which test items measure what they purport to measure, was calculated using Cronbach's alpha. Cronbach's alpha ranges from 0 to 1 where a value of 0 indicates no internal consistency and a value of 1 indicates perfect internal consistency. As can be seen in Table I–7, the ABCD-2 subtests have high internal consistency. As was the case with test-retest reliability, internal consistency analyses can be misleading if the test is either too easy or too hard. For example, the high alpha for Story-Retelling Delayed is due to the fact that almost every individual with AD scored 0. The Reading Comprehension (word) subtest and the Comparative Questions subtest are relatively easy and are associated with little variance in scores.

Validity of the ABCD-1 and ABCD-2

Criterion validity of ABCD-1 was determined in the original standardization study through correlation with three well-known measures of dementia severity: the Global Deterioration Scale (GDS; Reisberg, Ferris, de Leon, & Crook, 1982), the Mini-Mental State Examination (MMSE; Folstein, Folstein, & McHugh, 1975), and the Block Design subtest of the Wechsler Adult Intelligence Scale–Revised (WAIS-R; Wechsler, 1981). Correlations between these three measures and ABCD-1 subtests were high, ranging from .62 to .85 (Bayles & Tomoeda, 1993).

In a later, poststandardization study, Bayles, Tomoeda, Wood, Cruz, and McGeagh (1996) compared the ABCD-1 to five measures known to be sensitive to dementia to determine which was the best for discriminating individuals with early AD from normal elders: the Block Design subtest of the WAIS-R (Wechsler, 1981), the Modified Wisconsin Card Sorting Test (Hart, Kwentus, Wade, & Taylor, 1988; Jenkins & Parsons, 1978), a test of verbal fluency (Bayles, Trosset, Tomoeda, Montgomery, & Wilson, 1993), a verbal picture description test (Tomoeda & Bayles, 1993), and the MMSE (Folstein et al., 1975). The ABCD was the best measure for discriminating early dementia and for distinguishing mild from moderate Alzheimer's dementia.

The criterion validity of ABCD-2 was determined through correlation of the scores of the AD patients with their GDS rating and MMSE performance. As can be seen in Table I–8, the weighted average of the coefficients ranged from moderate to very large indicating high criterion validity. Some subtests, for example, Story Retelling-Delayed is less highly correlated because AD patients vary

Table I-6. Test-Retest Reliability Coefficients for ABCD-2 (n = 19)

ABCD-2 value	First Testing		Second Testing		
	M	(SD)	M	(SD)	r
Subtest Raw Score					
Mental Status	8.7	(3.1)	8.8	(2.9)	.88
Story Retelling-Immediate	8.2	(3.2)	8.3	(3.8)	.88
Following Commands	6.8	(2.0)	7.2	(1.7)	.86
Comparative Questions	4.8	(1.4)	5.3	(1.4)	.82
Word Learning: Free Recall	3.2	(2.6)	4.1	(2.8)	.75
Word Learning: Total Recall	8.0	(5.0)	8.8	(5.2)	.89
Word Learning: Recognition	30.1	(11.9)	31.1	(13.6)	.91
Repetition	46.7	(20.7)	50.0	(17.9)	.77
Object Description	5.4	(3.6)	6.1	(3.8)	.87
Reading Comprehension: Word	7.3	(1.4)	7.3	(1.6)	.57
Reading Comprehension: Sentence	5.1	(1.6)	5.5	(1.4)	.74
Generative Naming	6.4	(3.6)	6.2	(2.9)	.71
Confrontation Naming	13.5	(4.5)	14.1	(4.9)	.92
Concept Definition	26.4	(15.8)	27.1	(17.0)	.97
Generative Drawing	5.6	(3.9)	5.8	(3.4)	.72
Figure Copying	7.7	(2.8)	8.3	(3.0)	.80
Story Retelling-Delayed	3.6	(4.2)	5.6	(4.7)	.84
Domain Score					
Mental Status	3.1	(0.8)	2.9	(0.7)	.72
Episodic Memory	2.9	(0.6)	3.0	(0.7)	.94
Language Expression	2.9	(0.8)	3.1	(0.7)	.92
Language Comprehension	3.4	(1.1)	3.7	(1.0)	.89
Visuospatial Construction	2.5	(0.9)	2.6	(0.9)	.75
Total Score					
ABCD-2 Total	14.9	(3.5)	15.3	(3.4)	.95

Table I-7. Estimates of Internal Consistency of the ABCD-2 Subtests by Subgroup

ABCD-2 Subtest	Mild Cognitive Impairment (n = 143)	Alzheimer's Dementia (n = 111)	Other/Mixed Dementia (n = 75)	All Dementias	
				Mild (n = 88)	Moderate (n = 106)
Mental Status	.29	.81	.74	.45	.78
Story Retelling-Immediate	.76	.81	.70	.69	.79
Following Commands	.48	.74	.64	.40	.70
Comparative Questions	.08	.51	.54	.35	.56
Word Learning-Free Recall	.47	.49	.58	.62	.58
Word Learning-Total Recall	.37	.80	.78	.80	.78
Word Learning-Recognition	.64	.94	.95	.94	.95
Repetition	.74	.90	.90	.84	.92
Object Description[a]	–	–	–	–	–
Reading Comprehension-Word	.14	.73	.55	.64	.62
Reading Comprehension-Sentence	.50	.77	.64	.56	.71
Generative Naming[a]	–	–	–	–	–
Confrontation Naming	.69	.91	.80	.69	.87
Concept Definition	.96	.97	.95	.96	.95
Generative Drawing	.20	.81	.78	.73	.78
Figure Copying	.29	.87	.78	.77	.83
Story Retelling-Delayed	.90	.58	.90	.92	.90

[a]Subtest reliability is not calculable. Cronbach's coefficient alpha was used to estimate internal consistency for all other subtests.

Table I–8. Correlations of ABCD-2 Subtest Raw Scores with Criterion Measures for Alzheimer's Dementia Sample (Decimals Omitted)

ABCD-2 Subtest	Criterion test			Magnitude[b]
	GDS	MMSE-2	Average[a]	
Mental Status	75	89	83	Very large
Story Retelling-Immediate	53	58	56	Large
Following Commands	60	72	66	Large
Comparative Questions	46	61	54	Large
Word Learning-Free Recall	49	45	47	Moderate
Word Learning-Total Recall	58	59	58	Large
Word Learning-Recognition	53	54	53	Large
Repetition	57	71	64	Large
Object Description	56	60	58	Large
Reading Comprehension-Word	56	62	59	Large
Reading Comprehension-Sentence	58	69	64	Large
Generative Naming	60	72	66	Large
Confrontation Naming	69	69	69	Large
Concept Definition[c]	62	71	67	Large
Generative Drawing	64	75	70	Very large
Figure Copying	43	69	57	Large
Story Retelling-Delayed	31	33	32	Moderate

[a]Weighted average of the coefficients. [b]Magnitude of the average coefficients based on Hopkins's (2002) criteria.

little in performance. Thus, although the test is extremely effective in detecting AD, it is ineffective in quantifying dementia severity.

ABCD-2 Performance of Individuals with MCI

As can be seen in Table I–9, individuals with MCI were significantly poorer in performance than healthy older adults on every ABCD-2 subtest. The largest differences were on: word learning free recall, object description, generative naming, and story-retelling delayed. Individuals with MCI differed in performance from those with mild AD on all subtests but following commands, repetition, and reading comprehension (word and sentence).

ABCD-2 Performance of Mild and Moderately Severe AD Patients

The average performance of mild AD patients (mean age = 76.74) on ABCD-2 subtests is charted in Table I–9 and can be compared to the performance of healthy elders (mean age = 70.44) and healthy young adults (mean age = 20.29). Mild AD patients were significantly inferior to normal elders on all subtests.

Moderate AD patients in the ABCD-2 standardization study performed significantly

Table I-9. ABCD-2 Subtest Means (*M*) and Standard Deviations (*SD*) for Young and Old Normal Controls (*NC*), Individuals with Mild Cognitive Impairment (*MCI*), and Mild and Moderate (*Mod*) Alzheimer's Disease

ABCD-2 Raw Score	Sign. Diff. *p* < .05	Young NC (*n* = 72)		Old NC (*n* = 105)		MCI (*n* = 143)		Mild AD (*n* = 48)		Mod. AD (*n* = 63)	
		M	(*SD*)	*M*	(*SD*)	*M*	(*SD*)	*M*	(*SD*)	*M*	(*SD*)
Mental Status	2,3,4,5	12.9	(.3)	12.9	(.2)	12.6	(.8)	9.8	(2.6)	5.5	(3.1)
Story Retelling-Immediate	2,3,4,5	14.5	(1.9)	14.6	(1.8)	12.5	(3.1)	7.3	(3.9)	3.7	(3.6)
Following Commands	2,3,5	9.0	(.2)	8.9	(.3)	8.4	(.9)	8.2	(1.0)	6.5	(2.0)
Comparative Questions	2,3,5	5.9	(.4)	6.0	(.3)	5.8	(.5)	5.7	(0.7)	4.7	(1.2)
Word Learning-Free Recall	1,2,3,4,5	10.4	(2.5)	9.1	(2.3)	6.8	(2.5)	2.3	(1.8)	1.0	(1.3)
Word Learning-Total Recall	2,3,4,5	15.5	(1.0)	15.6	(.7)	14.7	(1.5)	7.8	(4.2)	4.0	(3.6)
Word Learning-Recognition	2,3,4,5	47.6	(1.0)	47.3	(1.3)	46.4	(1.9)	36.5	(7.2)	28.1	(9.9)
Repetition	1,2,3,5	71.8	(5.1)	68.5	(6.2)	59.8	(10.0)	58.1	(11.4)	39.5	(19.2)
Object Description	2,3,4,5	9.4	(2.3)	9.4	(2.2)	7.7	(2.6)	6.5	(2.9)	3.5	(2.0)
Reading Comprehension-Word	2,3,5	8.0	(.0)	8.0	(.1)	7.8	(.6)	7.8	(0.6)	6.3	(1.8)
Reading Comprehension-Sentence	2,3,5	6.8	(.5)	6.7	(.6)	6.2	(1.1)	5.9	(1.2)	4.0	(2.1)
Generative Naming	2,3,4,5	12.5	(3.3)	12.8	(3.3)	9.9	(3.0)	7.6	(3.3)	3.8	(2.8)
Confrontation Naming	1,2,3,4,5	17.7	(1.8)	19.0	(1.3)	17.5	(2.4)	15.6	(2.9)	10.1	(4.8)
Concept Definition	1,2,3,4,5	53.6	(8.0)	57.3	(3.8)	44.7	(12.8)	39.2	(11.3)	22.5	(13.3)
Generative Drawing	2,3,4,5	13.5	(1.0)	13.3	(1.1)	12.4	(1.9)	10.6	(3.2)	5.9	(4.0)
Figure Copying	2,3,5	11.7	(.7)	11.8	(.5)	11.4	(.9)	10.8	(2.1)	7.8	(3.9)
Story Retelling-Delayed	2,3,5	13.9	(3.0)	14.1	(2.1)	10.7	(5.1)	0.9	(2.5)	0.1	(0.5)

1 = Old NC vs. Young NC; 2 = Old NC vs. MCI; 3 = Old NC vs. Mild AD; 4 = MCI vs. Mild AD; 5 = Mild AD vs. Mod AD.

Source: Bayles and Tomoeda (2019).

poorer than mild AD patients and normal elders on every subtest. Their poorest performance was on the memory subtests.

ABCD-2 Subtests Most Sensitive to Mild AD

Of the 17 ABCD-2 subtests, Story Retelling–Delayed and Word Learning were those most sensitive to mild AD and thus are the best for screening individuals at risk for AD, the most common dementia-producing disease. As can be seen by comparing scores in Table I–9, the disparity in performance between normal elders and AD patients is greatest on these measures. The shorter of these subtests is Story Retelling, making it more appropriate for screening. Individuals are told a short story and asked to retell it immediately and again after a short delay. It is quick to administer and score. The examiner tells the patient: "I am going to tell you a short story. When I am done, I want you to tell it back to me." After the examiner tells the story, the patient retells the story and then again after a delay of 15 min or more. Examinees are advised to remember the story as they will be asked to retell it again later.

The story contains 17 units of information. In the ABCD-2 standardization study, normal elderly control subjects were able to retell, on average, 14.6 units of information immediately after hearing it (S.D. = 1.8) and 14.1 units of information after a delay (S.D. = 2.1). Individuals with mild AD averaged 7.3 units of information in the immediate condition (S.D.= 4.2) but only 1.1 units in the delayed (S.D. = 2.7).

The ABCD-2 Word Learning subtest involves five steps: controlled encoding of 16 words, a distractor task, free recall of the 16 words, use of category cues to facilitate the recall of items missed in the free-recall condition, and recognition of the 16 encoded words from among 48 words. Combining the free-recall and cued-recall scores results in a total recall score. The average total recall score of healthy elders was 15.6 (S.D. = .7); the average score of individuals with mild AD was 7.4 (S.D. = 4.6). For the recognition condition, normal elderly controls scored an average of 47.3 (S.D. = 1.3); individuals with mild AD scored 36.8 (S.D. = 6.8).

As an aside, the simple and reliable mental status subtest is increasingly being used, along with the memory tests, to screen at risk individuals. The subtest's 13 items evaluate orientation to time, place, and person, as well as general knowledge. It takes less than 5 min and requires no special training. The maximum possible score is 13. In the ABCD-2 standardization study, only 5% of the normal elderly had a score below 11.5; mild AD patients averaged 9.5 (S.D. = 3) and moderate AD patients averaged 5.3 (S.D. = 3.3).

Functional Linguistic Communication Inventory (FLCI) for Moderately and Severely Demented Individuals

The FLCI (Bayles & Tomoeda, 1994) characterizes the functional linguistic communication of moderately and severely demented individuals. Individuals who are severely demented find the ABCD-2 too difficult and are unable to do the majority of the subtests. The Functional Linguistic Communication Inventory (FLCI; Bayles & Tomoeda, 1994) was developed to document the functional communication abilities of moderately and severely demented individuals, important information for care providers.

Like ABCD-1, the FLCI evolved from NIH supported longitudinal studies of individuals with dementia and was standardized on 40 AD patients whose dementia severity was staged with a modified version of the Functional Assessment Stages (Reisberg, Ferris, & Franssen, 1985). Twenty individuals were tested twice with a one-week interval between administrations and high test–retest correlations were obtained for all FLCI subtests. The FLCI takes approximately 30 min to test the following skills:

- Naming and greeting
- Answering questions
- Participating in a conversation
- Comprehending signs and matching objects to pictures

- Reading and comprehending words
- Reminiscing
- Following commands
- Pantomiming
- Gesturing
- Writing

The FLCI score sheet enables clinicians to compare the performance of the examinee to that of AD patients in the standardization study. Also, the examinee's intact communicative functions can be charted (see Section V, "Reimbursement and Care Planning for Persons with Dementia" for typical FLCI profiles of individuals in the mild, moderate, moderately severe, severe, and very severe stages of dementia). Test results form the basis for functional maintenance programs and caregiver counseling.

Many Other Tests Are Available for Diagnosing MCI and Dementia

Tests of Mental Status

The Mini-Mental State Examination (MMSE; Folstein et al., 1975) is widely used (Shulman et al., 2006) and evaluates orientation to person, place, and time; general knowledge; memory; communication; and copying. It requires 5 to 10 min to administer. The total possible score is 30 and population-based norms by age and education level are available (Crum, Anthony, Bassett, & Folstein, 1993). Clinicians generally consider a score less than 24 as indicative of dementia (Desmond, 2002). Based on the results of our longitudinal studies, we suspect MCI in literate people with scores of 25 to 26 (Bayles, Tomoeda, Montgomery, Cruz, & Azuma, 2000). Similarly, Monsch et al. (1995) recommended that an MMSE score of less than 26 be used to indicate impairment.

Comprehensive reviews of the psychometric properties and uses of the MMSE have been reported by Tombaugh and McIntyre (1992) as well as Lezak, Howieson, Loring, Hannay, and Fischer (2004). Recently, Mitchell completed a meta-analysis of 34 dementia and five MCI studies to determine the accuracy of the MMSE for detecting dementia and MCI and reported that the MMSE had "very limited value in making a diagnosis of MCI against healthy controls . . . and similarly limited ability to help identify cases of Alzheimer's disease against MCI" (2009, p. 411). Mitchell concluded that the MMSE is best used to rule out a diagnosis of dementia in community and primary care settings.

Tests of Episodic Memory

A primary feature of AD is rapid forgetting of recent information; thus, it is unsurprising that the best measures for screening for AD are tests of episodic memory (Albert et al., 2011; Rentz & Weintraub, 2000). Reports from several comprehensive longitudinal studies indicate that *initial learning of information and loss of information over a delay interval* are the key characteristics that discriminate between nondemented elders and those with the earliest signs of AD (Grober & Kawas, 1997; Locascio et al.,1995; Robinson-Whelen & Storandt, 1992; Rubin et al., 1998; Welsh, Butters, Hughes, Mohs, & Heyman, 1991).

Examples of tests routinely used to measure a patient's ability to learn and recall information after a delay include the Logical Memory subtest (basically a story recall task) of the Wechsler Memory Scale–Revised (or other versions) (Wechsler, 2009) and the Buschke Selective Reminding Test (Buschke & Fuld, 1974), which requires learning, storing, and retrieving information after a delay via free- and cued-recall and recognition.

Verbal Fluency Tests

Tests of verbal fluency, also known as generative naming or category naming, are timed measures in which the subject must generate as many words as possible beginning with a letter (usually F, A, or S) or a semantic category (e.g., animals or fruits) in 60 s. In the Taler and Phillips (2008) review of over 70 studies involving patients with MCI, the majority of investigators reported differences between normal controls and those with MCI using a category fluency measure rather than a letter fluency measure. This finding was confirmed by Clark and colleagues (2009) who found greater longitudinal declines in category fluency than letter fluency in a cohort of normal, elderly, preclinical AD cases as well as AD patients followed for up to 5.9 years. Later, Mueller et al. (2015) examined the relation between phonemic and semantic verbal fluency and cognitive status and found that both phonemic and semantic fluency yielded lower scores in persons with evidence of psychometrically confirmed Alzheimer's-associated MCI compared with those who were cognitively healthy. The ABCD-2 has a category fluency subtest and comparison data on the performance of young and older healthy adults, individuals with MCI, mild and moderately severe AD patients, individuals with mixed dementia and individuals with Parkinson's disease.

Other Common Tests

To assess global cognition in individuals with dementia, Bossers, van der Woude, Boersma, Scherder, and van Heuvelen (2012) conducted a literature search to identify neuropsychological tests that were being used in randomized controlled trials to assess cognition in older individuals with dementia. Fifty-nine tests were identified and evaluated for their reliability and validity. As a result of their analyses the following recommendations were made:

- To assess global cognition, they recommended the Severe Impairment Battery (Saxton, McGonigle-Gibson, Swihart, Miller, & Boller, 1990), Mini Mental State Examination (Folstein et al.,1975), and the Alzheimer Disease Assessment Scale.
- To assess attention, they recommended Digit Span Forward, Digit Span Backward, and Trail Making Test–A.

- To assess executive functioning, they recommended verbal fluency, clock drawing, and Trail Making Test–B.
- They did not recommend a specific memory test. One to consider is the widely used Wechsler Memory Scale–Fourth Edition (WMS–IV; Wechsler, 2009). Another is the Rivermead Behavioral Memory Test–Second Edition (Wilson, Cockburn, & Baddeley, 1991).

Bossers and colleagues (2012) *did not evaluate measures for characterizing language skills*, an important omission given the evidence of early changes in language and cognitive function in AD and other dementing diseases. Naturally, the authors of this text recommend the ABCD-2 for evaluating language skills with the added bonus of also having tests for memory, mental status, and visuospatial construction. Another test that combines assessment of memory and verbal learning is the California Verbal Learning Test (CVLT; Delis, Kramer, Kaplan, & Ober, 2000). The CVLT is a standardized assessment of rate of word learning, retention after short- and long-delay intervals, semantic encoding ability, recognition memory, intrusion and perseverative errors, and response biases.

Broad-Based Assessments

Montreal Cognitive Assessment

The Montreal Cognitive Assessment (MoCA) Version 3 (Nasreddine, 2011) was developed as a quick screening tool for detecting MCI. It takes approximately 10 min and has items related to attention and concentration, executive function, memory, language, visuoconstruction, conceptual thinking, calculation, and orientation. One point is added to the sum of all subscores for an individual who has 12 or fewer years of formal education for a total maximum score of 30 points. MoCA scores of 26 or higher are considered normal. Using the cutoff score of 26 (with 25 or below indicative of impairment), Nasreddine et al. (2005) found the MoCA to be sensitive to detecting 90% of MCI subjects in contrast to the 18% detected by the MMSE.

However, that cutoff value was challenged as inflating the rate of false positives, especially for older or less educated individuals (Rossetti, Lacritz, Cullum, & Weiner, 2011). A meta-analysis by Carson, Leach, and Murphy (2017) of the several validation studies that have been carried out on the MoCA revealed that a *cutoff score of 23/30 resulted in better diagnostic accuracy.*

Repeatable Battery for the Assessment of Neuropsychological Status

The Repeatable Battery for the Assessment of Neuropsychological Status (RBANS) (Randolph, Tierney, Mohr, & Chase, 1998) was designed as a brief test to detect and characterize cognitive decline in adults between the ages of 20 and 89 who have neurological impairment from dementia, head injury, or stroke. The RBANS has parallel forms that allow for repeated evaluations to measure change in neuropsychological status over time. Five cognitive domains are evaluated: immediate memory, visuospatial/construction, language, attention, and delayed memory. Index scores adjusted for age for each of the five domains can be derived and summed for a total score.

The RBANS has been validated for use with persons with MCI (Karantzoulis, Novitski, Gold, & Randolph, 2013) and AD (Freilich & Hyer, 2007; Humphreys, Dempsey, O'Bryant, & Sutker, 2006; Randolph et al., 1998; Silva, Humphreys, Dempsey, O'Bryant, & Sutker, 2006). Duff, Hobson, Beglinger, and O'Bryant (2010) administered it to individuals with MCI and reported that they generally performed worse than cognitively intact peers. Although they reported good specificity for MCI, sensitivity was moderate to poor and caution was urged when using the RBANS to identify MCI (Duff et al., 2010).

Clark, Hobson, and O'Bryant (2010) suggested that greater diagnostic accuracy could

be achieved with the RBANS by using percent retention scores (delayed recall score on final learning trial). More recently, Karantzoulis et al. (2013) administered the RBANS to 81 individuals with MCI and compared their scores with those of healthy older adults. The MCI group was most impaired on the Delayed Memory Index and their performance was similar to that previously reported for mild AD patients. Thus, they concluded that it is a suitable battery for detecting and tracking MCI associated with AD.

Addenbrooke's Cognitive Examination (ACE)

The ACE was developed in 2000 by Mathuranath, Nestor, Berrios, Rakowicz, and Hodges and was revised in 2006 (Mioshi, Dawson, Mitchell, Arnold, & Hodges, 2006). The original version is a 100-point test designed to detect mild dementia and differentiate early AD from FTD. It incorporates and expands the MMSE memory, language, and visuospatial components, and adds letter and category fluency tests. In the Mathuranath et al. study, 139 new patients in a memory clinic were selected and classified into dementia or nondementia groups using the ACE. Using a cut-off score of 88, the ACE showed high reliability, construct validity for dementia, and sensitivity for identifying patients with dementia. The ratio of the scores of verbal fluency plus language (V + L) to orientation and recall memory (O + M) resulted in a VLOM ratio that differentiated mild AD patients from those with FTD. Larner (2007) confirmed that the ACE has good sensitivity, specificity, and predictive value for the diagnosis of dementia; however, it was less accurate in the differential diagnosis of AD and FTD.

The revised version (ACE-R; Mioshi et al., 2006) is easier to administer and was designed for cross-cultural use. It generates five subscores that are associated with the domains of attention/orientation, memory, fluency, language, and visuospatial skills and has a maximum score of 100. Results of administration of the ACE-R to subjects with AD, FTD, Lewy

Body dementia (LBD), MCI, and age-matched controls resulted in good reliability and concurrent and convergent validity. Changes to the ACE-R resulted in improved sensitivity, specificity, and positive predictive value for identifying patients with dementia. The VLOM ratio analysis of the ACE-R replicated results of the ACE (Mathuranath et al., 2000) for distinguishing AD from FTD, a finding that lead Mioshi and colleagues to advocate for its clinical utility.

Short Screening Tests

Although administering an array of tests in the specified cognitive domains is the best clinical practice, sometimes clinicians have to do a quick screening. The literature contains a number of reviews of two cognitive screening instruments for use in primary care settings (Brodaty, Low, Gibson, & Burns, 2006; Ismail, Rajji, & Shulman, 2010; Milne, Culverwell, Guss, Tuppen, & Whelton, 2008; Yokomizo, Simon, & Bottino, 2014): The Memory Impairment Screen and the 7-Minute Screen.

Memory Impairment Screen (MIS)

Buschke and colleagues (1999) developed the MIS that comprises a four-item delayed free- and cued-recall test that uses controlled learning to ensure encoding of information. The examinee is presented with four cards, each with a word from a different semantic category. The examinee is asked to read the word aloud (e.g., "potato") and associate it with its semantic category cue (e.g., "vegetable"). This is followed by a distracter task (counting from 1 to 20 forward and backward). Thereafter, the patient is asked to freely recall the four items (free recall). Category cues are provided only when the item is not retrieved during the free recall (cued recall). The MIS score is calculated as [2 × (free recall)] + (cued recall), resulting in scores ranging from 0 to 8. Scores of 4 or less are considered indicative of cognitive impair-

ment sufficient to warrant comprehensive assessment. Buschke et al. (1999) recommend that different cutoff scores be selected depending on whether the instrument is being used for clinical or research purposes. The MIS takes approximately 4 min to administer and equivalent, alternate forms are available.

7 Minute Screen (7MS)

The 7MS is an amalgam of 4 tests with previously demonstrated sensitivity to AD that are easy to administer and score (Solomon et al., 1998). It is called the 7-Minute Screen (7MS) because of the time it takes the average examinee to complete the test. The screen consists of Enhanced Cued Recall, Category Fluency, the Benton Temporal Orientation Test (Benton, 1983), and Clock Drawing. In the standardization study, the sensitivity of the screen was 92% and specificity was 96% for identifying individuals with AD in a population of patients referred to a memory disorders clinic and community-dwelling control patients (Solomon et al., 1998). Recently, Ijuin and colleagues (2008) reported that the sensitivity of the 7MS for detecting early-stage AD was 90.5% with specificity of 92.3%.

What About Aphasia Test Batteries?

Whereas many fine aphasia test batteries exist, they were not designed for individuals with dementia. Most are too easy for mildly and moderately demented Alzheimer's and Parkinson's patients and lack subtests of verbal episodic memory and mental status, important in differential diagnosis. For individuals with frontotemporal degeneration and vascular disease, aphasia batteries can be appropriate but they still need to be paired with tests of memory, mental status, and executive function to track the emergence and course of dementia. According to Kertesz, Davidson, McCabe, and Munoz (2003) behavioral quantitation is particularly sensitive to frontotemporal dementia.

ADAS-COG: Widely Used in Drug Trials

Finally, clinicians should be familiar with the previously mentioned Alzheimer's Disease Assessment Scale–Cognitive section (ADAS-Cog; Rosen, Mohs, & Davis, 1984, 1986) that was recommended by Bossers and colleagues (2012). The ADAS-Cog is a measure of cognitive function that is widely used in AD drug trials (Sevigny, Peng, Liu, & Lines, 2010) and the literature is replete with references to it (Doraiswamy, Kaiser, Beiber, & Garman, 2001; Sevigny et al., 2010; Verhey et al., 2004). The cognitive section is one of its two parts and consists of measures of word recall, spoken language, language comprehension, test instruction recall, word finding, following commands, naming, figure construction, ideational praxis, orientation, and word recognition. It is scored by errors, with a maximum error score of 70. The higher the score on the ADAS-Cog, the worse the performance.

The ADAS combines a mental status or cognitive portion with a behavioral rating portion (Weiner, 2003) and comprises 21 items. The entire ADAS takes approximately 45 min to administer and must be given by a professional trained in its administration.

Differentiating the Types of Dementia

Differentiating MCI and Mild Dementia from Delirium and Depression

Delirium

The diagnostic criteria for MCI and dementia specify that the cognitive deficits not be the result of *delirium*. Thus, clinicians need to know how to recognize delirium. Delirium is a confusional state that develops over a short period of time in which an affected individual experiences disturbances of consciousness, attention, cognition, and perception (American

Psychiatric Association, 1999). Fluctuations in symptoms are often reported (Cole et al., 2011; Downing, Caprio, & Lyness, 2013). Individuals with dementia are typically alert and do not have the disturbances of consciousness that characterize delirium, although individuals with Lewy Body often fluctuate in the level of their mental status.

A widely used clinical measure for identifying delirium is the Confusion Assessment Method (CAM) instrument (Inouye et al., 1990) that is designed to allow nonpsychiatry clinicians to assess the presence, severity, and fluctuation of nine features of delirium (see Wei, Fearing, Sternberg, & Inouye, 2008, for a systematic review of the instrument).

Depression

Depression is a disorder of mood in which an individual is preoccupied with negative thoughts. Although depressed individuals experience moments of happiness and laughter, overall their perspective is pessimistic. As previously mentioned, depression is particularly common in the elderly and associated with the following signs and somatic complaints:

- Poor appetite
- Loss of weight
- Constipation
- Fatigue
- Sleep problems
- Agitation
- Flat affect
- Irritability

In addition, certain behaviors are common in depressed individuals and include:

- Self-deprecatory comments
- Statements about feeling sad or helpless
- Failure to try
- Inattentiveness
- Indecisiveness
- Inconsistency in performance (better performance on some difficult tasks than would

Table I–10. Differentiating Dementia from Delirium and Depression

	Dementia	Delirium	Depression
Onset	Insidious	Acute	Acute
Conscious state	Impaired very late	Highly variable	Unusual
Mood	Stable	Variable consciousness	Depressed with diurnal variation
Duration	Long term	Short (Days)	Short (Weeks)
Cognitive Features	Reduced short-term memory greater than long-term memory	Short attention span	Reduced short- and long-term memory

Adapted and reproduced with permission from The Royal Australian College of General Practitioners from Popplewell, P., Phillips, P. Is it dementia? *Australian Family Physicians*, 2002; 31:319–321.

be expected, and poorer performance on some easy tasks than would be expected)
■ Worse performance in the morning
■ Slow speaking rate
■ Monotonous voice
■ Low volume

Popplewell and Phillips (2002) provide guidelines for distinguishing between dementia, delirium, and depression (Table I–10). The features best for identifying depression include the onset of the condition, the patient's conscious state, and mood.

The results of a meta-analysis by Ismail et al. (2017) of 57 studies that reported on the prevalence of depression in a combined MCI population of 20,892 individuals revealed that 32% of patients were depressed. Depression is also prevalent in individuals with dementia and a predictor of cognitive decline in older patients (Downing et al., 2013; Taylor, 2014). In fact, it is not unusual for *mild* AD patients, who realize that their memory and cognitive abilities are deteriorating, to become depressed. Similarly, delirium can complicate dementia, but it is typically triggered by another medical condition (e.g., high fever, bacterial infection, toxicity). If delirium is suspected, medical professionals should be alerted.

Differentiating Frontotemporal Dementias (FTD)

As described in Chapter 10, the consensus criteria for FTD described three forms (National Institute on Aging, 2017): (1) a *behavioral variant* in which early and progressive changes in personality and frontal executive functions are prominent (including Pick disease), (2) a *language variant* in which early and progressive changes in language function dominate the clinical picture (includes three variants of primary progressive aphasia), and (3) a *movement variant* in which movement disorders are the presenting symptom. The differences in clinical presentation described in Table I–11 can help distinguish individuals with mild AD from those with the behavioral and movement disorder variants of FTD.

Caregiver Questionnaires

Caregiver questionnaires have been developed for differentiating AD and the behavioral variant of FTD. These include the Neuropsychiatric Inventory (NPI; Cummings, 1997; Cummings et al., 1994), the Frontal Behavioral Inventory (FBI; Kertesz, Davidson, & Fox, 1997), and the

Table I–11. Comparison of Clinical Features of the Behavioral Variant of Frontotemporal Dementia (*bvFTD*) and Alzheimer's Disease (*AD*)

Feature	bvFTD	AD
Onset	Typically early (age 45–65 years)	Typically late (after age 65 years)
Personality changes	Appears early	Appears later
Affect	Blunted; unconcerned, indifferent	Concerned; may be anxious

Cambridge Behavioral Inventory (CBI; Wedderburn et al., 2008).

Neuropsychiatric Inventory (NPI). The NPI was developed to assess psychopathology in individuals with dementia (Cummings, 1997; Cummings et al., 1994). It evaluates the frequency and severity of 12 behavioral disturbances common in patients with dementia: delusions, dysphoria/depression, agitation/aggression, disinhibition, hallucinations, anxiety, euphoria/elation, irritability/lability, apathy/indifference, aberrant motor activity, nighttime behavior disturbances, and appetite/eating abnormalities. The NPI also evaluates the amount of caregiver distress generated by these behavioral disturbances. Cummings et al. (1994) demonstrated the content and concurrent validity, interrater reliability, test–retest reliability, and internal consistency of the NPI. Levy, Miller, Cummings, Fairbanks, and Craig (1996) reported that the NPI behavioral profiles are capable of differentiating patients with FTD from those with AD. A summary of the use of the NPI to measure frontal systems impairment in dementia can be found in Malloy and Grace (2005).

A shortened form, the NPI-Q, was developed to provide a brief, reliable version suitable for use in general clinical practice settings (Kaufer et al., 2000). The NPI-Q differs from the standard NPI in that it is a two-page, self-administered questionnaire rather than an interview, and each of the 12 symptom domains is assessed by a written question. If the informant indicates the symptom was present in the past 4 weeks, then the severity of the symptom is also rated. When the NPI and NPI-Q were administered to the informants of 60 AD subjects, symptom severity scores on both measures were highly correlated (Kaufer et al., 2000). Adequate test–retest reliability with the NPI-Q was also reported. More recently, Musa and colleagues (2017) examined the psychometric properties of the NPI-Q and reported positive and significant correlations between the NPI-Q and ACE-R as well as adequate reliability and validity for clinical use.

Frontal Behavioral Inventory (FBI). The FBI (Kertesz et al., 1997) is a 24-item questionnaire administered to caregivers. Half the items address *deficit* behaviors: apathy, indifference, disorganization, verbal apraxia, aspontaneity, inflexibility, personal neglect, alien hand, inattention, concreteness, loss of insight, and logopenia (paucity of speech). The other half address *excess* behaviors: perseveration, inappropriateness, restlessness, hypersexuality, irritability, impulsivity, aggression, incontinence, irresponsibility, excessive or childish jocularity, hyperorality, and utilization behavior (need to touch objects).

Each item is scored on a 4-point scale (none, mild, moderate, and severe). An optimal FBI cutoff score of 27 differentiates individuals with FTD from individuals with AD with 90% sensitivity and 100% specificity (Kertesz et al., 2003). The FBI was better than the Mini-Mental State Examination (Folstein et al., 1975) and the Mattis Dementia Rating Scale (Mattis, 1976) for differentiating FTD and AD patients (Kertesz et al., 2003), and a meta-analysis (Mathias & Morphett, 2010) also found the FBI to be excellent for distinguishing between AD and FTD. Moreover, researchers reported that FBI items can discriminate between individuals with the behavioral and language variants of FTD (Kertesz, Nadkarni, Davidson, & Thomas, 2000; Konstantiopoulou, Aretouli, Ioannidis, Karacostas, & Kosmidis, 2013).

Cambridge Behavioural Inventory. Based on previous work by Bozeat, Gregory, Lambon Ralph, and Hodges (2000), the Cambridge Behavioural Inventory (CBI; Wedderburn et al., 2008) is an 81-item, self-administered caregiver questionnaire to assess a patient's memory, orientation and attention, everyday skills, self-care, mood, beliefs, challenging behavior, disinhibition, eating habits, sleep, stereotypic behaviors, motivation, and insight. Caregivers rate these behaviors on a scale from 0 to 4, with higher scores reflecting more frequent problems.

A preliminary version of the CBI was found to have adequate test–retest reliability and concurrent validity (with the NPI) and discriminated patients with FTD and AD (Nagahama, Okina, Suzuki, & Matsuda, 2006). The FTD patients had more frequent symptoms of disinhibition, stereotypic behavior, elation/mood, anxiety, poor self-care, and changes in eating habits than patients with AD. Wedderburn and colleagues (2008) administered the CBI to carers of a large cohort of Parkinson's disease (PD), Huntington's disease (HD), Alzheimer's disease (AD), and behavioral variant FTD (bvFTD) patients and reported it to be useful and valid in discriminating between patients with a range of neurodegenerative diseases. However, Hancock and Larner (2008) reported that the CBI had limited diagnostic value in two separate samples of healthy adults and patients with dementia who varied in etiology. The CBI achieved only modest values for sensitivity, specificity, and positive predictive value (Hancock & Larner, 2008).

Recently, the CBI was revised (CBI-R; Wear et al., 2008) and shortened to 45 questions. Wear and colleagues reported that it differentiated patients with bvFTD, AD, PD, and HD and had high internal consistency.

Differentiating Primary Progressive Aphasia (PPA) and Mild AD

The SLP is often the first rehabilitation professional to see an individual with PPA because aphasia is a presenting symptom and the most prominent clinical feature. Impairments in memory and other cognitive functions do not occur until later; however, in AD they are the presenting symptoms (Warren, Harvey, & Rossor, 2005). The following are the key features of the variants of PPA and those of typical AD:

- *Logopenic variant*: Patients with the logopenic variant demonstrate difficulties with single word retrieval, sentence repetition, and semantic and phonological paraphasias.
- *Nonfluent agrammatic variant*: Patients with the nonfluent agrammatic variant produce agrammatic language and exhibit halting effortful speech.
- *Semantic dementia variant*: Patients with the semantic dementia variant demonstrate loss of memory for the meaning of words and objects. Their presenting complaint is usually difficulty finding or understanding words.
- *Typical mild AD*: Fluent noneffortful speech, normal grammar, occasional mild anomia, and severe episodic memory deficit.

It is important to note that the word "typical" was used to describe individuals with mild AD. This is because AD can present in atypical ways, and logopenic PPA may be a case in point. Individuals with logopenic PPA do have AD pathology, but the evolution of their cognitive symptoms differs in that the language disorder precedes the memory impairment so characteristic of typical mild AD patients. Consensus is lacking as to whether this form of PPA is an atypical form of AD or if logopenic PPA has a unique pathologic profile that includes some common pathologic features of AD (Beber, Kochhann, da Silva, & Chaves, 2014; Giannini et al., 2017; Madhavan et al., 2013). Regardless, to differentiate them, clinicians should administer both language and episodic memory tests.

Table I–12. Speech-Language Tasks Useful in Differentiating between Primary Progressive Aphasia (PPA) Variants

Speech-Language Function	Examples of Tasks	PPA Variant Impaired
Speech production–Grammar	Picture description, story retelling, etc.	Nonfluent agrammatic variant
Speech production–Motor speech	Motor speech evaluation, repetition of multisyllabic words, etc.	Nonfluent agrammatic variant
Confrontation naming	Single-word retrieval	Semantic variant severely impaired with semantic errors; logopenic variant moderately impaired with phonemic errors
Repetition	Oral repetition of words, phrases, sentences, etc.	Logopenic variant with phonologic errors
Sentence comprehension	Answering questions, following directions, etc.	Nonfluent agrammatic variant affected by grammatic complexity; logopenic variant affected by sentence length
Single-word comprehension	Matching word to picture or word to definition, etc.	Semantic variant
Object/people knowledge	Semantic associations, matching gesture to object, etc.	Semantic variant
Reading/spelling	Reading regular and irregular words or words from different word classes, etc.	Semantic variant with irregular words; logopenic variant producing phonologic errors

Source: Adapted from Gorno-Tempini et al. (2011).

In early semantic dementia, autobiographical (episodic) memory is typically preserved (Maguire, Kumaran, Hassabis, & Kopelman, 2010); in early AD, it is impaired. Le Rhun, Richard, and Pasquier (2006) reported that an analysis of responses on MMSE items aids in differentiating early PPA from AD. In their study, patients with PPA were significantly better on MMSE items related to word recall and constructional praxis, whereas AD patients were better on items related to word registration, object naming, sentence repetition, and following verbal instructions.

Snowden (2005) suggests careful testing of memory because semantic dementia is most commonly misdiagnosed as AD. He advocates the use of tests of word naming and comprehension and face and object recognition to aid in the differentiation of semantic dementia from AD. Gorno-Tempini et al. (2011) provide a summary of the language tasks that may be used to assess speech and language functions in PPA and how to identify the PPA variant in which the speech-language function is most impaired (Table I–12).

An Assessment for Differentiating Semantic Dementia: The Cambridge Semantic Memory Test

Adlam, Patterson, Bozeat, and Hodges (2010) reported on a test battery that is sensitive to mild semantic deficits called the Cambridge Semantic Memory (CSM) test battery. The CSM test battery (Adlam et al., 2010) consists of a collection of tests that use the same stimulus items to assess semantic knowledge via dif-

Table I–13. Comparison of Clinical Features of Vascular Dementia (*VaD*) and Alzheimer's Disease (*AD*)

	VaD	AD
History of hypertension	Usually present	Not necessarily present
Focal neurologic signs	Present	Generally absent
Brain areas involved	Cortical or subcortical dysfunction	Cortical dysfunction
Disease progression	Usually abrupt or stepwise deterioration, but may also be gradual	Gradual decline over time

ferent input and output modalities. Sixty-four items represent three categories of living things (animals, birds, and fruit) and three categories of manmade things (household items, tools, and vehicles). The test assesses category fluency, naming, word comprehension (word-to-picture matching), sorting by category using pictures at three levels (superordinate, basic and subordinate), and sorting by category at three levels to evaluate semantic association. The battery has two forms: one in which all stimuli are presented as pictures and another in which all items are presented in words. The patient is shown a stimulus item (target) and asked to select the one item, of four same-category items, that is associated with the target. For example, for the target "camel," the four choices are tree, sunflower, cactus (correct response), and rose.

The CSM test battery and a number of other neuropsychological tests were administered to a control group and seven patients with MCI, eight patients with AD, and 15 patients with semantic dementia (Adlam et al., 2010). Semantic deficits were most consistent and pronounced in the semantic dementia group, although some degree of semantic memory impairment was observed for all patient groups on the CSM test battery. The authors concluded that the CSM is sensitive but not specific, and cannot be used alone to differentiate MCI, AD, and semantic dementia. Use of the CSM test battery with large samples of patients are needed and are likely forthcoming.

Differentiating AD from Vascular Dementia

Researchers have documented that vascular pathology and AD often co-occur; therefore, it is helpful to know the medical/clinical features of both diseases. Tables I–13 and I–14 provide general summary information that can be useful in distinguishing the two patient populations and recognizing their co-occurrence.

Assessment Instruments for Vascular Dementia (VaD)

Neuropsychological assessment and rating scales have been used to determine the presence of VaD. The most widely used instrument is the Hachinski Ischemic Scale (HIS) (Hachinski et al., 1975).

Hachinski Ischemic Scale (HIS) (Hachinski et al., 1975). The HIS comprises 13 items that are considered typical of the dementia associated with multiple infarctions. Moroney et al. (1997) administered the HIS to neuropathologically confirmed patients with AD, VaD, and mixed dementia (AD and VaD) and reported that a score of 4 or less was typical of individuals with AD and a score of 7 or more was typical of those with VaD. Items that distinguished *VaD from AD* included:

- Stepwise deterioration
- Fluctuating course

Table I-14. Differences between Cognitive Profiles of Vascular Dementia (*VaD*) and Alzheimer's Disease (*AD*)

Feature	Difference between VaD and AD
Cognitive impairment	May be greater overall in VaD
Executive function impairment	Prominent in VaD
	Often early feature in VaD
	Manifests as relatively greater degree of impairment in frontal lobe functions in VaD, such as:
	Attention
	Working memory
	Planning
	Sequencing
	Abstraction
	Speed of mental processing
Perseveration	More prominent in VaD

Source: Modified from Ferris and Gauthier (2002).

- Focal neurologic symptoms
- Hypertension
- History of stroke

The two items that differentiated *mixed dementia from VaD* were stepwise deterioration and emotional incontinence and the two that *differentiated mixed dementia from AD* were fluctuating course and history of stroke.

Critical Analysis of Literature on Differentiating VaD and AD

Sachdev and Looi (2003) conducted a systematic computerized literature search of several bibliographic databases for articles published between January 1966 and December 2000 that reported a comparison of the performance of individuals with VaD and AD on neuropsychological tests. The studies were scrutinized to determine if they met strict criteria for inclusion in their analysis and 32 studies were selected for the final review. Studies were grouped according to the broad cognitive domain(s) that were assessed (e.g., intelligence, language, nonverbal memory, etc.). Sachdev and Looi (2003) reported that despite the relative heterogeneity of VaD pathology and diagnostic criteria used, group differences

were found in the neuropsychological profiles of the two groups:

- Individuals with VaD had relatively preserved long-term memory, greater impairment in frontal-executive function, and greater motor dysfunction than individuals with AD.
- No clear differences could be determined on tests of language, constructional abilities, memory registration, conceptual function, visual perception, and attention and tracking.

Based on these findings, Sachdev and Looi recommend tests of verbal long-term memory, such as the California Verbal Learning Test (Delis et al., 2000).

Matioli and Caramelli (2010) investigated the diagnostic value of brief cognitive tests in differentiating VaD and AD and concluded that the value of such instruments was very limited. The VaD patients performed worse on category and letter fluency and CLOX 2 and AD patients were worse in delayed recall.

In an effort to diminish the pervasive problem of heterogeneity among patients with vascular dementia, Graham, Emery, and Hodges (2004) focused on patients with subcortical vascular dementia and compared their cognitive performance to AD patients matched for age, education, and general level of cognitive function. After administering a range of neuropsychological tests, they found that the two groups could be discriminated using two tests: the Wechsler Memory Scale–Revised (WMS-R; Wechsler, 1987) logical memory–delayed recall test and a silhouette naming test. The WMS-R logical memory test is a story retelling task, and the silhouette naming test, a subtest of the Visual Object and Space Perception Battery (Warrington & James, 1991), requires subjects to name silhouette drawings of common animals and objects.

Differentiating Mild AD from Dementia with Lewy Bodies (DLB) and Parkinson's Disease with Dementia (PDD)

As described in Chapters 7 and 8, scientists now view Parkinson's disease with dementia (PDD) and dementia with Lewy bodies (DLB) as neurodegenerative conditions that share many pathological and clinical features, including a common disorder of α-synuclein metabolism (Emre et al., 2007; Tröster, 2008). The diagnosis of PDD is made when dementia develops in a patient in whom PD is well established, whereas a diagnosis of DLB is appropriate when the diagnosis of dementia precedes or occurs within a year of development of motor symptoms (Emre et al. 2007).

For at least three decades, researchers have recognized that DLB is associated with the presence of Lewy bodies in cortical and subcortical structures and neuronal loss; plus, 75% of individuals with DLB have the characteristic neuropathologic features of AD—particularly amyloid plaques (Hansen et al. 1990; Tröster, 2008). Both DLB and AD patients exhibit progressive decline in cognitive functioning; however, the other characteristic features of DLB that distinguish it from AD as can be seen in Table I–15. Undoubtedly, additional findings will emerge about the neuropsychological characteristics of each condition from investigations in which the revised diagnostic criteria for PDD and DLB are used; nonethe-

less, a review of past literature reveals that DLB is generally associated with greater deficits in attention, visuospatial, and executive function (Donaghy & McKeith, 2014; Hansen et al., 1990; Kemp et al., 2017; Noe et al., 2004). In comparison, AD is associated with greater episodic memory deficits than DLB. The clinical features that best differentiate DLB and AD in the early stage of dementia are visual hallucinations and visuospatial/construction impairments (Tiraboschi et al., 2006).

The neuropsychological profile of patients with PDD can be summarized as demonstrating deficits in memory, visuospatial, and executive functions (Emre et al., 2007). These three cognitive domains are affected early, even in patients with PD-MCI (Aarsland et al., 2010), with memory impairment being most common, followed by visuospatial, and then attention/executive function impairment. Language is reported to be less impaired in PDD than AD (Emre et al., 2007; Tröster, 2008), although we (Bayles & Tomoeda, 1993) found that the eight PDD subjects in our ABCD validation study to be similar to AD subjects in degree of impairment on most ABCD subtests. Then too, the sample of PDD subjects performed significantly worse than mildly demented AD subjects on four ABCD subtests (Object Description, Comparative Questions, Generative Naming, and Figure Copying).

Screening Instruments for PDD

The Parkinson Study Group Cognitive/Psychiatric Task Force reviewed a number of cognitive screening measures for potential use in clinical trials of individuals with PD (Chou et al., 2010). To be reviewed, all measures needed to be brief (less than 15 min to administer). The task force recommended the Montreal Cognitive Assessment (MoCA; Nasreddine, 2011) as a minimum cognitive screening instrument for PD clinical trials. Other investigators (Kehagia, Barker, & Robbins, 2010) reported that two simple bedside assessments—the pentagon copying task of the MMSE and a semantic fluency task—were sensitive to predicting cognitive decline in PDD 3 years and 5 years

Table I–15. Comparison of Clinical Features of Lewy Body Disease (*LBD*) and Alzheimer's Disease (*AD*)

Clinically, LBD patients are more likely than AD patients to have the following:

1. *Fluctuating cognitive impairment*—Fluctuation in cognitive function is common and apparent in the early stages of LBD (McKeith et al., 1996). The degree and frequency of fluctuation can vary between individuals and within the same individual.

2. *Visual and/or auditory hallucinations*—The visual hallucinations of LBD patients are typically detailed, well formed, and recurrent (McKeith et al., 1996), and occur in 93% of cases; whereas auditory hallucinations are less common, occurring in approximately 50% of cases (Bolla, Filley, & Palmer, 2000). Hallucinations appear early in the disease course (Luis et al., 1999).

3. *Confusional state and clouding of consciousness*—The fluctuation in cognitive status can be the result of transient confusion and variability in attention and alertness (McKeith et al., 1996).

4. *Symptoms of parkinsonism*—Parkinsonian features that can appear early in LBD include rigidity and bradykinesia, hypophonia, stooped posture, problems with balance, and a slow shuffling gait. In AD, parkinsonian features appear late in the disease.

5. *Shorter duration of illness*—Patients with LBD experience a shorter illness duration that is about half as long as for patients with AD (McKeith, Fairbairn, Perry, & Thompson, 1994).

6. *Sensitivity to neuroleptics*—LBD patients are extremely sensitive to neuroleptic drugs, such as risperidone or haloperidol, to the degree that the reaction can be life-threatening (Bolla et al., 2000).

later (Williams-Gray et al., 2009; Williams-Gray, Foltynie, Brayne, Robbins, & Barker, 2007). Parashos, Johnson, Erickson-Davis, and Wielinski (2009) used the Cognitive-Linguistic Quick Test (CLQT; Helm-Estabrooks, 2001) as a cognitive screening tool in PD patients with and without dementia and found the CLQT to be similar to the MMSE in sensitivity and specificity for dementia in PD. Memory was most affected in the PDD group and attention was most affected in the nondemented PD group.

Summary of Important Points

- Assessment of cognitive function is critical to the diagnosis of MCI and dementia because by definition these are conditions of cognitive impairment.
- Early identification of MCI and dementia is profoundly important because many cases are treatable and others will benefit from drugs that slow disease progression, cognitive stimulation, and lifestyle changes.
- Comprehensive evaluation of cognitive and language functions is needed to correctly di-

agnose the myriad conditions associated with MCI and dementia.

- Prior to testing: review the medical history; arrange for a good test environment; check hearing, vision, and literacy; and build rapport to reduce test anxiety.
- Be alert to possible depression and drug effects that can invalidate test performance and lead to an incorrect diagnosis.
- Depressed individuals typically have many somatic complaints and communicate a sense of helplessness and despair. Inconsistency of performance is a red flag for depression.
- Individuals with delirium typically have an acute medical condition that causes variability in their conscious state.
- Speech-language pathologists have an important role in screening for MCI and characterizing dementia because change in language performance is a common early symptom.
- To obtain valid and reliable information about a client's cognitive-communicative abilities, use tests that have been standardized on individuals with dementia (for whom etiology and severity are specified) and healthy adults.

- The behavioral diagnostic criteria for MCI include a performance on neuropsychological tests that is 1 to 1.5 SD below the mean of healthy elders with similar education.
- Comprehensive evaluation of cognition should include measures of language comprehension and production, attention, memory, visuospatial and visuoconstructive skills, mental status, and executive function.
- Presence of episodic memory impairment is a red flag for possible AD.
- Prominent visual spatial impairment is a red flag for possible LBD.
- Aberrant behavior is a red flag for the bvFTD.
- Progressive language impairment is a red flag for PPA.
- The Arizona Battery of Communication Disorders of Dementia (ABCD) is a standardized battery designed to evaluate cognition and language in individuals at risk for MCI and those with mild and moderate dementia.
- The ABCD has subtests for evaluating language comprehension, language expression, verbal memory, visuoconstruction, and mental status as well as screening tasks to rule out illiteracy or hearing loss.
- ABCD subtests can be given individually or collectively to obtain a construct score (e.g., Linguistic Expression Ability) or overall score.
- The Story Retelling subtests (Immediate and Delayed) of the ABCD are a time-efficient and sensitive method for screening for Alzheimer's dementia.
- Of the 14 ABCD subtests, the Repetition subtest is particularly sensitive to cognitive impairment in individuals at risk for MCI.
- The Story Retelling–Immediate and Delayed and Word Learning subtests are the ABCD subtests most sensitive to frank dementia.
- The Functional Linguistic Communication Inventory is a standardized battery for evaluating the ability to comprehend and produce language in individuals with moderately-severe and severe dementia.

- Dementia is not to be confused with delirium, a confusional state that develops over a short period of time and is characterized by a disturbance of consciousness.
- Frontotemporal dementia (FTD) has three variants—a behavioral presentation, a language presentation, and a motor disorders presentation.
- Individuals with behavioral variant FTD *present* with early changes in personality and executive functioning and relatively preserved memory and visuospatial skills.
- Individuals with the FTD language variant of nonfluent agrammatic aphasia *present* with effortful, halting speech with speech sound errors and impaired comprehension of syntactically complex sentences.
- Individuals with the FTD language variant of logopenic aphasia *present* with impaired naming and speech and impaired sentence and word repetition.
- Individuals with the FTD language variant of semantic dementia *present* with progressive loss of conceptual knowledge with relative sparing of episodic memory.
- Individuals with VaD typically have history of hypertension, focal neurologic signs, abrupt or stepwise deterioration, and impairment in executive function.
- The primary symptom that typifies AD is episodic memory impairment.
- Parkinson's disease and Lewy body disease share many pathological and clinical features. In PD, motor symptoms typically develop before dementia; in LBD dementia precedes or occurs early within a year of development of motor symptoms.
- Individuals with LBD often have fluctuating cognitive impairment, visual and auditory hallucinations, and parkinsonism features.
- The three primary features of individuals with PDD are memory, visuospatial, and executive function impairment.

II

Cognitive Intervention

A Treatment Model for Successful Clinical Intervention

Speech-language pathologists (SLPs) have a significant role in providing services at all stages of the cognitive impairment continuum in an effort to sustain abilities or delay the effects associated with dementing diseases. A clinician who knows a client's profile of processing deficits and strengths can design a person-centered care plan that can produce positive changes in the brain. The best outcomes occur if treatment is implemented in the earliest phases of the dementia continuum, when individuals retain the capability to learn and apply strategies for sustaining function. The following treatment guidelines are appropriate for individuals with mild cognitive impairment (MCI) and those with mild to moderate dementia. Individuals with severe dementia typically have a care program to sustain them at their highest level of functioning that does not usually include individual therapy.

This model is designed to be a patient-centered approach using the science-based principles of learning (Caeyenberghs et al., 2018; Kleim & Jones, 2008; Nudo & Bury, 2011) and the results of studies of cognitive stimulation programs (Belleville et al., 2018; Jean, Beregeron, Thivierge, & Simard, 2010; Li et al., 2011; Rebok et al., 2014; Simon, Yokomizo, & Bottino, 2012; Stott & Spector, 2011):

1. Make treatment person centered
2. Target client skills and behaviors that have the potential to improve
3. Provide individual and group therapy
4. Provide training of strategies that can improve function
5. Use repetition and repeated retrieval training to create and strengthen new learning
6. Include neuro-proactive education about physical, mental, and social health
7. Provide opportunities to support communicative engagement and socialization
8. Ensure that duration of treatment is sufficient to strengthen skills and create learning
9. Use objective and subjective measures of skill strength and learning

Cognitive Intervention for Mild Cognitive Impairment (MCI)

Mild cognitive impairment (MCI) is a recognized stage on the continuum of cognitive deterioration that is associated with dementia-producing diseases. At this stage, the cognitive deficits are insufficient to meet the criteria for dementia and do not prevent those affected from performing the basic activities of daily living. Language performance impairments are common because the production and comprehension of language is inseparable from cognition. Thus, SLPs have an important role in the early detection of MCI, as well as in providing services that can slow or prevent progression to dementia.

Individuals with MCI are ideal candidates for clinical intervention because they retain the capability to learn and therefore build "cognitive reserve." The fact is, the degree to which an individual can adapt to the effects of aging, brain injury, and disease depends on the individual's cognitive reserve: a term used to refer to brain resiliency. Individuals with greater cognitive reserve have richer and more extensive synaptic networks and are therefore better able to compensate for brain damage. The strength of cognitive reserve is related to brain size, level of education, and life experiences. Individuals with larger brains, more education, and who have had cognitively challenging careers have greater cognitive reserve and a reduced risk of dementia (Rouillard et al., 2017).

Cognitive Reserve Is *"Neuroprotective"*

The truth in the claim that greater cognitive reserve is neuroprotective is apparent from studies of individuals with Alzheimer's disease (AD). Consider that even though two individuals have the same degree of brain pathology, those with higher levels of cognitive

reserve display fewer clinical symptoms. Research has shown that some individuals with extensive brain pathology display few, if any, cognitive deficits in life (Arriagada, Growdon, Hedley-Whyte, & Hyman, 1992; Bennett et al., 2006; Driscoll & Troncoso, 2011; Katzman et al., 1988). In fact, approximately 25% of individuals with AD pathology, whose brains undergo postmortem examination, are symptom free in life (Bennett et al., 2006; Ince, 2001; Mufson, Malek-Ahmadi, Perez, & Chen, 2016).

Cognitive Intervention Strengthens Cognitive Reserve

Evidence now exists that cognitive intervention can produce positive changes in the brains of individuals with MCI (Belleville & Bherer, 2012; Hampstead et al., 2011; Hampstead, Towler, Stringer, & Sathian, 2018; van Paasschen et al., 2013). These changes include increased brain metabolism, cortical thickness, and density of white matter tracts (Belleville & Bherer, 2012; Engvig et al., 2010; Mufson et al., 2015). Or, said another way, cognitive interventions increase cognitive reserve. Therefore, it is widely accepted that cognitive therapy can slow cognitive decline and lessen functional disability in individuals with MCI (Belleville et al., 2011; Belleville et al., 2018; Hampstead, Stinger, Stilla, Giddens, & Sathian, 2012; Hampstead et al., 2018; Jak, Seelye, & Jurick, 2013; Jean et al., 2010; Li et al., 2011; Rebok et al., 2014; Simon et al., 2012; Stott & Spector, 2011). Cognitive interventions have also been reported to improve quality of life for individuals with MCI (Jelcic et al., 2012; Tesky et al., 2017; Woods, Aguirre, Spector, & Orrell, 2012). Unsurprisingly, the best outcomes from cognitive intervention programs (CIPs) occur when a program is implemented early.

Worthy of note is the recent recommendation by the American Academy of Neurology (Petersen et al., 2018) that individuals with MCI and their family members be provided with information about the potential benefit of cognitive intervention. This recommendation followed a similar statement from the National

---

Box II–1. Definitions of Neuroplasticity and Cognitive Reserve

Neuroplasticity: The brain's ability to continually change in response to stimulation. Positive changes in response to stimulation result in increased *cognitive reserve*.

Cognitive reserve: Neuroprotection that helps compensate for typical and atypical cognitive-communicative changes resulting from aging or pathology.

Academies of Sciences, Engineering, and Medicine (NASEM, 2017) and was soon endorsed by the Alzheimer's Association. In 2017, the World Health Organization (WHO) released a comprehensive action plan that emphasizes prevention as a key component in the global response to dementia (WHO, 2017).

Make Treatment Person Centered

Patient-centered care is "respectful of and responsive to individual patient preferences, needs, and values, and ensuring that patient values guide all clinical decisions." (IOM's Quality Chasm Report, 2001, p. 6). Epstein and colleagues remind us that patient-centered care is the right thing to do as it improves patient care and well-being, bridges socioeconomic and cultural disparities, and leads to better value in terms of the health care dollar (Epstein, Fiscella, Lesser, & Strange, 2010).

In 2001, the World Health Organization (WHO) adopted a framework (International classification of functioning, disability and health; ICF) for evaluating health and disability to foster the provision of person-centered care (Table II–1). This framework emphasizes the importance of evaluating the *physical* and *mental health* of individuals as well as their *social functioning* (World Health Organization, 2001). Taken together, these three components provide a full picture of the health of the individual. Clearly these components are interrelated, that is, impairment in one component has consequences for the other two. Because dementia-producing diseases affect all three components, therapy programs that are designed to support all three have the greatest positive impact and are most likely to be person centered.

The following are examples of why it is important to consider the physical, mental, and social state of your clients in planning intervention. Consider that individuals with probable Parkinson's disease MCI (PD-MCI) have significant physical challenges that individuals with probable AD-MCI do not have. For example, their bradykinesia makes them very slow in completing the basic activities of daily life and family members often become frustrated with their slowness. Additionally, their physical weakness often results in a soft, barely audible voice that makes it hard for others to hear them. Their slowness and soft voice are two examples of conditions that need to

Table II–1. International Classification of Functioning, Disability, and Health Framework for Intervention with Mild Cognitive Impairment (*MCI*)

Health Condition: MCI (i.e., performance on a standardized assessment [e.g., ABCD] of 1 to 2 SD below the mean of healthy elders)		Intervention Focus
Body Functions and Structures	Subtle impairments in memory, language, and executive functions.	Target client skills and behaviors that have the potential to improve.
Activity	Improve performance on cognitive-linguistic tasks.	Use repetition and repeated retrieval training to create and strengthen new learning.
Participation	Increase participation in life roles.	Provide opportunities to support communicative engagement and socialization.
Contextual Factors: Personal and Environmental	Address modifiable risk factors and modifiable protective factors.	Include neuro-proactive education about physical, mental, and social health.

be taken into consideration when planning intervention. Individuals with probable behavioral variant frontotemporal dementia MCI (bvFTD-MCI) have aberrant behavior early that creates social challenges that individuals with PD and AD do not typically have. The nature of their behaviors may prevent them from being candidates for group therapy. Hearing loss is prevalent in older individuals and often goes untreated. Individuals with MCI who have untreated hearing loss often become socially isolated. Clearly, they are likely to have difficulty in group therapy and fail to gain the full benefit of individual therapy. By using the approach to evaluation recommended by the World Health Organization, clinicians are better prepared to plan intervention.

Suggestions for How To Make Therapy Person Centered

- Be familiar with the culture of the client.
- Know the modifications in your behavior that you must make to gain the respect and trust of your client.
- Know how to correctly pronounce the client's name.
- Know the occupation of the client.
- Have a sense of the degree to which the client has a support system.
- Interview the client about hobbies and preferred leisure activities.
- Comprehensively evaluate the cognitive and linguistic abilities of the client.
- Ask the client what goals he or she would like to achieve.
- Work with the client to set therapy goals.
- Solicit feedback from the client after therapy sessions.

Target Skills and Behaviors that Have the Potential to Improve

By definition, those with MCI exhibit mild impairments and are most likely to benefit from intervention because they retain the capability

to learn. That being said, clinicians should pay careful attention to the results of objective measures of impairment as well as self-reported subjective complaints that persons with MCI perceive as negatively impacting their daily life. Complaints or inconveniences reported by individuals with MCI may include:

Remembering names of people

Remembering names of objects

Difficulty focusing

Problems in paying attention

Trouble concentrating

Self-reported memory and language complaints even without objective impairment can be a preclinical indicator of AD (Tripodis et al., 2017). Self-reported subjective complaints in the domains of attention, executive function, or visuospatial impairments may be preclinical indicators of non-AD dementias such as vascular disease or PD (Pistacchi, Gioulis, Contin, Sanson, & Marsala, 2015).

Taking into account both objective impairments and self-reported complaints, intervention should target skills that will improve day-to-day functioning. Skills and strategies that can be implemented daily will be perceived as more meaningful and are more likely to generalize and be maintained beyond the intervention program.

Provide Individual and Group Therapy

Most successful cognitive intervention programs (CIPs) provide individual *and* group training. Individual training is needed to meet a client's specific needs in terms of cognitive therapy; group therapy provides social stimulation and opportunities for skill practice and developing new relationships. The provision of both is easier if two clinicians are available; one can provide the individual treatments, while the other manages the group. Nonetheless, there are ways for both types of therapy to be provided by a single clinician. For example, a circuit of cognitive stimulation "stations" can be created using computers and/or paper and pencil tasks. Clients can move between them while the clinician works individually with the various group members. Another alternative is to have individuals come in alone for individual therapy but together for group sessions. Based on a meta-analyses of cognitive intervention programs, Sherman and colleagues report that a group format is most frequently used (46% of the time), followed by computer-based programs (38% of the time), and then individual plus small group training (15% of the time) (Sherman, Mauser, Nuno, & Sherzai, 2017).

Provide Training of Strategies that Can Improve Function

It is the role of the clinician to provide strategies that improve the client's function and opportunities for practicing them. Particularly troubling to many individuals with MCI is remembering to remember. This type of memory is called prospective memory. Examples of prospective memory include remembering to give a message to a friend, silencing one's cell phone in a doctor's office, and taking a medication on time (Devanand, Liu, & Brown, 2017). Providing strategies that enable individuals to remember include use of external memory aids (e.g., keeping lists, writing down important information) and self-generated approaches (e.g., visual imagery, forming associations, method of loci).

Memory strategy training is a common feature of reviews of cognitive intervention programs (Jean et al., 2010; Sherman et al., 2017). In fact, according to these reviews, nearly half of the programs reviewed emphasized them. Then too, statistically significant improvements on objective measures of memory were obtained after training. Moreover, memory training was reported to positively impact performance in other cognitive domains.

Belleville et al. (2011) provide empirical support for training-specific strategies as a treatment for memory impairment in individuals with MCI. They provided a 6-week program for small groups of four or five people; sessions lasted 2 hrs. The treatment focus was mnemonics and techniques to promote elaborate encoding and retrieval of information. Study participants underwent functional magnetic resonance imaging (fMRI) before and after training. Results revealed increased activation in a large brain network typically associated with memory. Moreover, the memory training appeared to normalize the brain activation deficits associated with MCI, because posttest activation levels in the MCI group were similar to those of the control participants. In sum, the study results are more evidence that the MCI brain remains plastic and improves with intervention.

Hampstead and colleagues (2012) conducted a study to evaluate the benefit of learning a mnemonic strategy for encoding the location of objects in a computerized virtual home with nine rooms and recalling them later. Twenty-eight individuals with MCI as well as healthy older adults ($n = 21$) participated and were randomly assigned to either a strategy training group or a repeated exposure group. In this design, some of the adults with MCI learned the mnemonic strategy and some only experienced the exposure. Similarly, there were some healthy adults who learned the mnemonic strategy and others who only experienced the exposure condition. The mnemonic strategy consisted of a series of steps in which participants identified a salient feature in each room that was close to the target object to be remembered. Thereafter, they were told to verbally link the object to the room. Next, they were told to create a detailed mental image (or "movie") of the object, the room feature, and the fact linking the object to the room. Participants in both the strategy training group and the repeated exposure group were given six opportunities to see the location of each object. Later, they were shown the objects and asked to identify their location. For both the MCI and healthy adults, the mnemonic strategy training condition proved superior

Table II–2. Commonly Taught Memory Strategies

Strategy	Description
Method of Loci	Mentally linking a place with an item to be remembered.
STOP mnemonic	"Stop, Think, Organize, Plan"
Mind Mapping/Semantic Feature Analysis	Connections between a central word or idea are made using a diagram.
Visual Imagery (e.g., face-name associations)	Mental images are created to facilitate learning and recall of material.
Categorization and Hierarchical Organization	Aimed at classifying information to be learned by semantic category or by order of importance.
Chunking	Grouping information to be remembered.
External Prospective Memory Aids	Teach use of calendars, datebooks, or other devices (apps on smart phones, tablets, etc.).

to the repeated exposure condition. All study participants had fMRI scanning before and after training. Scans conducted before training showed reduced volume in the medial temporal lobes during encoding and retrieval in the MCI group. Following the mnemonic strategy training, both MCI participants and healthy controls had increased volume in the medial temporal lobes during encoding and retrieval as well as improved delayed memory scores as measured by performance on the Repeatable Battery for the Assessment of Neuropsychological Status (RBANS). For the exposure group, both MCI participants and healthy controls demonstrated improvement on the RBANs, but increased volume in the medial temporal lobes was not observed.

Clare and colleagues (Clare, Evans, Parkinson, Woods, & Linden, 2011; Clare et al., 2009) reported good results with an intervention that allowed participants to select one or two strategies for achieving functional goals related to completion of household tasks, leisure activities, and self-care. Study participants were introduced to strategies for acquiring new information including verbal and visual mnemonics, semantic elaboration, and expanding rehearsal. Participants received eight weekly, 1-hr sessions and were encouraged to practice at home. All participants learned and practiced

all strategies and then chose a preferred strategy to implement in their daily lives (see Table II–2).

Simon and colleagues (2017) also reported benefits of mnemonic strategy training in individuals with MCI. In their study, 30 participants with MCI were randomly assigned to either a mnemonic strategy training group for face-name associations or an education group, which served as an active control. Both groups received eight 1-hr sessions. Positive results were observed for those in the mnemonic strategy training group on both objective and subjective measures. Further, fMRI neuroimaging results for the mnemonic strategy training group revealed greater brain activation in the regions of the brain associated with interpreting faces and social cues, perception of physical features and emotions, and semantic memory and associative thinking.

Use Repetition and Repeated Retrieval to Create and Strengthen New Learning

Repeated exposure to information or repeated practice of a skill, the better the skill; the more exposure to information, the more enduring the memory of it. Repetition programs to enhance skills or create new knowledge can be likened to a workout session at a gym. However, rather than targeting muscle groups, the focus is repeated practice of a specific skill or repeated use of new information. Rather than doing "reps" on gym equipment, clients get repetition through face-to-face drills with the clinician, completion of many paper and pencil tasks, or computerized practice.

Computer-Based Training

A decade ago, the typical elder did not know how to use a computer. Today, most clients own a computer, smartphone, or tablet and know how to access the Internet. Many clients enjoy playing computerized games and the popularity of commercial brain fitness products has skyrocketed. Brain fitness products are now a multi-billion dollar industry (SharpBrains.com, 2013). Naturally, they are popular with clinicians because of their many advantages:

- Cost effective
- Provide multiple training options
- Allow for standardized procedures
- Are easily accessed in the clinic and at home
- Provide instant feedback to the user and clinician
- Provide an objective review of performance
- Are graduated in difficulty

Types of Computer Programs

There are three basic types of computer-based programs (Kueider, Parisi, Gross, & Rebok, 2012). The first type consists of programs designed to address a *specific domain of cognition* (e.g., processing speed or memory) through guided practice on a task graduated in difficulty. Clinicians can find programs that are designed to improve attention, memory, perception, visuospatial skills, cognition, language, and executive functions. The second type is designed to enhance *multiple cognitive domains* simultaneously through a variety of tasks. These types of programs provide instant performance feedback and are self-guided to enable participants to progress at their own pace. This more global training approach has produced good results in the domains of memory and visuospatial ability, but is less effective for improving attention and executive function. The third type is *video games*. Players manipulate images on a screen to achieve a goal. Game playing can enhance reaction time, processing speed, executive function, and global cognition in older adults (Basak, Boot, Voss, & Kramer, 2008).

Barnes et al. (2009) investigated the efficacy and feasibility of using an intensive computer-based, home-training program to improve processing speed and accuracy in auditory processing. All program participants were provided an at-home computer and access to Posit Science Corporation software. Participants with MCI used the program for 100 min per day, 5 days per week, for 8 weeks. The software used by the intervention group was designed to target processing speed and auditory working memory. The control group was given computer-based assignments that included listening to audio books, reading online newspapers, and playing spatially oriented computer games. Individuals in the control group participated for 90 min per day, 5 days per week, for 8 weeks. The RBANS was the primary outcome measure of global cognitive functioning. Although no statistically significant differences in performance on the RBANS were observed between the intervention and control groups, the authors did note improvement in the performance of the intervention group on the verbal and visual working memory tests. In the control group, there was a trend for improvement on measures of language and visuospatial function. These results draw attention to the importance of including treatment activities and stimuli relevant to the client. In this study, the control group essentially had the same treatment schedule but more opportunities for selecting topics of interest.

Rosen, Sugiura, Kramer, Whitfield-Gabrieli, and Gabrieli (2011) conducted a similar study with six individuals with MCI using the same cognitive-training software program. Of interest was whether the effects of stimulation would be detectable through fMRI—they were. The authors reported enhanced left anterior hippocampal activation as well as a performance improvement on the RBANS. Results of this study are further evidence that individuals with MCI retain sufficient neuroplasticity to benefit from cognitive intervention.

Jak et al. (2013) conducted an extensive review of the effects of computer-based training and whether program gains generalized to improvements in daily life. Results of the review indicate that the most robust improvements are on specifically trained cognitive tasks. Currently, there are limited data to support generalization of improvements to real-world activities. However, some investigators (Cipriani, Bianchetti, & Trabucchi, 2006; Rozzini et al., 2007) report improvement in memory on both objective and subjective measures following computer-based training. Then too, some investigators (e.g., Kueider et al., 2012) report that participants often "feel" as though they have improved cognition as a result of the training. Brehmer, Westerberg, and Bäckman (2012) confirmed self-reported cognitive improvements in older adults 3 months following computerized cognitive training. The clinical observation of positive feelings and increased confidence regarding cognitive abilities should not be underestimated. This potential benefit may have important implications for everyday cognitive functioning in persons with MCI.

Regardless of program type, the expertise and skilled services of the SLP are needed to formulate goals, select the best activity for creating the desired effect, evaluate progress, and make program modifications.

When selecting a computer-based CIP, the following questions should be asked:

1. Does the client have access to a computer or suitable electronic device?
2. Does the program require Internet access?
3. What does the program cost?

4. What specific cognitive skill(s) does the program purport to train?
5. Are data available that document the program's effectiveness?
6. Can the program be tailored to individual needs?
7. Does the program measure progress?
8. Does the program continually adjust the level of difficulty?

Unfortunately, there are insufficient data to recommend one computer-based CIP over another. Virtually all come with a claim that the program will improve cognitive function. Some developers even claim that their product can delay the onset of AD. Nonetheless, few products have been rigorously tested in older adults with and without cognitive impairment.

Include Neuro-Proactive Education for Clients About Physical, Mental, and Social Health

Receiving a diagnosis of MCI can be devastating. Individuals experience anxiety, fear, and a loss of self-confidence. Some have a catastrophic reaction (Jean et al., 2010). Others feel they have lost control over their lives (Wolinsky et al., 2009). Clinicians who provide education about the brain's plasticity and explain specific ways to build and support cognitive wellness give individuals with MCI a sense of control over their lives as well as hope. Family members also benefit from cognitive-wellness education. *Education about how to develop a neuro-proactive lifestyle is empowering.* Thus, we recommend that clinicians include in their training programs education about the science-based benefits of:

- Physical activity and how to integrate it into one's lifestyle
- Brain-healthy foods
- Controlling hypertension
- Consistent and sufficient sleep
- Stress reduction

- Positive thinking
- Social activities
- Being mindful
- Learning new skills
- Trying new things
- Correcting sensory deficits in so far as possible

Sensory deficits can make individuals with mild cognitive impairment appear more cognitively impaired than they are. Then too, hearing loss is associated with accelerated cognitive decline (Lin et al., 2013). Among the nearly 1,200 participants in the Lin study (mean age 77.4 years), those with hearing loss were more likely to develop cognitive impairment as measured by performance on the Mini-Mental State Examination. Participants were followed for 6 years. Individuals with hearing loss at baseline had a 24% increased risk for cognitive impairment, and a 30% to 40% accelerated rate of cognitive decline. Clinicians should ensure that sensory deficits are corrected in so far as possible.

Researchers with the Finnish Geriatric Intervention Study to Prevent Cognitive Impairment and Disability (FINGER) implemented a 2-year multicomponent intervention focused on cognitive training, exercise, diet, and vascular risk. Over 1,200 participants at risk for cognitive impairment participated. They were divided into an intervention group ($n = 631$) and a control group ($n = 629$). The control group received general advice about healthy aging, whereas the intervention group received nutritional intervention, physical exercise training, monitoring and maintenance of metabolic and vascular factors, and cognitive training. Cognitive training took place in both individual and group sessions and included a computer-based, weekly homework component. Cognition, as measured by performance on a comprehensive neuropsychological test battery, was the primary outcome measure. Improvement on objective measures of cognition was 25% to 150% better in the intervention group than in the control group regardless of sociodemographic factors, socioeconomic status, baseline cognition, and level

of cardiovascular risk. These results confirm that all elders at risk for cognitive decline benefit from multidomain interventions (Ngandu et al., 2015; Rosenberg et al., 2017).

Provide Opportunities to Support Communicative Engagement and Socialization

An early sign of cognitive impairment is withdrawal from social activities and decrease in level of activity. These changes can be so subtle that family members and even the individuals with MCI are unaware of them. Kaye and colleagues (2011) studied the activity levels and degree of participation in social activities of 28 individuals with MCI and reported a decline in time spent out of the home compared with cognitively intact participants. Research results clearly demonstrate that quality social relationships contribute to good health (Mavandadi, Rook, & Newsom, 2007; Mendes de Leon, Glass, & Berkman, 2003) and that people who lack social connections, or report frequent feelings of loneliness, suffer higher rates of cognitive decline, depression, morbidity, and mortality (Shankar, McMunn, Demakakos, Hamer, & Steptoe, 2017; Yang et al., 2016).

To stimulate social opportunities that support communicative engagement, many investigators use a group format in their cognitive intervention program, among them Kurz and colleagues. They provided a 4-week, 4-hr group program to individuals with MCI and mild dementia. Together, participants planned leisure activities and discussed methods for strengthening their social network. They received group training on stress reduction and management, relaxation, improving their memory, exercise, and the use of external memory aids. After 4 weeks, the participants with MCI demonstrated significant improvements on outcome measures of activities of daily living, mood, and memory. Participants with mild dementia exhibited performance improvements in verbal memory, but no other changes (Kurz, Pohl, Ramsenthaler, & Sorg, 2009).

Positive benefits of group treatment for family members as well as those with MCI have also been reported. Kinsella et al. (2009) used a group format to teach individuals with MCI and their family members about memory use in daily life and strategies to improve and cope with declining memory. Intervention consisted of five weekly, 90-min sessions. A problem-solving approach was used in the sessions to explain common memory problems. Thereafter, participants had an opportunity to practice strategies to improve or prevent memory failure. Written material and assignments were provided to facilitate application of the skills to everyday activities. Although more participants with MCI reported greater contentment with their memory at a follow-up interview than control participants, the difference did not reach significance. However, almost universally, participants commented on the reassurance they felt knowing other individuals with similar problems. Many participants made friends with other group members and continued to meet them on an informal basis after the treatment program ended.

Moebs and colleagues interviewed caregivers and individuals with cognitive impairment to better understand the benefits of social engagement in a cognitive intervention program (Moebs, Gee, Miyahara, Paton, & Croucher, 2017). All participants valued the emotional support and opportunity to learn strategies in the group setting. Socializing with others facing similar challenges was reported to be especially comforting for the participants with cognitive impairment.

Ensure that Duration of Treatment Is Sufficient to Strengthen Skills and Create Learning

The duration of programs for which data have been published have varied significantly from 8 to 24 weeks. In most CIPs, sessions were 1 hr long, though some programs had 2-hr sessions. Based on a meta-analyses of cognitive intervention programs, Sherman and colleagues reported that treatment duration was evenly divided at either short (8 weeks or less, 46.15%) or long duration (greater than 8 weeks, 53.85%) (Sherman et al., 2017). Sherman and colleagues also reported that duration of intervention (short or long) did not have an effect on intervention outcomes.

Various program formats have been associated with positive outcomes, as measured by objective outcome measures as well as subjective outcome measures and self-reports (Belleville et al., 2006, 2018; Karow, Harvey, Helm-Estabrooks, Bloom, & Cuellar, 2011; Rebok et al., 2014). Belleville and colleagues (2018) assigned participants with MCI (n = 145) to one of three groups: cognitive training, psychosocial training, and a no-contact control group. Both the cognitive and psychosocial training were administered in *eight weekly sessions of 120 min*. The educational content of the sessions was as follows:

Session 1: Memory and healthy aging

Session 2: Attention training

Session 3: Visual imagery skill building

Session 4: Method of loci

Session 5: Learning names of new acquaintances

Session 6: The PQRST (Preview, Question, Read, State, Test) method

Session 7: Review of strategies from previous sessions as well as an introduction to external memory aids

Sessions 8: Review of material from previous sessions

Despite the short exposure, participants in the cognitive-training group demonstrated improved performance on outcome measures related to cognition, well-being, and generalization of strategy training to daily life. These improvements were still present at the 6 month follow-up. Participants in the psychosocial and no-contact groups did not demonstrate improved performance on the outcome measures. Interestingly, these authors also included a personality measure to describe participants. Self-confidence and an appreciation for structure in their lives were better predictors of success in cognitive training than education, age, or sex (Belleville et al., 2018).

Although the program protocol designed by Karow and colleagues (2011) was similar to that of Belleville and colleagues (2018), it differed in that attention, memory, strategy training, and education were addressed in every session. This program was administered weekly for *10 weeks and sessions lasted approximately 120 min*. Training was conducted in groups of five to seven participants. Participants in this study demonstrated performance gains on both objective and subjective measures.

Rebok and colleagues (2014) examined the effects of a cognitive-training program focused on cognition and everyday functioning. Approximately 2,800 participants at risk for cognitive impairment were divided into a control group and three training groups: memory, reasoning, and speed-of-processing. Participants were followed for 10 years after the conclusion of the intervention program. This program was administered for *5 to 6 weeks and the 10 sessions lasted approximately 60 to 75 min*. Four additional booster sessions were administered at 11 and 35 months for a total of *eight additional sessions*.

Ten years after the intervention, the participants in the three cognitive training groups demonstrated less decline in outcome measures related to activities of daily living compared to the control group. In comparison to the control group, participants in both the reasoning and speed-of-processing groups had performance scores at or above their initial baseline results on outcome measures related to the cognitive outcome measures. Although participants in the memory training group did demonstrate positive outcomes at the 5-year assessment, benefits were not observed at the 10-year assessment. These results provide further evidence of the long-term benefits of cognitive intervention

Because CIPs vary in content, intensity of training, and type of clients, it is impossible to say what duration of a program will be sufficient to strengthen skills and create durable learning. That decision should be made by the clinician based on client performance. There are, however, steps the clinician can take to optimize program success:

- Comprehensively evaluate clients before training
- Involve the client in goal setting
- Use therapies that are evidence based
- Track performance at each session
- Modify treatment if improvement is not apparent
- If the client is improving and the resources are available, maintain the program until goals are met (assuming the client is willing)
- Schedule periodic booster sessions to sustain improvements

Use Objective and Subjective Measures of Skill Strength and Learning

The first step in planning intervention is to obtain valid information about the cognitive, emotional, and physical status of the client. Then, administer standardized assessments of cognition (including language function) and mental/emotional state. Next, interview clients about their leisure activities, frequency of exercise, diet, sleep, and social life. Thereafter, inquire about any medication or combination of medications the client is taking that may cause adverse effects on communicative functioning such as fatigue, sleepiness, slowed thinking, or agitation. Then, identify strengths and weaknesses in each of these domains (physical, mental, and social). With that information, a plan can be developed to improve skills, enhance knowledge, and foster behaviors that support cognitive wellness.

At present, no standardized, consistent method for evaluating program effectiveness is specifically recommended. Most investigators (Belleville et al., 2018; Li et al., 2011; Rebok et al., 2014) report improvement on specific cognitive abilities as measured through pre- and post-testing with standardized measures. When the therapy includes social engagement and strategy training, clinicians should consider using subjective measures to determine generalization of performance in everyday functioning.

Few investigators have assessed the effects of their program on real-world functioning. Nonetheless, evidence exists that intervention can positively impact an individual's ability to manage real-life challenges (Belleville et al., 2018; Clare & Woods, 2004; Kurz et al., 2009; Rebok et al., 2014; Troyer, Murphy, Anderson, Moscovitch, & Craik, 2008). With pre- and posttesting using objective (i.e., cognitive domain test scores) and subjective (i.e., patient/family perception, mood improvement, and participation) measures, program outcomes can be reviewed and needed modifications made. Of particular value for refining a CIP is the client's perspective on the value of the intervention program.

Looking Forward

The public's growing awareness of the value of cognitive intervention to build cognitive reserve will increase the demand for cognitive-training programs. Speech-language pathologists have a role in the early identification of individuals with MCI and in providing cognitive interventions that can strengthen skills and build cognitive reserve. They also have a role in doing the research on how best to stimulate cognitive reserve. Clinicians are encouraged to advocate for early identification of MCI and to create programs to screen middle-aged and older individuals who are hospitalized, residents of assisted living facilities, and those who visit clinics for hearing tests or speech-language services. Some clinicians now partner with physicians who serve older adults to provide follow-up, comprehensive cognitive-linguistic evaluations when the physician suspects the patient may be impaired. Those with MCI are then given the option of therapy. Finally, it is worth repeating that language changes are among the very earliest signs of MCI and it is the SLP who is best qualified to identify them.

III

Treatment: Direct Interventions for Individuals with Mild Cognitive Impairment and Dementia

Introduction

Direct interventions are those provided through individual and group therapy and education that enable clients to *strengthen* their knowledge and cognitive skills to *maintain* their highest level of cognitive function. *Indirect* interventions are modifications of the physical and/or linguistic environments to support cognition and communication. Also included in indirect intervention is counseling of professional and personal caregivers. Indirect interventions are the focus of Section IV.

Clinical Strategies Supported by Neuroscience

The human brain is constantly reorganizing as a result of experience (Kolb & Gibb, 2017). This capability to modify neuronal connections and rewire itself is known as *neuroplasticity* (NP). Plasticity occurs at many levels, from molecular events such as changes in gene expression to changes in behavior (Kolb, Teskey, & Gibb, 2010). Although brain plasticity is greater in infancy and early childhood, it remains plastic throughout life. The factors that influence NP were introduced in Chapter 1 and are recapped

here in Table III–1. Consideration of each is recommended when planning intervention. Notice that many "principles" of NP are also strategies that clinicians and teachers employ to promote learning. In fact, a synonym for NP is learning. The focus of this section is on clinical strategies that are patient centered and supported by the science-based principles of NP (Table III–2). These are the pillars of good therapy. A review of the NP principles will show that they are inherently person centered, as are the clinical strategies that follow. The factors that influence NP, that are listed in Table III–1, are not all of the factors that neuroscientists know to be influential; however, they are ones that clinicians can influence. Examples of other factors are epigenetics, gonadal hormones, drug history, and use of anti-inflammatories (Kolb et al., 2010).

Strategy: Provide Stimulation Related to Clients' Needs

Underlying NP Principles

- Specificity
- Use or lose
- Use and improve

Table III–1. Recap of Principles of Neuroplasticity

Principles of Neuroplasticity
Attention
Reward
Stimulation
Use or lose
Use and improve
Specificity
Simultaneity
Repetition
Intensity
Duration
Constrain/forced use
Interference
Transference
Time
Positive Emotion
Sleep
Age
Challenge and Novelty
Diet
Exercise
Relevance
Relatedness

Without stimulation, NP is not triggered. The stimulation should be designed to (a) impart knowledge, (b) strengthen existing knowledge, (c) teach a skill, or (d) strengthen a skill that will benefit the client. To achieve any of these goals, intensive stimulation is needed over a lengthy period. To date, studies have not been done on how the intensity and duration of therapy affects the communicative functioning of individuals with cognitive impairments secondary to dementia-producing diseases. However, as noted in Section I of this guide, the behavioral responses of clients and their performance on standard-ized assessments provide evidence as to the adequacy of the intensity and duration of therapy.

Strategy: Personalize Tasks by Giving Clients Choices

Underlying NP Principles

- Positive emotion
- Attention

Offering clients choices is essential to providing patient-centered care. We all like having choices, and familiarity with the premorbid interests of the client enables clinicians to provide appropriate choices and rewards. Perlmutter and Monty (1989) observed that personalizing a task through patient choice increased engagement, motivation, and performance. Having a choice of activities gives persons with dementia a sense of control over their learning.

Bourgeois and colleagues conducted a study in which they trained nursing assistants who were working with residents who had severe dementia. The nursing assistants were trained to provide the residents with a choice of options in regards to commonly encountered situations in long-term care facilities (Bourgeois, Camp, Antenucci, & Fox, 2016). To facilitate communication, picture card sets were presented to the patients and they were given the opportunity to make a visual choice regarding practical needs. Topics included food items, activities, daily living, socializing/communication, and pain. Results indicated that using pictures could be helpful to both the nursing assistant and the person with dementia. For the most positive outcomes, clinicians are encouraged to offer choices that reflect the premorbid interests of the client.

Strategy: Involve Multiple Modalities

Underlying NP Principles

- Simultaneity
- Relatedness
- Intensity

Table III–2. Person-Centered Clinical Strategies that Are Patient-Centered and Supported by the Science-Based Principles of Neuroplasticity

Evidence—Based Clinical Strategies
Provide stimulation related to clients' needs
Personalize tasks by giving clients choices
Involve multiple modalities
Avoid having clients multitask
Engage clients through self-generation
Control task complexity
Work within schemas to increase knowledge and facilitate retrieval
Use stimuli that evoke positive emotion
Use reminiscence to stimulate recall, engage attention, and elicits emotion
Design stimulation to reduce errors
Use repetition to produce durable memory
Repeated retrieval: A potent form of repetition that profoundly affects learning
Spaced retrieval: Retrieval of information or acts over increasingly longer intervals
Use priming to facilitate memory and increase knowledge
Elaborated encoding produces stronger memory
Use reward to sustain attention, increase frequency of desired response, and elicit positive emotion
Provide education about how sleep, diet, and exercise support neuroplasticity and cognition

Perception typically involves multiple senses and how the senses interact. For example, a touch on the hand improves vision near the hand. Seeing a friend across a room helps you hear what she or he is saying. Remember, white matter tracts connect all sensory reception and association areas.

Providing stimulation through multiple modalities decreases the level of difficulty for the individual. Learning and comprehension improve when information is experienced in more than one modality. Hearing information and then being able to review it in written form is better than simply hearing it, because of the rapid forgetting that characterizes many types of dementia. Providing information in one sensory modality and then in another also capitalizes on the value of repetition for strengthening encoding. For example, to teach a name, it is better to explain the name, show the patient its written form, and then have the client read the name, write the name, and associate it with a face or picture that can be described.

Bettcher and colleagues (2011) report that providing a verbal description, a picture, and a video presentation of a task strengthens the recall of the task schema and may assist persons with dementia in completing daily tasks. Because persons with Alzheimer's dementia retain the ability to read words far into the course of the disease, it is generally helpful to use the visual modality in addition to the auditory modality for providing information. Similarly, because they have difficulty retaining information, it is better to provide the object being discussed (Hopper, Bayles, & Tomoeda, 1998).

Mahendra, Bayles, and Harris (2005) investigated the influence of presentation modality during story recall tasks in 30 participants with Alzheimer's disease (AD) and 30 healthy controls. Short stories were presented to participants in the following modalities: (a) auditory (the examiner told story), (b) visual (study subjects read the story silently to themselves), and (c) combined auditory-visual modalities (study subjects read the story silently while listening to the examiner tell the story). Participant recall was assessed immediately and after 15- and 30-min delays. Story recall was significantly influenced by presentation modality in the participants with AD. Their story recall was best after silently reading a story, compared to hearing an examiner tell the story or simultaneously hearing and reading the story. The results do not suggest that multimodal stimulation is bad, but rather that exposure to information in different modalities be done sequentially rather than in a combined format that requires divided attention. When the AD participants read the story silently, they were able to take the time they needed to process the story information; when they listened to the story being read, they had to process at the rate of the reader.

Strategy: Avoid Having Clients Multitask

Underlying NP Principle

- Interference

From personal experience, we know that tasks requiring division of attention or alternating attention are harder, and researchers have demonstrated that the neural activation associated with a given task decreases in healthy adults if a second task is done at the same time (Just et al., 2001; Rees, Frith, & Lavie, 1997; Vandenberghe et al., 1997). In short, the tasks interfere with each other. The same is true for individuals with dementia. Because of their deficits in attention and memory, persons with dementia have greater difficulty dividing their attention than healthy adults (Duchek, Hunt, Ball, Buckles, & Morris, 1997; McGuinness, Barrett, Craig, Lawson, & Passmore, 2010; Perry, Watson, & Hodges, 2000). Filoteo and colleagues (1992) reported that individuals with AD were better at focusing attention on a single aspect of a stimulus than dividing attention between two aspects of the same stimulus. Camicioli, Howieson, Lehman, and Kaye (1997) observed that persons with dementia slowed their walking speed when asked to perform a verbal fluency task (reciting male names) while walking. Gordon and colleagues used fMRI data to demonstrate that control of attention is diminished even in the preclinical stages of the disease (Gordon et al., 2015).

The popular activity of texting while doing something else is multitasking, and multitasking requires divided attention. Unsurprisingly, research has shown that the "timesaving" technique of multitasking makes healthy adults *less efficient* (Ellis, Daniels, & Jauregui, 2010; Newman, Keller, & Just, 2007; Ophir, Nass, & Wagner, 2009; Skaugset et al., 2016) and, in fact, *consumes more time*. The process of switching between tasks can take longer than doing one task to completion and then completing the next task because the brain must overcome the "inhibitions" it imposed to stop the first task and do the second task. Newman and colleagues (2007) had subjects listen to sentences while comparing rotating objects. When done together, the resources available for processing visual input dropped 29% and brain activation for listening dropped 53%. Ophir et al. (2009) found that media multitaskers are more susceptible to interference from irrelevant environmental stimuli and irrelevant representations in memory, and that they perform worse on task switching. In summary, multitasking causes attention gaps, stress, trouble concentrating, and problems with recent memory. To reduce task difficulty for persons with cognitive impairment, avoid multitasking.

Strategy: Engage Clients through Self-Generation

Underlying NP Principles

- Attention
- Relevance
- Intensity

Self-generation. Having clients "generate" a response during learning rather than just watching and listening increases their attention and actively engages them; thereby, facilitating their learning. This "generation effect" was first described by Slamecka and Graf (1978) who observed that young adults had better memory for words they generated in response to cues than for words they simply heard. Mitchell, Hunt, and Schmitt (1986) reported the same effect in both old and young adults and individuals with AD. In their study, participants read 30 sentences of subject–verb–object (SVO) form and generated the object in another 30 SVO sentences (e.g., "the gentleman opened the ___."). Later, they were presented with the verbs from the 60 sentences and asked to supply the objects associated with them. Study results showed that individuals with AD, like healthy young and older adults, better remembered the self-generated objects than those already present in the stimulus sentences they read.

Lipinska, Bäckman, Mäntylä, and Viitanen (1994) conducted a study in which they provided a 20-page booklet to participants with AD. On each page was the name of a concrete noun. Participants had to generate "general properties" for 10 of the nouns. For the other 10 items, they had to make yes/no judgments about whether the item was a member of the category provided by the experimenter. At recall, the participants with AD were provided their own self-generated cues for 10 of the words and the experimenter provided cues for the remainder. Recall was best when participants were provided with their self-generated cues.

More recently, researchers demonstrated that active involvement during the study phase of a word-stem completion task significantly improved performance (Millet, Le Goff, Bouisson, Dartigues, & Amieva, 2010). When participants with AD had to make semantic judgments about the words or generate words in the encoding phase, their performance was equivalent to that of healthy elders; however, when they only read or rated the words, word-stem completion priming was inferior to healthy elders.

Strategy: Control Task Complexity

Underlying NP Principles

- Attention
- Stimulation

Determinants of Task Complexity

- Type of demands on memory
- Time constraints
- Number of cognitive operations

Clinicians can reduce task complexity in many ways.

1. By using cued recall or recognition paradigms rather than free recall.

   Recall tasks, in which learners must search long-term memory for answers, are recognized as more difficult than recognition tasks (Anderson & Bower, 1972; Hasher & Zacks, 1979; Kintsch, 1970). This is true for healthy older individuals and those with cognitive impairment (Danckert & Craik, 2013). All students know the truth of this statement. A multiple-choice test is easier than an essay test because the correct answers only have to be recognized. Answering an essay question requires an effortful search of memory and the formulation and generation of a coherent, correct

Table III–3. Mean Raw Scores and Standard Deviations of Young and Older Healthy Control Participants, and Participants with Mild Cognitive Impairment (MCI), Mild and Moderate Alzheimer's Disease (AD) on the Word Learning Subtest of the Arizona Battery of Communication Disorders of Dementia-2

	Young Healthy	Older Healthy	MCI	Mild AD	Moderate AD
Word Learning–Free Recall	10.4 (2.5)	9.1 (2.3)	6.8 (2.4)	2.4 (2.0)	1.0 (1.4)
Word Learning–Total Recall	15.5 (1.0)	15.6 (.7)	14.7 (1.5)	7.4 (4.6)	3.6 (3.4)
Word Learning–Recognition	47.6 (1.0)	47.3 (1.3)	46.6 (1.9)	36.8 (6.8)	27.0 (9.7)

response. Like students, persons with cognitive impairment perform better on recognition tests. Table III–3 shows the performance of individuals with mild and moderate Alzheimer's as well as young and older healthy individuals on tests of free recall, cued recall, and recognition. As the data reveal, the ability to freely recall information diminishes with age. The performances of healthy adults and those with dementia were better in the cued recall and recognition conditions than in the free recall condition. (Note: to determine the effect of cued recall, subtract the free recall score from the total recall score.)

2. Work within the client's working memory span capacity.

Working memory span capacity, or the ability to hold incoming information in consciousness, attenuates slightly with age and markedly in individuals with dementia (Belleville, Peretz, & Malenfant, 1996; Cherry, Buckwalter, & Henderson, 1996). Reduction in span capacity can affect an individual's ability to comprehend task instructions or keep the necessary stimuli in consciousness. Although the client might be able to perform the task, an overload of working memory makes it impossible.

Daneman and Carpenter (1980) documented that a large span capacity for auditory–verbal information is associated with better language comprehension than a small span capacity. Having knowledge of the client's span capacity for verbal and

visual information is important in designing tasks that will not be so overwhelming. Often, when persons with cognitive impairment are given more information than they can process, they withdraw.

3. Reduce the number of mental operations.

Clinicians should match task demands to the ability of the client. Consider the number and type of mental operations required to complete the task and the level of complexity of the stimuli. Bayles, Tomoeda, Kaszniak, and Trosset (1991) conducted a research study that enabled them to compare the difficulty of a variety of communication tasks. They administered 11 different tasks to persons with AD dementia in the order shown in Table III–4. All tasks used the same 13 conceptual stimuli (see Table III–4); thereby, enabling them to make intertask comparisons of difficulty. The most difficult tasks were superordinate and coordinate naming that required recall of conceptual information. In superordinate naming, study participants had to grasp the relation between the stimulus concept and the larger category of things to which the stimulus concept belonged, retrieve the superordinate, and express it orally. This task placed demands on working memory span, attention, and decision making, as well as lexical and semantic memory. In coordinate naming, study subjects had to grasp the relation between the stimulus concept and other objects in the same category and then provide the names of coordinates. Like superordinate naming,

Table III–4. Tasks and Concepts Used in the Bayles, Tomoeda, Kaszniak, and Trosset (1991) Study

Tasks (*N* = 11)	Concepts (*N* = 13)
Confrontation Naming	Pencil
Auditory Comprehension	Comb
Dictation	Hanger
Oral Reading	Mask
Definition	Racquet
Reading Comprehension	Dart
Coordinate Naming	Harmonica
Superordinate Naming	Domino
Superordinate Identification	Knocker
Pantomime Expression	Stethoscope
Pantomime Recognition	Compass
	Tongs
	Abacus

this task taxed working and semantic memory systems.

Least difficult of the tasks were oral reading of words, auditory comprehension, and reading comprehension; the latter two being multiple-choice tasks that required recognition of the answer, rather than recall. Oral reading is a mechanical task that does not require comprehension of the words or manipulation of information.

Concept difficulty also affected performance. Less common concepts were those most likely to elicit an error. The concepts of compass, stethoscope, and abacus elicited the most errors, and pencil and comb elicited the fewest. In summary, remember that:

- Recognition is easier than recall
- Comparing features of items is harder than item recognition
- Expressing relationships is harder than confirming relationships
- The more cognitive manipulations needed to do the task, the harder the task

- Complexity of stimuli interacts with task complexity
- Visibility of instructions enhances performance

Strategy: Work within Schemas to Increase Knowledge and Facilitate Retrieval

Underlying NP Principles

- Specificity
- Stimulation
- Relatedness
- Simultaneity

Semantic memory comprises concepts, propositions, and schemas. Concepts are the elemental unit. Concepts have associations; for example, "soft" with "hard" and "pillow" with "bed." They can be used to form propositions; for example, "The soft pillow is on the bed" and "Texting while driving is dangerous." When propositions are associated with each other, schemas are formed. Some examples of schemas are:

- How to give a bridal shower
- How to check in at the airport
- How to play golf

Because our knowledge of the world is hierarchically organized, the activation of a concept stimulates an increase in activation of a related concepts (Arkin, Rose, & Hopper, 2000). Similarly, activation of a proposition results in an increase in the activation of related propositions. Schemas can also be related. This information is important when planning stimulation because concepts related to a target word, proposition, or schema advantage its retrieval.

Concepts have features that define them. For example, the concept of insect has the following features: well-defined head, thorax, and abdomen with wings and three pairs of legs. Common insects include flies, beetles, and ants. Research has shown that relearning a semantic category, like insects, is facilitated if therapy focuses on atypical category members, because atypical category members are associated with a broader array of category features (Kiran, 2007). In the case of insects, less typical are cicadas and walking sticks; more typical are ants and ladybugs.

Strategy: Use Stimuli that Evoke Positive Emotion

Underlying NP Principles

- Emotion
- Attention

Emotion affects perception, guides attention, and ultimately modulates behavior (Pessoa, 2009). Individuals are continuously in a state of allocating their finite attentional resources to particular stimuli and they do so according to how incoming stimuli are prioritized (Vuilleumier, 2005). Stimuli that are pleasurable, unique, and/or threatening attract our attention. Emotional memory enables us to recognize danger (Damasio, 1999; Darwin, 1872; Emery, 2003). Thus, events, people, and objects with emotional significance are more memorable and produce changes in brain chemistry that facilitate learning (Comblain, d'Argembeau, & Van der Linden, 2005; Haj, Postal, & Allain, 2012; Schaefer & Philippot, 2005; Talarico, LaBar, & Rubin, 2004).

LaBar, Mesulam, Gitelman, and Weintraub (2000) demonstrated that emotionally charged information captures the attention of participants with dementia better than neutral information. In the LaBar et al. study, participants with AD and normal controls were shown pairs of visual scenes: some emotionally charged, some neutral. Recordings of eye movements revealed that participants with AD, like normal controls, were more attentive to the emotionally charged scenes. Moayeri, Cahill, Jin, and Potkin (2000) presented stories accompanied by slides containing either emotionally charged or neutral elements to participants with AD. Although participants with AD were inferior to normal controls at recalling both types of story elements, emotional passages were better remembered than neutral ones. In sum, emotion captures attention and produces better performance.

Care should be taken to use stimuli that evoke positive emotion and action. Neither individuals with dementia nor their caregivers benefit from the creation of a negative emotion. Negative moods can persist long after the provoking stimulus is forgotten, thereby, increasing caregiver stress, staff time, and diminishing the individual's quality of life. If the form of stimulation causes the client to err more than 20% of the time, a negative mood can develop.

The best learning zone is one in which individuals are pushing just beyond their abilities but aren't overwhelmed. When individuals are overwhelmed, they can panic, and panic impedes learning.

Strategy: Use Reminiscence to Stimulate Recall, Engage Attention, and Elicit Emotion

Underlying NP Principles

- Attention
- Stimulation
- Emotion
- Relatedness

Reminiscence therapy stimulates recall (Thornton & Brotchie, 1987) and fosters active engagement. A systematic review of interventions found reminiscence therapy to be effective in reducing social isolation and depression in institutionalized older adults (Franck, Molyneux, & Parkinson, 2016). When participants with dementia and healthy adults are presented with pictures, newspaper articles, video clips, clothes, and props associated with a theme, their personal experiences related to the theme come to mind (Hellen, 1992). Sheridan (1995) recommends using a variety of materials to trigger all the senses. A synergy often develops in reminiscence sessions in which group members aid each other in the recall of past events. When one member of the group shares a memory, it stimulates memories in other group members.

Good Reminiscence Sessions Require Planning (Gillies & James, 1994)

1. Select a theme.
2. Obtain related tangibles.
3. Develop a list of questions that probe for the obvious and less obvious recollections individuals are likely to have.
4. Make a plan to include all group participants. For example, have some individuals describe a tangible item and then ask other members what they think about the tangible.
5. Have group members share responsibility for reading newspaper articles or article headlines.
6. Pair reminiscence with a stimulus for physical activity such as food preparation (Boczko, 1994), exercise, or music.

Suggested Themes for Reminiscence Sessions

- Culturally appropriate holidays
- Personal milestone events (getting married, graduation)
- Notable world events
- Weather events
- National traditions
- Geography

Music and Reminiscence

Music is a potent tool for engaging patients and stimulating reminiscence. It has been shown to reduce agitation and anxiety (Sherratt, Thornton, & Hatton, 2004; Svansdottir & Snædal, 2006), loneliness, and depression (Summer, 1981), and stimulate participation in activities (Christie, 1992).

Music elicits emotion (Cuddy & Duffin, 2005; Foster & Valentine, 2001; Haj et al., 2012; Irish et al., 2006) and emotional memories are easier to recall than unemotional (Comblain et al., 2005; Haj et al., 2012; Schaefer & Philippot, 2005). These facts formed the basis of a study of the effect of music listening on autobiographic recall and the number of emotional words used in the recounting of autobiographic memories in participants with AD and healthy older adults (Haj et al., 2012). Haj and colleagues reported that autobiographic recall was significantly improved after listening to music; particularly, music chosen by the participants, as compared with Vivaldi's "Four Seasons" and silence. Significantly more memories were recalled after listening to music than after silence, and significantly more were remembered after listening to chosen music than "Four Seasons." Also, more emotional words were produced by participants with AD than healthy elderly adults, especially in the chosen condition.

Helmes and Wiancko (2006) reported that playing quiet baroque music significantly reduced noisemaking behavior in individuals with dementia. Gerdner and Swanson (1993) observed that music preferred premorbidly by persons with dementia produced a beneficial effect on behavior. The results of a more recent randomized controlled trial (Ridder, Stige, Qvale, & Gold, 2013) of music therapy with 42 nursing home residents with dementia indicated reduced agitation and disruptiveness in those who had 6 weeks of music therapy compared to those who received standard care. This reduction in agitation and disruptiveness prevented the need for increased medication to treat behavioral and emotional symptoms.

Strategy: Design Stimulation to Reduce Errors

Underlying NP Principles

- Repetition
- Emotion
- Attention

Persons with dementia who have episodic memory deficits typically forget their error responses. Consequently, they do not self-correct as neurologically normal adults do in trial-and-error learning (Baddeley & Wilson, 1994). When an error response is repeatedly given, its engram is strengthened, making it more accessible in the future. A substantial body of evidence demonstrates that errorless learning (EL) procedures can be used to teach a variety of tasks to individuals with memory problems (Ehlhardt et al., 2008; Fish, Manl, Kopelman, & Morris, 2015).

For individuals who do not have a serious episodic memory deficit, making a high number of errors is nonetheless upsetting. Thus, to avoid creating a negative mood and reluctance to participate in therapy, minimize error responses. The probability of error responses can be reduced by manipulating the characteristics of the stimuli and response contingencies. Some techniques for reducing errors are vanishing cues, errorless learning, and retrieval cues that reflect the support given at encoding.

Vanishing Cues. The technique of vanishing cues is frequently used to reduce the production of errors in amnesic individuals (Baddeley & Wilson, 1994; Clare et al., 2000; Wilson, Baddeley, Evans, & Shiel, 1994; Winter & Hunkin, 1999). In this technique, learners are given strong cues at first. Gradually, cue strength is reduced until the target response is given in the absence of cues. For example, to teach the patient that the name of the night nurse is Janet, you present the name in its full form on a card and ask the patient to read the card when you ask the question, "What is the name of your night nurse?" The client simply reads the name printed on the card. Thereafter, the letters in the name are reduced on succeeding cards that are given to the client until the last card is blank (Jane_, Jan_ _, Ja _ _ _, etc.).

The vanishing-cues method has been used successfully in persons with dementia (Fontaine, 1995; Wilson & Moffat, 1992) and persons with memory impairments as a result of injury (Glisky, Schacter, & Tulving, 1986; Leng, Copello, & Sayegh, 1991; Van der Linden & Coyette, 1995).

Errorless Learning (EL). Errorless learning (EL) procedures are those that provide sufficient cueing or scaffolding to minimize errors through gradual fading of cues as the target is learned. Guessing is discouraged. Whereas trial-and-error learning requires self-insight and monitoring, EL is less effortful. Researchers note its usefulness for individuals with diminished prospective memory, poor error monitoring, and executive function deficits (Clare & Jones, 2008; Fish et al., 2015).

Haslam, Moss, and Hodder (2010) successfully taught face–name associations to individuals with dementia using a combination of vanishing cues and errorless learning. They began by showing a picture of a face and telling the subject the name of the individual. After a short delay, they asked the subjects to recall the name of the pictured individual. If the subject's response was incorrect, the clinician provided phonological and semantic cues as needed. Gradually, the strength of the cueing was reduced.

Use Retrieval Cues that Reflect Support Given at Encoding. The amount of informational overlap between a retrieval cue and the memory engram established at the time of encoding is vital to memory proficiency. This is known as the *encoding specificity principle* (Tulving & Thomson, 1973). A substantial literature exists demonstrating that recall is improved when retrieval cues reflect support given at encoding (Diesfeldt, 1984; Herlitz & Viitanen, 1991; Karlsson et al., 1989). All of us are familiar with detectives having witnesses return to the scene of a crime as a memory trigger. Many of us experienced the same phenomenon at high school and college reunions. Back at our alma maters, surrounded by old friends, we recall events we likely never would have thought of again had we not returned to the setting in which they occurred. Also, most of us are familiar with the phenomenon of being at a loss for how to answer a test question if the question is worded differently from how the information was presented in class; therefore, to facilitate recall, use retrieval cues that reflect support given at the time of encoding.

Kirk and Berntsen (2017) conducted an interesting study in which they compared the level of autobiographical recall of individuals with AD and healthy elders in two conditions: object-cued recall and word-cued recall. They found that relative to word-cueing, object cueing produced more memories with a higher degree of episodic content. Moreover, the AD patients benefitted more from object cueing. The authors suggest using objects associated with an individual's past to stimulate recall of autobiographical memories.

Strategy: Use Repetition to Produce Durable Memory

Underlying NP Principles

- Repetition
- Use and Improve
- Use or Lose

Repetition is needed to create new long-term memory. Repetition causes electrochemical changes in neuronal networks that ultimately lead to the structural changes (synaptogenesis, dendritic arborization, more receptors in synapses) needed for the creation of long-term memory. When individuals repeatedly access information and bring it to conscious awareness, the engram for the information is strengthened, making it more accessible for future recall (Green, 1992). All of us learned the importance of this fact as students. The more frequently we thought about the information presented in lectures and class exercises, the more likely we were to recall it on a test. Just as repetition is essential to creating long-term

learning in healthy individuals, it is also essential for the creation of strong engrams in memory-impaired individuals (Glisky, 1997). Many researchers have demonstrated that repetition facilitates learning in persons with dementia (Heun, Burkart, & Benkert, 1997; Little, Volans, Hemsley, & Levy, 1986; Mahendra, 2001; Small, Kemper, & Lyons, 1997).

For some persons with dementia, new fact learning is impossible. When this is the case, the clinical focus will be on maintaining preserved knowledge (e.g., names of grandchildren, how to make a 911 call) through repeated opportunities to use it.

Repeated Retrieval: A Potent Form of Repetition that Profoundly Affects Learning

Underlying NP Principles

- Repetition
- Transference
- Simultaneity
- Intensity

"Repeated retrieval" (RR) is a term that cognitive scientists and educators know well because it has been shown to be superior to traditional forms of learning (Karpicke, 2017). It is a cognitively intense activity in which the learner periodically actively retrieves the information to be learned. Traditionally, educators have focused on facilitating the encoding of new information with little attention given to the effects of information retrieval. In fact, retrieval of information was not thought to change the strength of the knowledge. That has changed. Cognitive scientists have produced a wealth of data that show that the act of retrieving knowledge, like taking a test, produces large effects on learning (Blunt & Karpicke, 2014 Karpicke, 2012). Moreover, when the information is retrieved and associated with previously known information, new associations are formed. For a review of the impact of repeated retrieval, see Karpicke (2017).

Repeated retrieval is best accomplished by:

1. An initial learning phase in which the learner is acquainted with the information to be learned.
2. Thereafter, the information is set aside for a period.
3. Later, the learner engages in active retrieval through tasks like:
   a. completing a quiz that engages recall rather than recognition
   b. drawing a concept map of the new information
   c. devising a method of self-checking their recall of the information
   d. linking the new information, that they can recall, to previously known related information
   e. analyzing what they remembered and forgot after a retrieval session
4. Thereafter, the client is regularly asked to retrieve the information through a test or other means.

Whereas asking dementia patients with episodic memory deficits to freely recall and reconstruct information they have recently been exposed to may be beyond their ability, repeated retrieval will benefit those with mild cognitive impairment (MCI) and those with mild dementia whose episodic memory is spared.

Spaced Retrieval: Retrieval of Information or Actions Over Increasingly Longer Intervals

Underlying NP Principles

- Repetition
- Duration

Whereas the emphasis of repeated retrieval is *active recall*, the emphasis of spaced retrieval training (SRT) is on *increasing the spacing* of information recall (Brush & Camp, 1998a). Individuals are asked to recall information (e.g., a name, procedure, location) over increasingly longer intervals of time. Spaced retrieval is a simple procedure requiring little cognitive effort from the patient (Schacter, Rich, & Stampp, 1985) and can be contrasted with RR, which is cognitively effortful. Clinicians control the type of target response, duration of the intervals between retention probes, and the number of learning trials. The first intervals between recall probes are very short, sometimes just seconds, and are gradually extended. When an incorrect response is given, the clinician returns to the length of interval that last produced a correct response. Activities during the intervals between retention probes can be related to the desired response or unrelated.

Originally described by Landauer and Bjork in 1978, SRT was not used with a patient with dementia until 1985. Since then, its efficacy has been explored by many investigators who report success in teaching face–name associations (Abrahams & Camp, 1993; Bier et al., 2008; Camp & Schaller, 1989; Hopper, Drefs, Bayles, Tomoeda, & Dinu, 2010; Moffat, 1989; Vanhalle, Van der Linden, Belleville, & Gilbert, 1998), object location (Camp, 1989), object names (Abrahams & Camp, 1993; Jacquemin, Van der Linden, & Feyereisen, 1993; McKitrick & Camp, 1993; Wilson & Moffat, 1992), personal information (Materne, Luszcz, & Bond, 2014), and various verbal and motor responses (Bird, 2000; Camp, Bird & Cherry, 2000; McKitrick & Camp, 1993).

The SRT technique has been extensively used with dementia patients and its efficacy with them is thought to result from spared nondeclarative memory processes that enable them to learn associations even though they may not remember the event of learning (Erkes, Raffard, & Meulemans, 2009; Haslam, Hodder, & Yates, 2011; Thivierge, Simard, Jean, & Grandmaison, 2008). SRT can be nested in other activities such as conversation, reminiscence, physical therapy, or doing a craft project, and can be used by both personal and professional caregivers (Brush & Camp, 1998a).

Brush and Camp (1998b) used SRT to teach seven participants with dementia and two participants with memory impairment, as a result of stroke, three pieces of information: the therapist's name, a fact important to the person (e.g., room number, spouse's birthday), and a compensatory technique for improving communication. Five participants with dementia completed the study and learned the three pieces of information, as did the two participants who had suffered a stroke; however, participants had varying levels of recall a month later.

Davis, Massman, and Doody (2001) tested the efficacy of using spaced retrieval to teach previously known but forgotten personal information in a randomized placebo-controlled study of 37 participants with AD. Cognitive stimulation served as the placebo and consisted of home-administered attention exercises. Participants with AD in the intervention group improved in the recall of personal information during the 5-week intervention, whereas the performance of participants in the placebo group remained constant.

More recently, Materne et al. (2014) applied the same principles previously reported by Brush and Camp. Thirteen dyads of community-dwelling participants with dementia and their caregivers received hour-long sessions of SRT once weekly for up to six weeks with the goal of teaching personally relevant information. At the end of the intervention, 12 participants correctly recalled and used the taught information. Six months post intervention, five participants retained the information.

A modified SRT approach in which either related or unrelated information was discussed during recall intervals has also been investigated (Hopper et al.,2010). In the first condition, the recall intervals were filled with activities unrelated to the information being learned (unrelated condition). In the second condition, the recall intervals were filled with related activities (modified condition). Thirty-two individuals with mild to moderate

dementia participated. Most were able to learn the associations in fewer than four sessions and retained the information for up to six weeks. The modified SRT format, in which the within-session recall intervals were filled with information related to the target association, did not result in faster learning or longer retention of learned associations. Participants learned previously known associations in the standard SRT format (with unrelated information in the recall intervals) significantly faster than new associations taught in the modified SRT format.

A commonly asked question is, "How long does a dementia patient remember what is learned through SRT?" Researchers have reported retention of information for many months in some individuals. In these cases, the individuals had frequent occasions to use the learned information. If the information to be learned is not needed, and therefore never accessed, it will not be retained long. Additional "booster" training sessions may be needed periodically to maintain the information (Hopper et al., 2005). Others have reported that effectiveness of SRT decreases as the severity of dementia increases (Oren, Willerton, & Small, 2014).

Examples of Uses for SRT

Previously known but forgotten fact knowledge can be refreshed through SRT in individuals with mild dementia who have episodic memory impairment but spared nondeclarative memory.

Examples of valuable fact knowledge:

- Personal information
- Name–face associations of caregivers and family members
- Location of important objects
- 911 as an emergency number

Individuals with preserved episodic memory but impaired procedural memory can be taught new information through SRT.

Examples of useful procedures:

- Making a phone call for help
- Making a safe transfer
- Finding an important location (e.g., bathroom, bedroom, nurses' station, dining room)
- Increasing volume of voice
- Operating a faucet
- Inserting a hearing aid

Individuals with intact declarative and nondeclarative memory systems can learn both facts and procedures through RR and SRT.

Strategy: Elaborated Encoding Produces Stronger Memory

Underlying NP Principles

- Association
- Intensity
- Specificity
- Relatedness

Elaboration enhances encoding and healthy adults show improved learning when they have to engage in *greater depth of processing* of to-be-remembered material (Arbuthnott & Kratzig, 2015; Hattie & Donoghue, 2016; Levin, 1988).

Some methods for creating elaborated encoding include having the client:

- Restate newly learned information
- Answer questions about the new information
- Link new information to related information
- Use the information/skill in a new context

Strategy: Use Priming to Facilitate Memory and Increase Knowledge

Underlying NP Principles

- Stimulation
- Relatedness
- Simultaneity

Priming is a widely used evidence-based technique for facilitating retrieval of information.

Priming refers to the phenomenon of "advantaging" a response by virtue of prior exposure to the target or a related item. Priming is demonstrated empirically by an increase in the frequency, speed, or accuracy of a response as a consequence of prior exposure to a particular stimulus (Ochsner, Chiu, & Schacter, 1994; Tulving & Schacter, 1990). Recent exposure to a word, concept, or proposition makes the word, concept, or proposition more likely to come to mind. For example, if you have recently seen the word "desert," you will recognize it more quickly on tasks requiring you to make judgments about it (for example, whether it is a real word). You will also make faster judgments about the words "hot" and "dry" because they are associated with the concept of desert. The prior exposure to the word "desert" heightened the level of activation of the concept "desert" and its lexical representation. It also heightened the level of activation of related concepts and their lexical representations. The heightened activation of "desert," "hot," and "dry" occurred without your awareness and are the result of the spreading activation of energy within semantic and lexical memory.

Storms (1958) conducted one of the early studies that fueled interest in the phenomenon of priming. Students were asked to study a list of words (List A) all of which elicit high-frequency associations. For example, the word "eagle" typically elicits the word "bird." Then, Storms presented the students with a second list of words (List B) that were high-frequency responses to the words on List A, but which do not usually elicit words on List A. For example, the List A word "eagle" elicits "bird," but the word "bird" (List B) does not usually elicit the word "eagle." Storms observed that the production of words on List A, as responses to the words on List B, was significantly higher when List A was previously seen. Cofer (1960) subsequently labeled this phenomenon as "priming of associations."

Types of Primes

- Associative: Learner has prior exposure to an item **associated** with a target response.

■ Repetition: Learner has prior exposure to the **target**.

Repetition or Direct Priming. *Repetition* or *direct priming* refers to the paradigm in which an item presented in the training phase (or study phase) of an experiment is identical to, or composed of, fragments of the target item to be produced. For example, exposure to the word "boat" in the training phase will result in faster judgments about the word "boat" when it is seen again, or prior exposure to the word "boat" will result in individuals saying "boat" when later shown the fragment "bo_ _." Repetition, or direct priming, is perceptual; that is, it is modality specific and independent of the meaning of the item. Commonly used repetition priming tasks require subjects to complete a word, make a decision about a word, or identify previously seen words.

Associative or Indirect Priming. *Associative* or *indirect priming* refers to the paradigm in which the item presented in the training phase is associated with the item to be produced. Associative, or indirect priming, is conceptual or semantic. Commonly used indirect, associative priming tasks are word association, category production, and general knowledge tests. In word-association tasks, a word presented in the training phase produces a preference for an associated word. For example, the word "water" produces a preference for "wet."

In category-production tasks, the participant is presented with items from a particular category; for example, vegetables. Later, he or she is asked to generate as many exemplars of vegetables as possible. The prior exposure to items from the category increases the likelihood that they will be produced later in the category-production task.

In a general-knowledge task, the prior presentation of a word increases the probability of it being given as the answer to questions related to the word. For example, prior exposure to the word "saguaro" will increase the probability that saguaro will be given as an answer to the question, "What is a large cactus that grows in southern Arizona?"

Using Priming Clinically

Many priming techniques exist, among them verbal cueing, use of graphic material to stimulate recall, use of music to prompt, and use of context and routines as cues.

Verbal Cueing/Prompting

Many SLPs are unfamiliar with the term "priming" but routinely use priming to facilitate the performance of clients (by providing cues). Clinicians often give an associate of a word to facilitate its recall ("use it to cut through wood" for "saw"). Often they provide the name of the larger category the target word belongs to ("it's a form of transportation" for "car"). Sometimes they provide the opposite of a word to stimulate the target ("happy" for "sad"). Clinicians use more than words to prime desired behavior, among them routines, memory books, music, and contexts.

Using Visual and Graphic Materials to Cue/ Prompt. Wallets and memory books with photographs of past events and loved ones, together with text, have been demonstrated to improve the meaningfulness of verbiage produced by dementia patients in conversation (Bourgeois, 1990, 1991, 1992, 2007). The photographs and text in the memory wallets and books activate memories and prime information associated with the pictured events and people.

Using Music and Context as a Cue or Prompt. All of us have memories and emotions associated with music; thus, music used as a prime can transport us to a past event. If the event is positive, our mood improves. Music is a tool clinicians can use because evidence shows that musical memory is better preserved than other types of semantic memory (Cuddy et al., 2012; Cuddy, Sikka, Silveria, Bai, & Vanstone, 2017). Some investigators argue that musical semantic memory appears to be an "island" of cognitive preservation (Omar, Hailstone & Warren, 2012; Vanstone, Cuddy, Duffin, & Alexander, 2009). Foster and Valentine (2001) used music to facilitate autobiographic recall in individuals with dementia. They observed increased arousal and interest when background music was played during recall. Mahendra (1999, 2001) also used music to stimulate the recall of autobiographic events with individuals with dementia and observed greater animation, increased verbal output, and greater physical action (imitating drum playing, toe tapping, and, in one case, dancing).

Using Context and Routines as Cues. Context also cues behavior and routines are important for creating context. A routine is a behavioral chain in which each behavior functions as a discriminative stimulus for the next behavior and a conditioned reinforcer for the previous link (Halle & Spradlin, 1993). Ylvisaker and Feeney (2002) described routines as concrete structured event complexes that become organized mental representations that cue behavior. Recognition of this fact has led clinicians to train individuals in the contexts in which the desired behavior is needed. This is important because skills acquired in a clinical context often do not transfer to real-world contexts (Martin & Pear, 1996).

Strategy: Use Reward to Sustain Attention, Increase Frequency of Desired Response, and Elicit Positive Emotion

Underlying NP Principles

- Attention
- Emotion

Clients learn faster when they are rewarded for learning. In deciding on the type and frequency of reward, remember that reward and emotion are related. Merzenich notes that if the consequence of a target behavior is a little rewarding or a little punishing, it can take many

trials to learn. But, if it is something really desired or really hated, it is learned quickly (Merzenich, Van Vleet, & Nahum, 2014).

Strategy: Provide Education About How Sleep, Diet, and Exercise Support Neuroplasticity and Cognition

Underlying NP Principles

- Sleep
- Diet
- Exercise

Sleep. Sleep is essential to memory, learning, and neuroplasticity (Gorgoni et al., 2013; Landmann et al., 2016). Kuhn and colleagues (2016) characterize the effect of sleep on learning as a period for "recalibrating homeostatic and associative synaptic plasticity." Said more simply, both declarative and procedural memories are consolidated during sleep (Ellenbogen, Payne, Stickgold, 2006; Walker, 2009) and linked to prior knowledge. Whereas the awake brain functions to encode memories, the sleeping brain functions to optimize memory consolidation. Many researchers have demonstrated that when humans are given new material to learn and then sleep, their recall of the new information is better than if they are asked to recall the information later but have not slept (Rasch & Born, 2013). Potkin and Bunney (2012) randomly assigned 40 male and female healthy adolescents to a sleep or no-sleep condition. The subjects in the no-sleep condition were trained on a paired-associate declarative memory task and a control working memory task at 9AM and tested 12 hours later at 9PM. The subjects in the sleep condition were trained on the paired-associate task at 9PM and tested 12 hours later at 9AM following sleep. The group who slept between learning and recall had a 20.6% increase in recall of the new information compared to the group that did not sleep. Researchers think that the electrical activity and connectivity that is stimulated between neurons during the day is cleared during sleep enabling the brain to reset and be ready for the next day's stimulation (Kuhn et al., 2016).

Diet. The brain comprises highly metabolic activity and needs a constant and stable supply of glucose. However, the brain does not store glucose; it is supplied by food. When glucose enters the blood stream from digestion, the pancreas releases insulin to keep blood sugar under control. Refined sugar causes glucose levels to rise too high too fast. Thus, the body commences to rid itself of this sudden excess by releasing more insulin to pull the blood sugar level down as fast as possible. This creates a "crash" of sorts. When the level of blood sugar drops below normal, neurons starve and rob glucose from nearby fluids. That cascade of events has negative effects on attention and memory. If there are many vacillations in glucose levels over time, the kidneys and liver suffer. The best ways to stabilize blood sugar at a healthy level is to control your intake of carbohydrates, increase fiber, choose foods with a low glycemic index, and exercise regularly.

Particularly important to brain health is the consumption of foods high in antioxidants. These foods combat free radicals, the toxic atoms with an uneven number of electrons that are by-products of oxygen metabolism. Once created, they search for molecules from which they can steal an electron. Their victims then become free radicals. Left unchecked, a chain reaction results that creates more and more oxidative damage to brain cells. Free radicals often injure the cell, damaging the DNA and making the cell vulnerable to disease. Fortunately, we can repair brain cells that have suffered oxidative damage by eating foods that are high in antioxidants. The following is a listing of foods that are particularly high in antioxidants: dark green vegetables, sweet potatoes, raspberries, blueberries, dark skinned grapes, walnuts, and pomegranates.

Also important to brain health is the consumption of healthy fats (e.g., salmon, sardines, olive oil, and nuts) rather than bad fats (meats and cheeses that contain saturated fats) and

maintaining hydration. The National Institute on Aging (2017) recommends a diet that consists of vegetables and fruits, whole grains, lean meats, fish and poultry (in modest amounts), low-fat or non-fat dairy products, limiting solid fats, sugar and salt, controlling portion sizes, and 8 cups of liquids daily, though not those with sugar.

Exercise. Evidence from animal and human studies indicate that vigorous physical exercise facilitates neuroplasticity of many brain structures; thus, enhancing cognitive function (Budde, Wegner, Soya, Voelcker-Rehage, & McMorris, 2016; Hotting & Roder, 2013). Our brains are compromised by inflammation, hypertension, hyperglycemia, glucose intolerance, free radicals, and insulin insensitivity. Exercise relieves all of these. It increases heart rate that results in increased oxygen. This causes the release of hormones that nourish cells and increases growth factors that promote neurogenesis and neuronal connections. Cotman, Berchtold, and Christie (2007) reported that the parts of the brain that control thinking and memory, namely the prefrontal cortex and medial temporal cortex, have greater volume in people who exercise.

Providing information to individuals with MCI or mild dementia about the benefit of exercise to cognitive function is strongly recommended. In 2008, the U.S. Department of Health and Human Services recommended the 2015–2020 physical activity guidelines for Americans 65 years and older:

- Engage in at least 150 min a week of moderate aerobic activity or 75 min a week of vigorous aerobic activity, or an equivalent combination of moderate- and vigorous-intensity aerobic activity. Aerobic activity should be performed in episodes of at least 10 min and preferably spread throughout the week.
- For additional and more extensive health benefits, older adults should increase their aerobic physical activity to 300 min (5 hr) a week of moderate intensity, or 150 min a week of vigorous-intensity aerobic physical activity, or an equivalent combination of moderate- and

vigorous-intensity activity. Additional health benefits are gained by engaging in physical activity beyond this amount.

- Include muscle-strengthening activities that involve all major muscle groups on two or more days a week.
- Do exercises that maintain or improve balance if they are at risk of falling.
- Determine their level of effort for physical activity relative to their level of fitness.

Summary: Science and Clinical Practice

- Early intervention is better than late.
- Attention is critical to learning.
- Stimulation must be provided to create brain change.

- The type of stimulation determines the kind of change in the brain.
- Novel and challenging tasks result in greater synaptogenesis.
- Positive emotion advantages learning.
- Repeated retrieval produces large learning effects.
- Reward increases the frequency of the desired behavior.
- Repetition is essential to the formation of long-term memory.
- The intensity and duration of therapy need to be sufficient to create observable learning.
- Sleep is crucial to memory consolidation and normal executive functioning.
- Food is medicine.
- The physical byproducts of exercise nourish the brain and body.

IV

Indirect Interventions for Individuals with Dementia

Overview

Indirect interventions are linguistic, environmental, and technological modifications that can facilitate the functioning of individuals with dementia, improve their safety, and enhance quality of life. Speech-language pathologists (SLPs) teach them to caregivers, recommend them in care plans, and oversee their implementation.

Linguistic Modifications

Numerous linguistic modifications help persons with dementia communicate by facilitating cognitive processing. They can be classified according to their impact on language comprehension and production.

Improving Language Comprehension

Language comprehension is a complex, multistage process (Rochon, Waters, & Caplan, 2000). Listeners must analyze the form, content, and context in which an utterance is spoken to derive the proposition(s) being expressed; thus, techniques for facilitating comprehension can be subcategorized according to whether they primarily involve the form, content, or use of language.

Form

Use a Slower than Normal Rate of Speech. As previously mentioned, the brain damage associated with dementing diseases results in slower information processing, as does normal aging. By slowing speech rate, the load on memory is reduced because fewer words are spoken per minute, resulting in fewer concepts that the individual must process. The average rate of speech is 160 to 170 words per minute, but fast speakers produce 200 or more words per minute. Calculate your normal rate of speech and if you are a fast speaker, slow your rate to slightly less than average.

Limit the Number of Conversational Partners. Keeping track of the topic and who said what to whom when several people are conversing can overwhelm persons with dementia because of deficits in attention and memory (Baddeley, Baddeley, Bucks, & Wilcock, 2001; Collette, Van der Linden, & Salmon, 1999). Many caregivers fail to appreciate this fact and are surprised when the person with dementia becomes agitated at large family gatherings. Persons with dementia do best communicating one on one.

Use a Pleasant and Accepting Vocal Tone.
Everyone becomes uncomfortable when someone speaks in an unfriendly tone. Clinicians and caregivers who use an accepting vocal tone evoke a positive reaction from the person with dementia. People who use a condescending or threatening tone create emotional distress that interferes with comprehension.

Content

Reduce the Number of Propositions in Sentences. The greater the number of propositions, the more cognitive resources listeners must garner to interpret the message. Rochon et al. (2000) administered a battery of working memory and sentence comprehension tests to participants with AD and age-and education-matched elders. Individuals with AD were found to have reduced spans and impaired central executive processes. Rochon and colleagues observed that the number of propositions in stimulussentences affected the performance of participantswithAD.Whensentencescontained a single proposition, AD patients performed like healthy elders; when they contained two propositions, the performance of AD patients was significantly inferior to that of healthy elders. By simplifying syntax, the number of propositions can be reduced. Consider the differences in cognitive demand between the following sentences:

1. One proposition: The woman arrived late.
2. Two propositions: The woman, who was coming from Charlotte to Boone, arrived late. (Proposition 1: The woman was late; proposition 2: The woman was coming from Charlotte to Boone.)
3. Three propositions: She was traveling from Charlotte to Boone on a recently refurbished airplane that took off late. (Proposition 1: She was traveling from Charlotte to Boone; proposition 2: The airplane was recently refurbished; proposition 3: The airplane took off late.)
4. Four propositions: The airplane that was coming from Charlotte was late, but the airplane that was coming from Connecticut was early. (Proposition 1: The airplane was late; proposition 2: The airplane was coming from Charlotte; proposition 3: The airplane was early; proposition 4: The airplane was coming from Connecticut.)

Simple subject-verb-object sentences, like sentence one, require the fewest cognitive resources because they are the least demanding on memory. When embedded clauses are added, as in sentence two, memory load is increased. Embedded clauses interrupt the main clause (who was coming from Charlotte to Boone) and the listener must hold part of the main clause (woman) in memory while processing the embedded clause (who was coming from Charlotte to Boone). Sentence three contains multiple propositions and embedding. In sentence four, two main clauses are conjoined by a conjunction and both contain an embedded relative clause. Four propositions are expressed. Conjoining propositions increases memory load as does embedding. Left-branching sentences with an initial dependent clause, such as, "When she was traveling from Charlotte to Boone, she developed air sickness," are harder to process than right-branching sentences, such as, "She developed air sickness when she was traveling from Charlotte to Boone." Dependent clauses occurring before the main clause must be held in mind until the listener/reader comes to the main clause.

Talk About the Here and Now. Because persons with dementia have difficulty recalling episodic information, they do best when the conversation concerns something they can see and feel. In other words, something to which they can refer. Doing an activity with the patient gives the patient something to talk about. Many clinicians have observed that patients talk more when doing an activity. Examples of "here and now" activities that provide a topic for conversation include:

- Arranging flowers
- Building an object
- Sewing

- Painting
- Playing musical instruments
- Coloring pictures
- Sorting playing cards

Simplify Vocabulary. All of us have stronger engrams for simple, high-frequency words than infrequently used words. The same is true for individuals with dementia; thus, it is important to share information using common, high-frequency words. Although sentences A and B express the same meaning, sentence B is easier to comprehend:

A. The philatelist was a centenarian.
B. The stamp collector was 100 years old.

Replace Pronouns with Proper Nouns. All pronouns have antecedents that must be remembered for pronoun and sentence comprehension. Persons with dementia who have episodic memory deficits have difficulty remembering antecedents. By repeating the proper noun, rather than using a pronoun (as in sentence one that follows), memory load is reduced and comprehension is facilitated (Almor, Kempler, MacDonald, Andersen, & Tyler, 1999):

1. Pat and Jim went to see Gary before he left for college. They wanted to wish him well.
2. Pat and Jim went to see Gary before *Gary* left for college. *Pat and Jim* wanted to wish *Gary* well.

Revise and Restate that which Was Not Understood. Occasionally, more than one explanation of a phenomenon or event is needed for us to comprehend. All of us know that some explanations are more comprehensible than others. When a person with dementia fails to comprehend, revising and restating the information may improve comprehension, especially if done in a noncondescending way.

Use

Ask Multiple-Choice or Yes/No Questions. Some question forms are less cognitively demanding than others. Open-ended questions like "What did you do last night?" place your conversational partner in a free-recall situation. With a moment's reflection, healthy adults can mentally reconstruct the events of the previous night; however, individuals with AD and other dementias associated with episodic memory impairment cannot. Although questions like "What do you want for dinner?" do not place individuals in a free-recall situation, they nonetheless pose difficulty because they require the generation of possibilities. Generating ideas is another cognitive ability impaired early in dementia. Choice questions like "Would you like chicken or pasta for dinner?" do not place patients in a free-recall situation or require them to generate possibilities. They must simply make a choice. Table IV–1 provides examples of difficult and easy types of questions.

Use Direct Rather Than Indirect Speech Acts. Indirect speech acts are best explained by example. Frequently used examples are when person A says to person B, "Can you pass the salt?" or "Why can't I ever find my charger?" In both examples, person A *is* making a request of the listener *indirectly* by asking a question. Being indirect is a way of being polite. When people are direct and say, "Pass the salt" or "Find my charger," they can be perceived as demanding and rude. Nonetheless, direct statements, politely worded, are often easier for persons with dementia to understand; for example, "Please pass the salt" or "Please help me find my charger."

Avoid Teasing and Sarcasm. Many forms of teasing and sarcasm involve exaggeration or being nonliteral. For example, the nurse who said, "You look so good today that I'll bet all the girls will be asking you for a date" to a confused nursing home patient was exaggerating. The interpretation of exaggeration, teasing, and sarcasm require sensitivity to context, an activity that is beyond the capacity of many individuals with dementia.

Table IV–1. Difficult and Easy Types of Questions

Difficult Types of Questions	
Open-ended free recall	Open-ended generative
"Of the movies you have seen, which is your favorite?"	"What should we buy Maddie for her birthday?"
Easy Types of Questions	
Two choices	Yes–No
"Would you like Mexican or Chinese food for dinner?"	"Do you like to travel?"
"Do you want to buy Maddie a watch or necklace for her birthday?"	"Do you want to buy Maddie a watch for her birthday?"

Avoid Talking to the Person with Dementia Like a Child. Talking to the person with dementia like a child is demeaning and provides a poor model for other caregivers. Many persons with dementia are offended by this, even if they are unable to articulate their perceptions.

Try Amplifying the Voice of the Speaker. Many caregivers report the effectiveness of assistive listening devices (Figure IV–1) in communicating with AD patients. Assistive listening devices look similar to a conventional body-worn hearing aid and serve to provide general sound-level gain. They improve the speech-to-noise ratio and help patients focus their attention (Doherty & Brangman, 2011). This is especially true if the caregiver has a soft voice.

Improving Language Production

Provide Something Tangible, Personal, and/or Visible to Stimulate Conversation.

This strategy is similar to talking about the here and now and helps both production and comprehension of language because it gives the patient and caregiver a point of reference. Furthermore, the tangible/visible personal object causes concepts related to the object to be activated through the process of spreading activation. This often results in the patient being able to call to mind other information that can be shared in the conversation. Memory wallets and books containing information about the patient stimulate language production and are an excellent example of this technique. Bourgeois (1992, 2007) wrote a book about conversing with individuals who have dementia through these memory assistive devices.

Memory Wallets and Books. Bourgeois has shown that some persons with dementia are more likely to make meaningful utterances

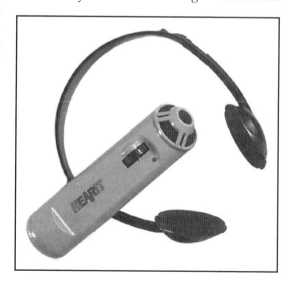

Figure IV–1. Example of an assistive listening device. (Courtesy of Hearit LLC, a division of Speech Banana Therapies, http://www.hearitllc.com)

and provide more factual information when a memory wallet or book is the stimulus to conversation (Bourgeois, Dijkstra, Burgio, & Allen-Burge, 2001; Hoerster, Hickey, & Bourgeois, 2001). The memory wallet is a compilation of pictures and sentences about the patient's life. The person with dementia does not have to actively recall the pictured events, merely recognize them. Bourgeois observed that pictures and sentences enabled participants in her studies to recall related information. The memory book is a larger version of the memory wallet. Memory books include biographic information and facts about people important to the patient simply stated and paired with pictures and other memorabilia. According to Bourgeois, individuals with mild dementia, those who score 19 to 24 on the Mini-Mental State Examination (MMSE), receive excellent benefit from the wallets and books. Moreover, individuals with mild dementia are aware that they have the wallets and books and refer to them on their own. Moderately impaired individuals with dementia, whose MMSE scores range between 12 and 18, typically require caregiver prompting to use the aids. Severely impaired individuals with dementia, whose MMSE scores are lower than 12, may not benefit from these aids.

Hopper, Bayles, and Tomoeda (1998) used a single-subject experimental design with replications across participants to investigate the efficacy of using dolls and stuffed animals to stimulate meaningful communication in four females with AD who were moderately demented. Study participants produced more relevant information units when the dolls and stuffed animals were used as conversational stimuli than when questions alone were used. Also, the participants with AD clearly enjoyed the dolls and stuffed animals as evidenced by their increased animation when they were presented with the dolls and how they hugged and talked to them.

Provide Food to Increase Sociability and Talking among Patients. Refreshments create a social atmosphere and are a cultural trig-

ger for conversation. Many long-term-care facilities have programs in which residents gather daily to make breakfast and talk about world events (Figure IV–2).

One program called "The Breakfast Club" has been described by Boczko (1994) and Santo Pietro and Boczko (1998); others have afternoon teatime. Many persons with dementia enjoy preparing food and if done with supervision, food preparation can be a useful and pleasurable stimulus for socialization and conversation.

To Facilitate Letter Writing, Supply the Materials, News Items, and a Picture of the Intended Recipient. This type of support makes it easier for the person with dementia to be successful in producing a letter. Even healthy adults have trouble thinking of things to write. Having a few news items written down eliminates the need for the patient to remember and may stimulate related memories. Also, being able to see the person for whom the letter is intended sharpens the patient's focus.

Avoid Placing Patients in a Free-Recall Situation

Two of the authors of this text recall a good example of preserving the dignity of the individual with memory problems that occurred in an interaction between a caregiver and patient when the authors visited their home. Both the caregiver and the patient greeted them at the door and the caregiver said to the patient, "You remember Cheryl and Kathryn, dear, they are here to test your memory." The patient responded, "Oh, yes, nice to see you again." Had the caregiver not provided the names and explained the purpose of our visit, the patient would have floundered and been embarrassed. The sensitivity of this caregiver to her spouse's inability to freely recall our names and appointment spared him embarrassment. Clinicians should counsel caregivers to avoid placing the patient in a free-recall situation, especially in the presence of other people.

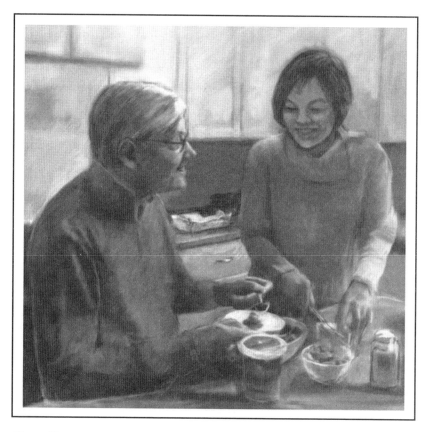

Figure IV–2. Providing refreshments or serving a meal creates a social context for communication. (Courtesy of the National Diabetes and Digestive and Kidney Disease, National Institutes of Health, Image N01164.)

When the Patient Forgets the Topic, Summarize What Has Been Said

A classic problem for individuals with dementia is forgetting what they intended to say; thereby causing the communicative interchange to fail. The thoughtful listener can summarize what has been said to enable the person to continue. This strategy helps the person with dementia save face. The following is an example of the benefit of this strategy:

> *Context*: An individual with dementia and her friend were talking during lunch that consisted of salad.
> *Patient*: I used to have a garden and raise tomatoes. We would go out to the garden with a salt shaker you know and . . . (here the patient forgot what she was going to say) let me see, oh my, uh . . .

> *Caregiver*: Going to the tomato garden with a salt shaker was a good way to get a snack.
> *Patient*: Yes, we picked tomatoes and ate them right in the garden.

Have the Patient Read Aloud

Because the mechanics of reading remain intact for many AD patients late into the disease course, reading aloud is a language production activity they can do. One caregiver friend of ours had her husband read popular novels aloud while she worked in the kitchen preparing food. He felt useful and she enjoyed the stories. We have heard many reports of elders with dementia who read storybooks to children in daycare centers or to their own grandchildren.

Do Not Repeatedly Correct the Patient

Persons with dementia often make erroneous statements and, too often, caregivers embarrass them by correcting misinformation, particularly when other people are present. Once a person is put on the defensive, agitation and hostility may result and he or she loses the desire to talk.

A strategy for indirectly correcting a patient with an erroneous idea is to provide the correct information in the patient's memory wallet or scrapbook. Frequent use of the wallet or book may help the patient stay informed. One moderately impaired individual with AD repeatedly told caregivers that her son was coming home from school and she needed to make supper. The caregiver put her son's picture in his navy uniform on her nightstand and every day reviewed the fact that he was at sea. In a few days, the patient's confusion about her son's whereabouts diminished and she told people that her son was in the Navy.

Environmental Modifications

A critical component of person-centered care is consideration of the environment. The environment affects cognitive function, behavior, communication, activities of daily living, and quality of life. This section contains valuable material about how to use the environment to improve the ability of patients with dementia to communicate, create positive behavior, and support quality of life.

Facilitate Perception of Stimuli

Aging significantly affects human sensory systems and perception. Diminished perception impedes learning because perception is the first step in information processing. The sensory systems most influential in information processing are the visual and auditory systems. An awareness of how aging affects sensory systems is needed to help elders compensate.

Environmental manipulations that facilitate perception advantage learning.

Vision and Aging

According to the 2015 National Health Interview Survey, vision loss is reported by 3.3 million U.S. adults ages 65 to 74, and four million age 75 and older (National Center for Health Statistics, 2015).

Common Vision Problems:

Presbyopia

Cataracts

Open-angle glaucoma

Age-related macular degeneration

Presbyopia

The most common age-related change is *presbyopia*, more simply defined as age-related farsightedness (National Institute on Aging, 2005). Although the eye stops growing in adolescence, the lens continues to grow in adulthood, becoming denser and less elastic after the age of 40 (American Academy of Ophthalmology, 2017). As a result, many elders experience:

- Increased sensitivity to glare
- A need for more light to perform activities
- A need for more time to adjust to lighting extremes
- Temporary blindness when moving from areas of dark to light
- An increased need for significant contrasts
- Decreased color sensitivity (Duffy, 2016)

Cataracts and Glaucoma

With cataracts, vision becomes blurred. People say that looking through a cataract is like looking at the world through a cloud or thick haze. Glaucoma refers to a group of eye disorders that damage the optic nerve. Symptoms include blurred vision, a blind spot in the visual field, pain in the eye, and loss of peripheral perception.

Macular Degeneration

Macular degeneration is the leading cause of visual impairment (American Macular Degeneration Foundation, n.d.). In this condition, degeneration occurs in the center of the retina, the back layer of the eye that records images that are sent to the optic nerve. The result is a blind spot in the center of the visual field. In the initial stages, most people do not report vision loss. However, progression can lead to wavy and/or blurred vision, and eventually the complete loss of central vision resulting in legal blindness (American Macular Degeneration Foundation, n.d.).

Individuals with AD are at higher risk for age-related macular degeneration and poorer overall visual function (Nolan et al., 2014). Those with visual deficits are impaired in their ability to read lips, recognize facial expressions, interpret contexts, follow directions, communicate, and perform on tests. Consequently, they may appear more cognitively impaired than they are. Even young adults, who wear glasses, often remark that they have trouble hearing and thinking without their glasses.

Unfortunately, the need for accommodations to enhance vision is underappreciated by many professional and personal caregivers. Clinicians should obtain information about the vision status of clients and consider environmental modifications that will maximize the abilities of those who are impaired.

Managing Problems with Vision to Facilitate Learning

First and foremost, clinicians need to screen for vision problems. A simple screening technique is included in both editions of the ABCD. Clinicians without access to the ABCD can easily create a similar one. Begin by typing a variety of letters in the four quadrants of a sheet of paper turned sideways. Repeat one letter, such as "A," several times in each quadrant of the page. The goal of the test is to see if the examinee can see and circle the occurrences of a particular letter; for example, all the "As." Also note whether the individual moved the paper to find the "As." If so, a visual field defect may be present and the client should be referred to an opthamologist for evaluation.

The following are steps clinicians can take to advantage visual perception:

- Use printed materials that are in large font size.
- Use colors that provide strong contrast (black on white or vice versa) to make print perceptible.
- Always identify yourself when greeting a client, even when a prior introduction has been made. Although elders may be able to see you, they may be unable to discern your facial features to sufficiently recognize you.
- Avoid standing or sitting in front of a window or bright light when talking as glare can reduce the perceptibility of your face.

Be on the Alert for "Sunlight Starvation"

Sunlight benefits the body's immune system and stimulates the production of vitamin D that is essential for bone health. Residents of nursing homes and homebound elders often have limited exposure to sunlight (Campbell, Kripke, Gillin, & Hrubovcak, 1988; Clark, 1975). As a result, they develop "sunlight starvation" and are at risk of vitamin D deficiency (Verhoeven, Vanpuyenbroeck, Lopez-Hartmann, Wens, & Remmen, 2012). Lack of sunlight also disturbs circadian rhythms that regulate a host of biologic processes (Brawley, 1997; Salgado-Delgado, Osorio, Saderi, & Escobar, 2011; Smolensky, Sackett-Lundeen, & Portaluppi, 2015), among them body temperature, hormone release, heart rate, blood pressure, and the sleep-wake cycle.

In addition to the negative effects of sunlight deprivation on bioregulatory processes, victims of sunlight starvation are at greater risk for depression and sleep disorders that can diminish cognitive functioning. Increased agitation is yet another by-product of light deprivation (Satlin, Volicer, Ross, Herz, & Campbell, 1992).

Results of some studies, though not all, demonstrate that exposure to bright light can reduce agitation and improve sleep-wake cycles in persons with dementia, likely due to the consolidation of circadian rhythms (Ancoli-Israel et al., 2003; Figuerio et al., 2014; Hanford & Figueiro, 2013). Brawley (1997) recommended the following guide for lighting in long-term-care facilities. Her recommendations are of value to SLPs and other personnel responsible for the care of elders:

Raise the level of illumination.

Provide consistent, even light levels.

Eliminate glare.

Provide access to natural daylight.

Provide gradual changes in light levels in transition spaces.

Provide lighting that can be focused on the task at hand.

Improve color rendition from lamps or light sources so as to avoid distortion of the environment and people in it.

Color and Vision

As previously noted, the lens of the eye thickens with age and yellows; thereby filtering out the short wave lengths. The consequence is distortion of color perception, particularly after the age of 60 years (Nguyen-Tri, Overbury, & Faubert, 2003; Schneck, Haegerstrom-Portnoy, Lott, & Brabyn, 2014). Discriminating along the blue–yellow axis is particularly affected as is discriminating among light colors. Individuals with AD are less able to distinguish between blue and green hues and between blue and violet hues.

Most resistant to age effects is the ability to discriminate the red hue (Schneck et al., 2014) and the brightness of color (Cooper, 1994). By providing high contrast, clinicians can increase function (Figures IV–3 and IV–4). For example, tabletops and countertops should contrast

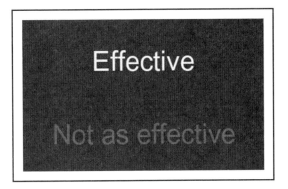

Figure IV–3. Example of high and low letter contrasts.

strongly with the color of the floor. Dishes that contrast with the color of the table facilitate eating. *The best contrast is provided by using a dark color against a light background, or vice versa* (e.g., black against white, light yellow against dark blue). Poor contrasts result from dark green against bright red, yellow against white, blue against green, and lavender against pink.

Hearing and Aging

Hearing loss is the most prevalent sensory disability in the elderly (Ciorba, Bianchini, Pelucchi, & Pastore, 2012). According to the National Center for Health Statistics (2017), presbycusis affects approximately 18% of individuals in the United States age 65 years or older. However, when all causes of hearing loss are considered, the percentage is higher. Lin, Niparko, and Ferrucci (2011) reported that 30% of individuals age 65 to 74 and 40% to 60% of people age 75 and older have a loss. Among long-term-care residents, the percentage approaches 90% (Hull, 2011).

Just as a deficit in vision can make individuals with dementia seem more intellectually and functionally impaired than they are, so can a deficit in hearing (Gates et al., 1996; Ohta, Carlin, & Harmon, 1981; Uhlmann, Larson, Rees, Koepsell, & Duckert, 1989; Weinstein & Amsel, 1986). Then too, those with hearing loss often experience further deterioration of hearing with advancing age (Cruickshanks et al., 2003). Hewitt (2017) reports that the risk

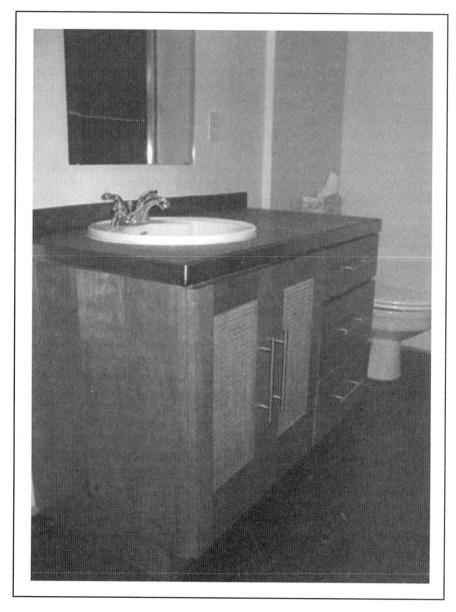

Figure IV–4. Example of bathroom with high contrast between sink and countertop and between toilet and floor.

of cognitive impairment increased with progressively greater amounts of hearing loss.

There is growing evidence that a relation exists between hearing loss and Alzheimer's disease (AD) (Hung et al., 2015). Gold, Lightfoot, and Hnath-Chisolm (1996) documented hearing loss in 94% of a sample of individuals

with AD. Moreover, in those with a hearing loss, cognitive decline accelerated (Kiely, Gopinath, Mitchell, Luszcz, & Anstey, 2012; Lin et al., 2011b; Lin et al., 2013; Nirmalasari et al., 2017). Using longitudinal data from individuals with AD, Ulhmann (1989) observed that cognitive decline over a 1-year period was almost twice as great in the group of hearing-impaired AD than in the nonhearing-impaired AD group.

Unsurprisingly, when individuals with dementia receive amplification devices, their cognitive and behavioral functioning improves (Acar, Yurekli, Babademez, Karabulut, & Karasen, 2011; Allen et al., 2003; Dawes et al., 2015). Palmer, Adams, Bourgeois, Durrant, and Rossi (1999) documented reduction in problem behaviors, as reported by caregivers, for all eight participants with dementia in their study after hearing aids were introduced. Similarly, Allen and associates (2003) reported improvement on measures of hearing handicap over 24 months of hearing aid use in their study of 31 participants with dementia.

Before making a judgment about the existence and severity of dementia in an individual, hearing should be tested. If a comprehensive assessment of hearing is impossible, clinicians should consider following the procedures recommended by Mahendra, Bayles, and Harris (2005):

Otoscopy

Pure-tone threshold testing

Word-recognition testing

Completion of the Hearing Handicap Inventory for the Elderly–Screening Version (Ventry & Weinstein, 1983)

Also, clinicians can screen hearing by simply administering a speech discrimination test (having client repeat spoken words or judge whether two spoken words are the same) in the environment in which the testing will occur. Regardless of dementia severity, most individuals can complete a simple speech discrimination test (Bayles & Tomoeda, 1993).

Strategies for Facilitating Hearing

Have clients wear their hearing aids.

Eliminate noise.

Look at hearing-impaired persons when talking to them.

Amplify your voice.

Facilitating Mood and Behavior

The physical characteristics of an environment influence how people feel and respond. Analyze the environment of each person with dementia in relation to what it evokes in terms of mood, language, and action. This analysis is particularly important for clients who exhibit negative behavior and/or are highly agitated. The following environmental features help create a happy mood and encourage positive behavior:

Accessibility of familiar objects

Pleasant smell

Sufficient lighting

Culturally appropriate decor

Availability of well-liked foods

Choices of food

Minimal visual distractions

No extraneous noise

No clutter

Pictures of past happy events

An energy outlet space where individuals can safely walk

Accessible craft materials and worktables

Music premorbidly preferred

Opportunities to do common tasks like folding laundry, raking leaves, setting the table

A consistent daily flow of events

Visibility of needed objects (e.g., comb and brush)

No mirrors (persons with dementia may not recognize themselves and become alarmed at the presence of a "stranger")

Orientation signs (e.g., bathroom, bedroom)

A visible calendar of daily events; for example

9:00AM Get newspaper

10:00AM Haircut at Sam's Barber Shop

11:00AM Grocery store for milk

12:00PM Lunch (egg salad sandwich and tomato soup)

1:00PM Rest

3:00PM Walk in the neighborhood

4:00PM Visit from granddaughter Isabella

6:00PM Dinner (chicken and rice)

Provide Something to Nurture

A highly successful approach for designing nursing homes is the provision of something for residents to nurture; for example, pets and plants. Thomas (1996) revolutionized the long-term-care industry with his Eden Alternative system of care that he developed in response to the isolation and inactivity he observed in nursing home residents. Thomas advocated for nursing homes to be "human habitats" where residents feel useful and needed and even thrive, as opposed to a place where they go to wait to die. A fundamental principle of the Eden Alternative model is for persons with dementia to be given the opportunity to give as well as receive care. Using this approach, Thomas reported that residents experienced fewer urinary tract infections, a decrease in upper respiratory infections, a decrease in medication use, and fewer deaths. Additionally, use of the Eden Alternative model has resulted in decreased staff turnover. Resnick and Ransom (2001) documented fewer behavioral incidents and decreased restraint use in Eden nursing homes compared with traditional nursing homes, and Bergman-Evans (2004) reported lower levels of boredom and helplessness over a 1-year period in a certified Eden Alternative facility compared with residents of a non-Eden facility.

Montessori Method

A clinical approach that combines several of the direct and indirect interventions discussed thus far is the Montessori method. This method promotes choice of activities and hands-on learning. Positive outcomes in social interactions

(Camp et al., 1997; Camp & Mattern, 1999) and active engagement (Ducak, Denton, & El-liot, 2018; Judge, Camp, & Orsulic-Jeras, 2000) have been observed in individuals with dementia who are provided with the opportunity to participate in purposeful tasks. To facilitate engagement and interest, activities that are functional and of interest to the person with dementia are recommended. With guidance from the clinician, the level of difficulty for each task can be modified. Examples of activities include:

- Making sure the bird feeder is full
- Planting and caring for flowers
- Brushing or combing a pet's hair
- Taking care of a fish tank
- Helping with meal preparation

Reduce Verbal Perseveration and Disruptions

Admonishing repetitious persons with dementia to quit repeating is ineffective because their episodic memory problems cause them to forget admonitions; however, changing the activity, especially to one that is physical, may eliminate the cues that elicit the ideational repetition.

When a person with moderate or late-stage dementia produces disruptive vocalizations, such as screaming and repeatedly calling out, it may be a sign that they are experiencing physical discomfort, emotional distress, are under- or overstimulated, or have an unmet need (Sloane et al., 1997; Takechi, Kokuryu, Kubota, & Yamada, 2012; Woods & Dimond, 2002). Caregivers should be trained to consider these possibilities. Smith and Filips (2009) have an excellent summary of the causes of disruptive vocalizations and strategies to reduce them:

Understimulation: Involve patient in enjoyable activities.

Overstimulation: Simplify environment, have quiet periods.

Pain: Reposition, exercise, medication.

Fatigue: Have rest periods.

Depression: Reduce sources of stress and fear.

Immobility: Take on outings.

Psychosis: Minimize sensory input.

The Environment Should Promote Safety

An important aspect of patient-centered care is the creation of a safe environment. The following steps improve safety:

Remove guns or other weapons.

Lock up poisons, insecticides, solvents, paints, and medications.

Put a nightlight in the patient's bedroom and bathroom.

Install a safety gate at stairwells.

Fasten edges of rugs.

Secure sliding glass doors.

Place decals on glass doors.

Secure electric cords to prevent tripping.

Install door locks that will prevent the person with dementia from wandering away; however, be sure the individual has an exit in the event of fire.

Place a sturdy light by bed with a remote switch.

Put nonslip mats in tub and shower areas.

Have an identification bracelet made with the individual's name, address, and note about being memory impaired.

Give police a current photo or videotape of the person with dementia.

Keep an article of worn clothing wrapped tightly in a plastic bag to be used to help track the lost person with dementia.

Deter the person with dementia from driving.

Driving is a safety issue for individuals with dementia and others. Connors, Ames, Woodward, and Brodaty (2017) conducted a large study of driving to determine what influenced individuals with AD to stop driving. Results showed that individuals stopped driving for the following reasons: older age, being female, severity of cognitive impairments, and amount of decline over time. Persons with dementia should be regularly monitored to ensure they can drive safely.

The short-term and episodic memory deficits that are present in early AD cause affected individuals to get lost easily. Then to, disorientation and visuospatial and visuoperceptual problems can lead to judgment errors. The Mayo Clinic website (2017) lists the following warning signs that individuals with AD should stop driving:

- Difficulty navigating to familiar places
- Inappropriate lane changing
- Confusing the brake and gas pedals
- Failing to observe traffic signals
- Making slow or poor decisions
- Hitting the curb while driving
- Driving at an inappropriate speed (often too slow)
- Becoming angry or confused while driving

Caregiver judgment as to the fitness of the individual with AD to drive is generally valid. Often, however, caregivers are met with resistance from the AD patient and need support from a physician, lawyer, or insurance agent. Counsel caregivers not to give in once the decision is made because the consequences of having an accident can be tragic.

Technologies to Support Cognition and Communication

Assistive technology for cognition (ATC) is increasingly being used to support the function of individuals with cognitive impairment. ATC refers to "cognitive prostheses" and "cognitive orthoses" (LoPresti, Mihailidis, & Kirsch, 2004; van Walsem, Howe, Frich, &

Andelic, 2016) that are extrinsic environmental supports for memory, engagement, and safety and independence.

Technologies to Support Memory

Commonly used devices and technologies can be adapted to serve the needs of the person with dementia. They can provide reminders and cue and monitor performance. For best results, use devices that the person with dementia already has experience using. The following are examples of devices and technologies that can be adapted to support memory:

- Cell/smartphones
- Tablets/pads
- Smart watches
- Clocks and calendars
- Apps

Imbeault et al. (2016) trained three participants with AD to use an organizer/planning application on their smartphone to complete daily activities. All three participants learned many of the functions associated with the application and applied them in their daily activities. These positive effects were maintained several months after termination of the training.

El Haj, Gallouj, and Antoine (2017) investigated whether an external memory aid (i.e., Google Calendar) would facilitate prospective memory in a participant with mild AD. During the baseline phase, the participant was instructed to perform three targeted events (e.g., attend her weekly bridge game) and three control events (e.g., buy her weekly magazine). Then, in the intervention phase, the three targeted events were cued by Google Calendar but the three control events were not. Results indicated that the participant was more likely to remember to complete the events cued by Google Calendar.

Technologies to Support Engagement

Many technologies now exist to help individuals with dementia engage with friends and rel-atives, among them smartphones, tablets, and apps such as Skype, Google Hangouts, and Facetime. Digital photo frames also help sustain memory of family.

Clinicians are incorporating these technologies in their therapy and educating caregivers about their potential for engaging family members with dementia. For example, clinicians and caregivers can use smart technology to stimulate reminiscence, provide amusing games, support video chatting, and create digital memory books.

In Europe, elders with no previous computer experience are using flat, touchscreen computers to obtain reminders about how to do basic tasks, stay oriented, and have Skype calls with family (Abreu & Almeida, 2012). Computers are also being used to stimulate cognition and entertain. Individuals with mild AD who received 24 weeks of computer-based cognitive stimulation plus psycho-stimulation had improved outcome scores on the MMSE and Alzheimer's Disease Assessment Scale-Cognitive subscale (ADAS-Cog) compared with those who only had psycho-stimulation (Tárraga et al., 2006). Many apps for game playing and stimulation are being used by individuals with mild to moderate dementia; for example, a simplified version of Scrabble and puzzles. The iPad touchscreen and intuitive operations are within the capacity of many persons with dementia.

Robotic animals are also being widely used to provide social stimulation to individuals with dementia at all levels of severity (Mordoch, Osterreicher, Guse, Roger, & Thompson, 2013). Best known is Paro, the baby harp seal that responds to touch and sound and can learn the patterns of response of the individuals who interact with it. Wada, Shibata, Musha, and Kimura (2005) reported that 20 minutes with Paro increased cortical neuronal activity significantly. Mordoch et al. (2013) provide an excellent review of the literature on the use of social-commitment robots in the care of elders with dementia. In fact, there are many reports of the positive response of nursing home residents to Paro and other robotic animals, among them increased social interaction, social well-being, and elevated mood (Bemelmans, Gelderblom, Jonker, & de Witt, 2012; Birks, Bodak, Barlas, Harwood, & Pether, 2016; Broekens, Heerink, & Rosendal, 2009; Libin & Libin, 2004; Topo, 2012). Improvement in communication and social interactions has also been reported following 4 weeks of group robot-assisted therapy for 30 min twice weekly (Sung, Chang, Chin, & Lee, 2015).

Researchers (Wilkinson, Charoenkitkarn, O'Neill, Kanik, & Chignell, 2017) in Canada are developing a tool called Ambient Activity Technology (AAT). The goal of this technology is to provide stimulation to individuals with varying levels of cognitive and physical abilities. AAT can be programed to offer personalized content for users. These devices are mounted to the wall and look like old-time radios with knobs, switches, and buttons that are easily accessed by persons with dementia.

Virtual reality-based (VR) interventions are being explored by many researchers (see García-Betances et al., 2015, for a review). With this technology, participants can be transported to "real-life" environments (e.g., grocery store, kitchen, outdoors) chosen by the participant or clinician. Serino and colleagues (2017) investigated a VR-based training protocol focused on improving visual-spatial memory in 20 participants with AD who were randomly assigned to either VR-based training or a control group. The training program consisted of 10 sessions about 20 min in duration for 3 to 4 consecutive weeks, with approximately three sessions a week. During each session, participants entered a virtual city and attempted to find one, two, or three hidden objects (i.e., a bottle of milk, a plant in a vase, and a trunk). Participants were specifically instructed to memorize the positions of these objects, which were each on different parts of the virtual city. Based on pre- and post-neuropsychological assessment, improvements in long-term spatial recall were observed for the VR-based intervention AD group. The VR-based control AD group did not show improvement.

Technologies to Support Safety and Independence

The use of Intelligent Assistive Technology (IAT) in dementia care can reduce caregiver burden, improve safety, and promote independence. Gagnon-Roy and colleagues (2017) conducted a literature review and identified several types of IATs:

- Monitoring technologies (including robots)
- Tracking and tagging technologies
- Smart homes

Robots can monitor daily activities and provide needed reminders (Petersen, Houston, Qin, Tague, & Studley, 2017; Ramakrishnan & Pollack, 2000). Additionally, their sensing systems have the capability to detect problems and alert caregivers. Sensors make it possible to locate misplaced objects that are radio-frequency identification tagged. Sensors can also be programmed to call 911 if no movement by the person with dementia is observed. Location trackers using GPS technology can be used for those individuals who may wander or get lost (Yang & Kels, 2017). Use of these location trackers may increase independence for the person with dementia. However, families should determine whether the safety and independence of the person with dementia outweighs the potential loss of privacy and autonomy associated with these devices.

Dem@Care (Lazarou et al., 2016) is one example of a multisensor smart home system that monitors the environment and the physiological status—including sleep, levels of activity, sociability, and mood—of the person with dementia. Collectively, the sensor data can inform caregiver decision making regarding safety and independence for the person with dementia. This system is currently being tested in Europe.

The following are recommendations for successfully providing technological support to individuals who have dementia:

- Ask the client and caregiver about their experience with technology.
- Educate the client and caregiver about technology options.
- Assess the level of support the client and caregiver will need to use the technology.
- Match the needs of the client and caregiver to the technology.
- Introduce technological support as early as possible.
- Provide sufficient training to enable clients and caregivers to effectively use the technology.
- Be aware of privacy issues related to use of technology.

Support of Feeding

Speech-language pathologists are frequently asked for help with the challenges of feeding persons with dementia. Moderate and demented patients often require eating assistance to ensure adequate nutrition and hydration. Environmental manipulations can improve nutrition and functional feeding. The following suggestions are based on the research of Van Ort and Phillips (1992) who studied nursing home practices related to meals and feeding:

- Have the same individual feed the person with dementia when possible.
- Feed persons needing assistance in the same place at each meal.
- Assistants should feed just one person at a time.
- Do not allow interruptions during the feeding (e.g., taking vitals, loud speaker announcements).
- Position the food so persons with dementia can see it.
- Use finger foods when possible.
- Place a spoon in the person's hand.
- Provide a model of scooping food and taking it to the mouth.
- Pace feeding so that the time between bites is about the same.

- Avoid mixing and stirring foods.
- Pair touch with the initiation of feeding and use it consistently as a cue.
- Watch for cues from the person that he or she wants another bite.
- Offer drinks frequently.
- Eliminate distractions such as a blaring television.
- Provide social reinforcement for feeding such as hugs, touching, and compliments.

Caregiver Education and Support

Clinicians have an important and long-term role in the education of caregivers. The course of dementing diseases spans years and the degree of cognitive-communicative impairment changes with time. Because disease duration is generally long (exceeding eight years on average for individuals with AD), the challenge caregivers face in providing quality care to their family member and ensuring their own health cannot be overstated.

The majority of Americans with dementia are cared for at home by family members. Mace and Rabins (2017) appropriately titled their book for caregivers *The 36-Hour Day*. Schumock (1998) reported that caregivers of persons with AD often spend 60 to 100 hours per week providing care. According to the Alzheimer's Association (2018), there are over 16 million unpaid caregivers of individuals with AD who provide 18.4 billion hours of care per year, valued at more than $323 billion. These hours include supervising medical treatments, assisting with activities of daily living, giving social support, and eventually assisting in their physical care (McCleary, Munro, Jackson, & Mendelsohn, 2005; Smale & Dupuis, 2004).

Caregiving has been characterized as a role that is "devoid of formal training, choice, and compensation" (Pruchno, Kleban, Michaels, & Dempsey, 1990). Schulz and Martire describe caregiving as "The provision of extraordinary care, exceeding the bounds of what is normative or usual in family relationships. Caregiving typically involves a significant expenditure of time, energy, and money over potentially long periods of time; it involves tasks that may be unpleasant and uncomfortable and are psychologically stressful and physically demanding" (2004, p. 240).

Dementia caregiving is recognized as the most stressful type of family caregiving (Ory, Hoffman, Yee, Tennstedt, & Schulz, 1999). Family caregivers have less time for themselves and other family members and have more work-related problems. Many caregivers of persons with dementia are themselves elderly and coping with one or more chronic diseases. If a spouse is not available for caregiving, the responsibility is often assumed by a middle-aged child of the individual with AD; and in many cases, this means leaving the workforce (Biegel, Sales, & Schulz, 1991; Schulz, 2000).

Health Risks of Caregiving

The chronic stress of caregiving takes a toll on the psychological and physical health of caregivers and can lead to early death (Gouin, Hantsoo, & Kiecolt-Glaser, 2008). Caregiving is associated with burden and depression (Arthur, Gitlin, Kairalla, & Mann, 2017; Kiecolt-Glaser, Dura, Speicher, Trask, & Glaser, 1995; Schulz et al., 1997; Schulz, O'Brien, Bookwala, & Fleissner, 1995; Teri, Logsdon, Uomoto, & McCurry, 1997; Yeager, Hyer, Hobbs, & Coyne 2010). Zarit (2006) estimated that 40% to 70% of caregivers of older adults have clinical symptoms of depression, and of these, one-quarter to one-half meet diagnostic criteria for a depressive disorder (Zarit, 2006). Arthur and colleagues (2017) report that 44% of participants in their study were at risk for clinical depression and 70% were at risk for being overburdened. Stalder et al. (2014) discovered elevated hair cortisol (HCC) levels in dementia caregivers as compared to noncaregiver controls. HHC levels are thought to reflect long-term cortisol levels and have been proposed as an endocrine marker for chronic psychological

stress. Additionally, there was a positive association between elevated HCC levels and both self-reported burden and depressiveness.

Caregivers have more serious illnesses (Kiecolt-Glaser, Glaser, Gravenstein, Malarkey, & Sheridan, 1996; Shaw et al., 1997), greater cardiovascular reactivity (King, Oka, & Young, 1994), slower wound healing (Kiecolt-Glaser, Marucha, Malarkey, Mercado, & Glaser, 1995), and an increased risk of mortality (Schulz & Beach, 1999). According to the Alzheimer's Association (2018), caregivers of spouses with dementia are more likely to have lower immune functioning, new hypertension, and new coronary heart disease. Schumock (1998) reported that caregivers use 71% more prescription drugs than individuals of a similar age and have 46% more visits to the doctor. When compared with people of the same age who do not have the responsibilities of caregiving, caregivers use more psychotropic medications (George & Gwyther, 1986).

More alarming are the alterations in the immune system that are suffered by caregivers (Allen et al., 2017; Kiecolt-Glaser et al., 1987; Mills, Yu, Ziegler, Patterson, & Grant, 1999; Vedhara et al., 1999). Compared with noncaregivers, caregivers often experience psychological, behavioral, and physiologic effects that contribute to impaired immune system function, coronary heart disease, and early death (Gouin et al., 2008; Hantsoo & Kiecolt-Glaser, 2008). They also have more days of infectious illness and reduced cellular immunity (Kiecolt-Glaser et al., 1991). Caregivers with the lowest levels of social support and the highest levels of distress have the greatest immune system dysfunction. The Alzheimer's Association reports that caregivers face approximately $9.7 billion in their own health care costs (2014).

Gender and Caregiving

The gender of caregivers appears to affect vulnerability to caregiving stress, depression, and loneliness. Women provide most of the care of individuals with dementia (Sharma,

Chakrabarti, & Grover, 2016); and female caregivers have been reported to experience more stress and burden than male caregivers (Cantor, 1983; Sparks, Farran, Donner, & Keane-Hagerty, 1998; Yeager et al., 2010; Zarit, Reever, Bach-Peterson, 1980; Zarit, Todd, & Zarit, 1986), though some investigators challenge this finding (Sharma et al., 2016). Furthermore, female caregivers are more likely to experience depression than males (Beeson, 2004; Schulz et al., 1995; Stuckey, Neundorfer, & Smyth, 1996; Yeager et al., 2010); however, some investigators dispute sex as a primary predictor of depression (Caspar & O'Rourke, 2009; O'Rourke et al., 2010; Pinquart & Sörensen, 2006). Nonetheless, females also report significantly higher levels of loneliness (Beeson, 2004). Male caregivers appear to be more likely to seek outside help and approach the problem of caregiving as they would a problem at work. Geiger, Wilks, Lovelace, Chen, and Spivey (2015) report that male caregivers often implement task-focused coping strategies as opposed to emotion-focused or avoidance-focused coping.

Younger wives and older husbands report the greatest burden in caregiving (Fitting, Rabins, Lucas, & Eastham, 1986). The association between health variables and caregiving appears to be stronger among spousal caregivers than child caregivers (Baumgarten et al., 1992). Yeager and colleagues (2010) obtained somewhat different results in that greater caregiver burden was associated with gender (female), presence of depressive symptoms, and being an adult child of the care recipient.

Family Strife and Violence

An infrequently recognized problem associated with caregiving is strife with other family members. The fact is that the existence of a person with dementia in a family often produces family conflict. In a study by Chenoweth and Spencer (1986), 60% of caregivers report that relations among family members deteriorated. Poulshock and Deimling (1984) and Cantor (1983) observed that increased burden is associated with adverse effects on caregiver–patient relations as well as relations between the caregiver and other members of the family and friends.

Wharton and Ford (2014) report that there is substantial risk to the safety and well-being of caregivers. Violence increases in families that have persons with dementia (Wharton & Ford, 2014). Paveza et al. reported that violence is a "significant clinical challenge in families living with a relative diagnosed with Alzheimer's disease or a related dementia" (1992, p. 493). More than half of all persons with dementia exhibit aggressive behavior. Paveza and associates indicate that 15% of their sample of 184 families witnessed severe violence by the person with dementia in the previous year and 5.4% of caregivers had been severely violent toward the person with dementia. The overall prevalence of violence was 17.4%.

Researchers have identified triggers for violence, among them pain, reduced vision or hearing, changes in the environment, excessive noise or activity, locked doors, limited privacy or space, and quality of relationship with caregivers (Enmarker, Olsen, & Hellzen, 2011; Kunik et al., 2010). Aggression is a significant predictor of institutionalization (Orengo et al., 2008). However, having said that, it can be difficult to place aggressive individuals in care facilities (Wharton & Ford, 2014). According to Pillemer and Suitor (1992), the predictors of violence on the part of the caregiver include physical aggression by the care recipient, disruptive behaviors, and a shared living situation. Spouses and older individuals appear more likely to become violent than other relatives.

Factors that Influence Caregiver Burden and Stress

Behavior problems by persons with dementia are reported to be more strongly related to caregiver burden than the physical and cognitive impairments, the duration of caregiving, or the intensity of care demands (Pinquart & Sörenson, 2003). Arthur et al. (2017) report that four or more behavioral and psychological symptoms of dementia (BPSD) create a "tipping point" for caregivers. At this point, they develop clinically-meaningful distress. Similarly, Gallicchio, Siddiqi, Langenberg, and Baumgarten (2002), in their study of 327 caregiver–patient dyads, found a high association between behavioral disturbances and caregiver burden. A review conducted by Adelman, Tmanova, Delgado, Dion, and Lachs (2014) specified a number of risk factors for caregiver burden:

Female sex

Low educational attainment

Reside with the care recipient

High number of hours spent caregiving

Depression

Social isolation

Financial stress

Lack of choice in being a caregiver

Ethnic Minority Groups and Caregiver Burden

The responsibility of family members to relatives with dementia is significantly influenced by their culture (Parker, Young, & Rogers, 2010; Williams & Harvey, 2013). Research results suggest that caregiver burden is higher in the Hispanic population than in non-Hispanic whites (Llanque & Enriquez, 2012). Hispanic Americans are the fastest-growing ethnic group in the United States (Humes, Jones & Ramirez, 2015), and have the fastest-growing dementia population (Thies & Bleiler, 2011). Upwards of 27% of Latino families informally care for a friend or family member (Talamantes, Trejo, Jimenez, & Gallagher-Thompson, 2006) and spend 30 hr per week doing so, while non-Hispanic whites spend an average of 20 hr per week (Alzheimer's Association, 2013).

Arévalo-Flechas and colleagues studied the perceptions and psychosocial impacts of caregiving on Latinos and compared them to those of non-Hispanic white caregivers (Arévalo-Flechas, Acton, Escamilla, Bonner, & Lewis, 2014). They reported that Latinos had significantly higher scores on the objective caregiver burden scale, lower scores on general health and social function, and more bodily pain. The authors describe several cultural values that likely contribute to their higher levels of burden:

Familismo (strong attachment to the nuclear and extended family)

Respeto (preservation of the dignity of parents and elders)

Marianismo (the suffering and sacrifice experienced reflect that of the Virgin Mary and fulfill God's will)

Additionally, the following common Latino cultural beliefs about dementia and caregiving contribute to caregiver burden:

(1) A good caregiver can control the behavioral changes associated with dementia.
(2) Dementia is shameful and embarrassing.
(3) Dementia is a private family matter and care is the responsibility of the family.
(4) Female family members are expected to assume the caregiver role.

A study of Hispanic caregivers of persons with dementia who live in New York City was conducted by Luchsinger et al. (2015). They reported that most Hispanic caregivers are women, with the majority being daughters, followed by wives. The majority of families interviewed reported a net household income of less than $30,000. Depression was reported by 16.8%, with 10.2% being treated with antidepressants. According to the Global Depression Scale (GDS), 34.8% met criteria for mild depression and 16.7% for severe depression. Higher satisfaction with social networks was related to lower caregiver burden and depression, and the researchers suggest that interventions to improve social networks for Hispanic caregivers of persons with dementia are needed. Additionally, helping caregivers find positive meaning in caregiving can improve their well-being (Farran, Miller, Kaufman, Donner, & Fogg, 1999; Quinn, Clare, & Woods, 2010).

The prevalence of both Alzheimer's disease and dementia are higher in the African American population than in non-Hispanic whites (Wells et al., 2017). There is research to suggest that African American caregivers provide more hours of care, more physically-demanding caregiving tasks, and more frequently report insufficient support services (Froehlich, Bogardus, & Inouye, 2001; Sörensen & Pinquart, 2005). Wells and colleagues (2017) pointed out that while there is research to suggest that African American caregivers experience higher levels of reward and lower levels of depression compared to non-Hispanic whites (Knight & Sayegh, 2010; Pinquart & Sörensen, 2005; Roff et al., 2004; Sörensen & Pinquart, 2005), this does not indicate a lack of compromised physical health or a variety of other significant and unique problems and challenges.

Asian American caregivers provide more direct care, use less formal support, and report higher degrees of depression and poorer physical health as compared to their white counterparts (Pinquart & Sörensen, 2007). In fact, they are less likely to use resources and services than other ethnic groups. The literature related to Asian American caregivers of persons with dementia indicates that cultural expectations regarding family responsibility influence burden. Some researchers purport that the strong sense of familism and filial responsibility by Asian American cultures lead to caregivers' reluctance to bring in the assistance of others (Lee & Bronstein, 2010). A study of four focus groups of 23 Korean American family caregivers of elders with dementia revealed common themes among caregivers:

Feeling overwhelmed

A need to fulfill cultural roles and responsibilities

Lack of outside help

Limited knowledge and misconceptions regarding dementia and AD

Barriers to services that are culturally responsive

Casado, Lee, Hong, and Hong (2015) reported that many caregivers lack understanding of the different types of dementia, share a belief that personality type is associated with the development of dementia, and hold the belief that pathological cognitive impairment is a normal part of aging. Casado and colleagues stressed the importance of providing dementia education and information about available resources to members of this population. According to Meyer and colleagues (2015) Vietnamese families have views similar to Koreans. They generally lack education about the diseases associated with dementia, their symptoms and course, and they are reluctant to access helpful resources.

A Medicare guidebook for navigating the dementia journey (https://www.medicare.gov/Pubs/pdf/02174-Nursing-Home-Other-Long-Term-Services.pdf) is an easily accessible resource that can be shared with all caregivers. It provides an overview of long-term-care options, resident rights and protection, how to pay for health care costs as well as information on how to choose a nursing home. Caregivers should consider the following:

- Is the nursing home Medicare/.Medicaid certified and currently licensed?
- Are current residents clean, well groomed, and appropriately dressed?
- Does the nursing home appear clean and well kept?
- Do residents have a choice of food items at each meal?
- Does the relationship between staff and residents appear to be warm, polite, and respectful?
- Is my primary language spoken by staff and fellow residents?
- Can residents, including those who are unable to leave their rooms, choose to take part in a variety of activities?

- Does the nursing home have specific policies and procedures related to the care of individuals with dementia? If so, does the policy include the use of non-medication-based approaches to care as a first response to behavioral symptoms?

Family Counseling

Dementia is a family affair, and clinicians should consider the patient and caregiver as a unit because their health and well-being are interdependent. The American Medical Association (AMA), the American Psychiatric Association (APA), and the American Association for Geriatric Psychiatry (AAGP) all strongly recommend partnering with the patient and caregiver in managing dementia. The AMA has even developed an assessment tool for obtaining information about the caregiver called the Caregiver Self-Assessment Questionnaire (Health in Aging, 2015). It comprises 18 questions about the caregiver's level of stress, health, and support. The AAGP views caregiver counseling as medically necessary.

When an individual is diagnosed with dementia, a family conference should be scheduled. This is especially true if the individual with dementia is living at home because in-home care has been reported to greatly increase the risk of detrimental health effects for the caregiver (Pinquart & Sörensen, 2003; Vitaliano et al., 2005). When the diagnosis is recent, the caregiver may be in shock or denial. If so, much of what is said at the initial conference may not be comprehended or accepted. Therefore, a follow-up conference may be needed after the family has absorbed the diagnosis. *The fact is, families caring for an individual with dementia benefit from periodic counseling.* A good schedule is every 6 months or at least annually because new challenges arise as the disease progresses. To appropriately counsel family, the clinician needs considerable information about the family including:

- Their understanding of the patient's disease
- Their methods of communication

- The degree of cooperation among members
- The existence and nature of major physical illness in other family members
- Their economic status
- Their cultural orientation

Kleinman (1988), a Harvard psychiatrist and medical anthropologist, recommends that clinicians ask patients and their caregivers for an explanation of the cause of the illness or disability to uncover potential differences between the explanatory models of the patient, caregiver, and clinician. With this knowledge, the clinician can negotiate with the patient and caregiver about possible treatments and expected outcomes. Although these questions were developed for use by physicians (Kleinman, Eisenberg, & Good, 1978), they are of value to any health professional:

1. What do you think has caused your problem?
2. Why do you think it started when it did?
3. What do you think your sickness does to you? How does it work?
4. How severe is your sickness? Will it have a short or long course?
5. What kind of treatment do you think you should receive?
6. What are the most important results you hope to receive from this treatment?
7. What are the chief problems your sickness has caused you?
8. What do you fear most about your sickness?

Culture Matters in Counseling

To counsel effectively, the clinician needs to understand and respect the culture of the client. What is culture? Culture is a shared way of perceiving the world. Lustig and Koester define it as "a learned set of shared interpretations about beliefs, values, norms, and social practices, which affect the behaviors of a relatively large group of people" (2013, p. 26). How can a clinician become familiar with the culture of the client? The simple answer is by asking the right questions of a cultural informant. Brislin (1994) identified critical features that distinguish the cultures of the world and the following questions are those clinicians should ask:

- Who is involved in decision making, the individual or the group?
- What are the roles of men, women, and children?
- How are time and space viewed?
- What is the primary language?
- What are important rituals and superstitions?
- What is the significance of work?
- How important is class and status?
- What is the religion and its basic tenets?
- What are the key values of the culture?
- How are health and illness viewed?

Emphasize What the Patient Can Do

Regardless of the cultural orientation, emphasize what the patient can do. Avoid focusing solely on the patient's deficits. The following is a summary of retained abilities and problem areas by stage of dementia that can be used to counsel families (after Hopper et al., 2001).

Early-Stage AD and Mild Dementia

This has been called the *forgetful* stage. The classic symptom is forgetting a recent experience. Individuals often comment that they are having difficulty remembering and finding objects. They may accuse family members or housekeepers of taking the lost object. Mistakes are more frequent, often they are related to money. Moreover, individuals with mild AD frequently experience depression. Sometimes subtle personality changes are evident, such as apathy, increased irritability, and suspiciousness.

Retained Abilities

Retained abilities are as follows:

- Can sustain attention and selectively attend to stimuli

- Able to follow a three-stage command
- Good recognition memory
- Responds to cueing
- Retains motor procedures and habits
- Semantic knowledge is generally intact
- Good grammar, syntax, and social language
- Able to read and comprehend at the sentence level
- Can write single words and comprehend gestures
- Independent in basic activities of daily living (ADLs) (e.g., toileting, bathing, feeding, and transferring)

Mid-Stage AD and Moderate Dementia

Mid-stage AD has been called the *confused* stage. Disorientation for time generally appears first followed by disorientation to place. Confusion results in poor job performance, money management difficulties, bad driving, and a deteriorating household. New environments are perplexing and travel becomes anxiety producing. Many persons with mid-stage dementia fatigue easily. Individuals with moderate dementia may withdraw from social gatherings, especially with nonfamily members. Personality changes are common and can take many forms (e.g., paranoia, hostility, and aggressiveness). Well-practiced skills are usually maintained, but caregivers observe the loss of functional ADLs, particularly bathing and grooming. Also, during this stage, individuals become unaware of their deficits. Sleep–wake cycles may be disrupted. Some individuals are awake at night and prone to restless wandering. It is not uncommon for them to become lost.

Retained Abilities

Retained abilities are as follows:

- Can sustain attention for limited amounts of time in a low-distraction environment
- Can follow a two-step command
- Fair recognition memory
- Responds to cueing

- Retains many motor procedures and habits
- Content of semantic memory may be accessible with recognition strategies and cues
- Good grammar, syntax, and social language
- Can comprehend simple statements, yes/no questions, and most choice questions
- Can reminisce about tangible stimuli
- Generally able to perform basic ADLs with minimal assistance

Late-Stage AD and Severe Dementia

Individuals in the advanced stages of dementia evolve to *global intellectual deterioration*. No longer do they have the capacity to reason and they may fail to recognize family and even themselves. They require constant supervision and are unable to carry out the routines of life. They become totally dependent on the caregiver. The images on television may confuse them as do new environments and unfamiliar persons. In the very late stage, these individuals are typically nonambulatory, incontinent, unable to feed themselves or chew, and they often have swallowing problems. Susceptibility to infection increases and pneumonia is a common cause of death.

Retained Abilities

Retained abilities are as follows:

- May attend to positive stimuli for short periods
- Sometimes responds to cues
- Generally recognize own name
- Often can contribute to a conversation
- Retains some aspects of social language (greeting, leave taking, responding to a compliment)
- May read at the word level
- May answer simple yes/no and choice questions
- May feed self with minimal assistance

Caregiver Education and Training

The National Institute on Aging and the National Institute on Nursing Research have supported studies of the value of caregiver intervention (Belle et al., 2003; Czaja, Schulz, Lee, & Belle, 2003). Results of these studies indicate that the best interventions are those that target the five types of risk to caregivers:

Safety

Social support

Health and self-care

Emotional well-being

Care-recipient problem behaviors

Several investigators have studied the effect of formal caregiver education and training programs on patient care and caregiver burden (Bourgeois, Dijkstra, Burgio, & Allen, 2004; Dijkstra, Bourgeois, Burgio, & Allen, 2002; Irvine, Ary, & Bourgeois, 2003; McCallion, Toseland, & Freeman 1999; McCallion, Toseland, Lacey, & Banks, 1999; Orange & Colton-Hudson, 1998; Ripich, 1994; Ripich, Wykle, & Niles, 1995; Ripich & Ziol, 2000; Shulman & Mandel, 1988). Results of these studies were reviewed by the Academy of Neurologic Communication Disorders and Sciences and the American Speech-Language-Hearing Association Committee to Establish Practice Guidelines for the Management of Dementia. The committee reported that educating caregivers on communication strategies may contribute to:

(a) more successful conversational exchanges;
(b) reduced caregiver burden;
(c) improved quality of life for patients;
(d) maintenance of patients' language skills; and
(e) an increase in caregiver understanding of how and why communication breaks down (Zientz et al., 2007).

Based on their review of the methodologic rigor of these studies, committee members recommended that an educational program have at least four sessions that include an opportunity for actual practice of strategies with individualized feedback.

V

Reimbursement and Care Planning for Persons with Dementia

Introduction

Before providing reimbursable services, clinicians must understand the regulations governing the provision of services and the rules for their documentation. This section begins with an overview of the Medicare regulations and is followed by a discussion of how performance on the Arizona Battery for Communication Disorders (ABCD) (Bayles & Tomoeda, 1993, 2019) and Functional Linguistic Communication Inventory (FLCI) (Bayles & Tomoeda, 1994) can be used to develop care plans and treatment goals.

Federal Law Mandates Care

With the "graying" of America, the demand for nursing home services has dramatically increased as has scrutiny of the nursing home industry. Consumers became outraged by the prevalence of dirty, unsafe facilities whose personnel were negligent in their care of residents. Congress responded and legislation was passed that set new, higher standards for nursing homes. This legislation is known as the Omnibus Budget Reconciliation Act (OBRA 1987). Its stated objective was the establishment of practices that maintain the highest level of function of long-term-care residents and that promote quality of life.

This legislation requires that residents be comprehensively evaluated upon admission and care plans be developed that will enable them to function at their highest level of ability. If improvement is expected and the special *skills of the speech-language pathologist (SLP)* are needed, claims reviewers will approve *"restorative/rehabilitative therapy"* and the clinician will be reimbursed (ASHA, 2015; Centers for Medicare and Medicaid Services, 2014).

When a patient has had a trial period of restorative therapy with no improvement in function, the clinician can develop a *skilled maintenance program* (MP). This plan is only appropriate if *skilled* care is needed to maintain the patient's current condition or to slow further deterioration of cognitive-communicative functioning. Clinicians can be reimbursed for the time involved in:

(a) Care plan development

(b) The time needed to instruct supportive personnel in carrying it out

(c) Periodic oversight to ensure the plan is followed as intended

Medicare's Comprehensive Assessment

A comprehensive assessment tool was created to comply with the OBRA regulation of assessment on admission and development of care plans. This tool is called the Resident Assessment Instrument (RAI) and it is composed of the Minimum Data Set (MDS), a screening tool, and the Care Area Assessment (CAA), a process that specifies "triggers" or issues to be addressed in care planning. These measures and more information about them can be found at https://www.cms.gov/Medicare/Quality-Initiatives-Patient-Assessment-Instruments/NursingHomeQualityInits/MDS30RAIManual.html.

Minimum Data Set

The Minimum Data Set (MDS) is a clinical assessment of an individual's physical and mental health status, behavior, functional abilities, and special needs. Sections of the MDS that are of particular importance to SLPs include:

Section B: Hearing, Speech, and Vision

Ability to hear and use of hearing aid

Speech clarity

Makes self understood

Ability to understand others

Vision and use of corrective lenses

Section C: Cognitive Patterns

Memory (short term and long term)

Memory/recall ability

Cognitive skills for daily decision making

Signs and symptoms of delirium (periodic disordered thinking/awareness)

Section K: Swallowing/Nutritional Status

Swallowing disorder

Height and weight

Weight change

Nutritional approaches

Percent of intake by artificial route

Section O: Special Treatment and Procedures Received in the Last 14 Days

Medical treatments

Therapies (including speech therapy, audiology, physical therapy, occupational therapy, psychology).

Although nurses generally oversee completion of the MDS, other health professionals may provide input related to their specialty. When they do, they sign the MDS form. Unfortunately, someone other than an SLP generally completes the MDS sections related to cognitive-communicative functioning and swallowing. This is a serious concern because they lack the training necessary to make valid judgments. Hopper, Bayles, Harris, and Holland (2001) reported that in a sample of 57 individuals with dementia, with deficits in communication and hearing as measured by objective testing, the majority were rated by a nurse as having normal or adequate communication and hearing. *Furthermore, it was reported that of those participants who had MDS-identified impairments in communication and hearing, none was referred for further evaluation!* Hopper, Slaughter, Hodgetts, Ostevik, and Ickert (2016) conducted a similar study and found that only half of the participants were appropriately referred for hearing impairment. Clearly, speech-language pathologists should make the evaluations of communication and hearing.

Care Area Assessment (CAA) Process

Care Area Assessment (CAA) summaries are used in partnership with the MDS. Each CAA identifies specific MDS responses that "trigger" the need for further evaluation of the resident so as to identify problems that can be remediated. Four of the 20 CAAs that are of interest to SLPs include:

- Cognitive loss/dementia
- Communication
- Nutritional status
- Feeding tube

A patient weakness that results in a CAA being triggered has to be addressed in the resident's plan of care unless justification to the contrary is entered in the medical record. For example, assume that the individual who completed the MDS checked that a resident "rarely/never understood," this would trigger the communication CAA and require the facility to address the resident's comprehension problem, unless a suitable explanation could be given as to why it should not be addressed. CAAs are used at the initial assessment, when there is a significant change in a resident's condition, or annually. Unfortunately, when the individual who completes the MDS fails to recognize a problem with cognition, communication, hearing, and/or nutritional status, the person with dementia receives no follow-up.

Wiener, Freiman, and Brown from RTI International prepared a document that assessed how the passage of OBRA 1987 influenced nursing home care. They reported improvement in care planning, an increase in the size of the nursing staff, more rigorous staff training, and a decline in the average number of deficiencies. Also, by 2007, fewer than 6% of the residents in long-term-nursing facilities had been restrained during the previous seven days. Nonetheless, in spite of progress, issues remain that need addressing, among them providing more information to consumers and reforming Medicaid and Medicare reimbursement. Moreover, nonresidential facilities/programs that offer day care should have minimum standards and compliance monitoring (Wiener, Freiman, & Brown, 2007).

Implementation of the 2014 Improving Medicare Post-Acute Care Transformation Act (IMPACT Act) has resulted in a more comprehensive MDS that includes additional sections. Of particular importance to the SLP are the sections relating to functional status and cognitive function. Functional status includes mobility and self-care. CMS currently defines cognitive function as the ability to express and understand ideas. Each facility must collect and submit these data or face a financial penalty. Because the MDS is now longer, SLPs and other health professionals may be called on to assist with the completion of sections related to their scope of practice (Warren, 2017).

Centers for Medicare and Medicaid Services

Under the executive branch of the federal government, the United States Department of Health and Human Services oversees the Medicare program. Within this agency are the Centers for Medicare and Medicaid Services (CMS). The CMS has 12 Medicare Administrative Contractors (MACs) that are regional offices responsible for disseminating the regulations, guidelines, and coverage rules. The CMS established the following process that must be followed for individuals admitted to long-term-care facilities:

- Residents must be comprehensively evaluated on admission to determine their level of functioning, needs, and patterns of activity.
- A care plan must be created based on the results of the comprehensive assessment. The plan must be designed to ensure the ability of the resident to attain/maintain his or her highest level of function and quality of life.
- Residents must be reviewed and reassessed by the MDS no less than every 3 months.
- A comprehensive reassessment (RAI) must be carried out after a significant change in a resident's mental and/or physical health status, but no less than every 12 months.

Basically, the passage of OBRA and IMPACT obligate care facilities to ensure that a resident's ability to carry out activities of daily living does not diminish unless the individual's clinical condition indicates that the loss of function was unavoidable. Inspectors visit nursing homes to ensure compliance with CMS regulations.

Role of the SLP

SLPs provide services at all stages of the cognitive impairment continuum for sustaining function and delaying the negative effects of dementing diseases. Because cognitive and communicative disorders profoundly affect an individual's ability to function, as well as quality of life, persons with dementia in long-term-care facilities require skilled interventions from SLPs. Therefore, clinicians routinely evaluate residents, develop care plans, and conduct periodic reassessments. As previously noted, care plans may be restorative; that is, involve direct therapy with residents who have the potential to improve, or may be maintenance programs to sustain current level of function. When a restorative/rehabilitative plan is developed, the clinician must:

- Provide objective evidence, or a clinically supportable statement of expectation that the patient has the potential to improve
- Demonstrate that the patient's maximum improvement is yet to be attained
- Show that the anticipated improvement is attainable in a reasonable and predictable period of time.

The proposed therapy must require the special skills of the SLP, be necessary, and physician approved. The provision of this documentation to claims' reviewers makes obvious the need for information about the patient's deficits and any retained abilities that can be used to improve function. It also necessitates that the clinician be knowledgeable of best practice techniques that can improve function in a reasonable period of time.

The requirements regarding maintenance programs (MPs) are that they be:

- Based on results of a comprehensive evaluation of the resident
- Developed by the SLP
- Explained to the resident and support personnel
- Executed by support personnel or the resident
- Signed by the referring physician.

A Relevant Question

Because individuals with dementia have progressive diseases and their dementia will inevitably worsen, one can reasonably ask whether they ever have the potential to improve. The answer is "yes," but with a qualification. Although behavioral therapy will not arrest the ultimate worsening of their dementia, it may enable individuals to use spared abilities to compensate for impaired abilities and therefore support them at the highest level of function of which they are capable, as the law requires.

Can SLPs Be Reimbursed for Cognitive Therapy?

Most techniques for improving the learning and retrieval of information are "cognitive" and, historically, SLPs have had difficulty gaining approval from Medicare claims reviewers for providing cognitive therapy. Fortunately, that has changed as Medicare personnel and claims reviewers now understand that communication is a cognitive enterprise and to improve it, one often has to work on the cognitive abilities that make communication possible. Today, Medicare policy statements support coverage of cognitive therapy services provided by SLPs. However, payers are carefully reviewing cognitive-related services, so clinicians should be vigilant about documenting medical necessity and the need for skilled services (Havens, McCarty, Sampson, & Warren, 2017). When cognitive therapy coverage by an SLP is denied, Kander (2006) recommends citing the following MDS memorandum:

> Dementia is the general loss of cognitive abilities, including an impairment of memory and may include one or more of the following: aphasia, apraxia, agnosia, or disturbed planning, organizing, and abstract thinking abilities . . . throughout the course of their disease, patients with dementia may benefit from pharmacologic, physical, occupational, speech-language pathology, and other therapies, according to CMS program memorandum AD-01-135, September 25, 2001 (p. 3).

Fortunately, group treatment is a covered service under Medicare (ASHA, 2015). However, in order to bill for group services the following requirements must be met:

- The group intervention must be appropriate to the patient's plan of care

- The skilled services of an SLP must be required to effectively implement the intervention
- The group consists of four or fewer individuals (Medicare recommendations)
- All of the "reasonable and necessary criteria" listed under Indications and Limitations of Coverage are met (Centers for Medicare and Medicaid Services, 2009).

Medicare Review Threshold for Therapy Claims

The Balanced Budget Act of 1997 required CMS to impose caps on outpatient physical, speech-language, and occupational therapy services. The unfortunate therapy cap is shared between speech-language pathology and physical therapy, and in January 2018 was $2,010. In February 2018, Congress passed legislation to permanently repeal the therapy cap and replaced it with a targeted medical review threshold of $3,000. Thus, no more than this amount can be paid for speech-language pathology and physical therapy services combined; however, a process to permit exceptions and exceed the threshold allows clinicians to provide additional services that are medically necessary.

The rules regarding exceptions are detailed and can be found on the CMS website (http://www.CMS.hhs.gov/Manuals/ioM/list.asp#). It is wise to periodically consult the American Speech-Language-Hearing Association's (ASHA) Billing and Reimbursement web page for updates on current reimbursement levels and other Medicare rulings (http://www.asha.org/practice/reimbursement/medicare/). Also, ASHA accepts requests for specific information. Send requests to: reimbursement@asha.org.

Using Test Performance to Develop Treatment Plans

CMS has standard forms for filing a treatment plan and reporting progress. Both require specification of the long-term and short-term treatment goals. The long-term treatment goal is more general and specifies the *end state* to be achieved. For example:

- The resident will be able to express needs with minimal cues 80% of the time.

Short-term treatment goals are the means for *achieving the end state* and may be numerous. For example:

- The resident will learn to identify the features of a communication board to 100% accuracy through errorless learning techniques in daily 15-min sessions for 2 weeks.
- Thereafter, the resident will learn to use the communication board to make requests with 80% accuracy through spaced retrieval training in daily 15-min sessions for 2 weeks.

Proposed treatments must be related to the functional level of the person with dementia. Additionally, the clinician must compare treatment effects to the person's pre-treatment functional level. The functional level of a person with dementia is best discovered using standardized measures that have been demonstrated to yield reproducible results. Clinicians should specify the standardized measure used in assessment on the treatment plan form. Finally, the clinician must provide evidence of the patient's potential to improve.

Planning Intervention

Planning intervention requires an understanding of the client's preserved knowledge and skills. This is as important to intervention planning as identifying deficits because spared systems and knowledge can be used to compensate for those impaired. Also, because memory-deficit profiles change with disease progression, periodic reevaluation is needed. For example, in individuals with Alzheimer's disease (AD), the primary problem for early-stage patients is impaired episodic memory;

Table V–1. Summary of Cognitive Deficits of Individuals with Mild Alzheimer' Disease (AD)

Mild AD		
Functions	**Deficits**	**Residual Abilities**
Orientation	Disoriented for time; confused.	Oriented to place and person.
Memory	Rapid forgetting of recent events; misplaces objects; gets lost easily.	Excellent recognition memory; average span; can reminisce; preserved procedural/habit memory.
Attention	Distractible; difficulty concentrating.	Follows three-step commands.
Associating	Difficulty with complex associative reasoning.	Simple associative reasoning of part to whole, function to object, color with objects, items in a class.
Sequencing	Trouble ordering components of complex activities and events.	Can order components of simple familiar activities.
Cognitive-Linguistic (Comprehension-Expression)	Diminished reading comprehension; spelling errors in writing; mild lexical retrieval problems; vocabulary shrinking; difficulty composing letters; forgets what she or he wants to say; reduced output.	Grammar and syntax intact; can express needs; can answer choice and yes/no questions; conversant; generates examples; describes objects, feelings; comprehends language; copies.
Perception	Mild visual perceptual deficits. Diminished sense of smell.	Generally good for ADLs.
ADLs	Difficulty with finances, housekeeping, shopping, travel, keeping track of medications, and some difficulty with telephone.	Can bathe, feed, and dress self; continent.
Reasoning	Difficulty with complex reasoning, implied information.	Able to solve routine problems.

thus, demands on it need to be reduced. Other declarative memory systems (semantic and lexical) are relatively functional in the early and middle stage of the disease but gradually deteriorate. Although working memory is compromised, environmental supports help individuals maintain orientation and focus their attention. Best preserved throughout AD are nondeclarative memory systems (conditioning, procedural learning, priming), which can be used to teach new behaviors (Salmon, Heindel, & Butters, 1992; see de Vreese, Neri, Fioravanti, Belloi, & Zanetti, 2001, for a review). Tables V–1, V–2, and V–3 provide an overview of cognitive impairments and abilities for mild, moderate, and severe dementia as related to ABCD scores.

A Case-Based Example of a Restorative Care Plan

Mrs. Jane Doe is a resident of Foley Ridge Care Community who was admitted with a diagnosis of mild dementia. In the 6 months of her residency, the staff has observed that Mrs. Doe rarely participates in activities, initiates conversation, expresses her needs, and is hard to

Table V–2. Summary of Cognitive Deficits of Individuals with Moderate Alzheimer's Disease (AD)

	Moderate AD	
Functions	**Deficits**	**Residual Abilities**
Orientation	Disoriented for time and place.	Oriented to person; knows name and spouse's name.
Memory	Rapid forgetting; decreased knowledge of current events.	Good recognition memory; attenuated span; can reminisce with assistance; preserved procedural/habit memory.
Attention	Highly distractible; drifts from topic and activity.	Can specify examples; can repeat.
Associating	Unable to carry out complex associative reasoning.	Retains simple associations; can do simple categorization; specification of attributes.
Sequencing	Difficulty sequencing even familiar activities.	Can do simple sequencing with assistance.
Cognitive-Linguistic (Comprehension-Expression)	Poor comprehension of written material; dysnomia and lexical retrieval problems; dwindling verbal output; difficulty generating a series of meaningful ideas; poor writing skills; tangential; misses the point.	Grammar and syntax intact; reads at word level; expresses needs with assistance; recognizes meaning of common words; follows 2-stage commands; can copy. Usually understands gestures.
Perception	Moderate visual perceptual deficits. Diminished sense of smell.	Usually sufficient for ADLs.
ADLs	Unable to handle finances, house-keeping, shopping, transportation, medications and laundry; difficulty dressing; dangerous driving.	Can bathe with assistance; generally continent; feeds self.
Reasoning	Problem-solving skills significantly diminished.	Can solve simple problems with cueing.

hear because of a barely audible voice. Staff are concerned because she is socially isolated. Her physician reports that she has no vocal pathology. The SLP administered the Arizona Battery for Communication Disorders (ABCD) that contains a speech discrimination hearing test (Figure V–1) to evaluate her cognitive-communication functioning. Additionally, a speech and voice evaluation was conducted. The SLP used Mrs. Doe's ABCD performance to complete the sections of the MDS related to cognitive-communicative functioning, as can be seen in Table V–4.

Mrs. Doe's performance on the ABCD, together with results of the hearing screening and speech and voice examinations, were used by the SLP to formulate the following long-term and short-term goals for Mrs. Doe.

Long-Term Goal

The long-term goal is for the resident to produce comprehensible language to express needs, and to participate in recognition-memory based activities through vocal loudness training to reduce social isolation.

Table V–3. Summary of Cognitive Deficits of Individuals with Severe Alzheimer's Disease (AD)

	Severe AD	
Functions	**Deficits**	**Residual Abilities**
Orientation	Disoriented for time, place, environment, and sometimes body parts.	May know own name; usually responds to greeting.
Memory	Devastated episodic memory; degraded knowledge of concepts; agnosia and apraxia common.	Some preserved recognition memory; often preserved procedural/habit memory.
Attention	Very limited, highly distractible; diminished sensitivity to context; unable to track multiparty conversation.	Will attend to pleasant stimuli for variable periods of time.
Associating	Confusion about common associations: part to whole, object with function, category membership, attributes of objects.	Often can match like objects; retains knowledge of simple associations.
Sequencing	Difficulty sequencing even familiar activities.	May carry out some highly routine procedures without assistance.
Cognitive-Linguistic (Comprehension-Expression)	Utterances often nonsensical; unable to write meaningfully; greatly diminished vocabulary; concrete; dysnomia; diminished output; poor reading comprehension of sentences.	Form of language generally intact; limited ability to express needs. May answer yes/no and choice questions; often can read at word level; often can add to a conversation. May retain some social aspects of communication.
Perception	Poor sense of smell. Moderate visual perceptual deficits.	Responds to stimuli if within visual field.
ADLs	Cannot perform any instrumental ADLs; incontinent of bladder, later bowel; unable to bathe and dress self.	Often can transfer; sometimes feeds self.
Reasoning	Unable to solve most simple problems.	Little, if any, reasoning capacities.

Short-Term Goals

The short-term goals are as follows:

- Spaced and repeated retrieval training daily to learn techniques for increasing vocal loudness by 50% for 3 weeks in 15-min sessions.
- Three times weekly participation in one 30-min group reminiscence program that uses recognition paradigms and priming to stimulate participation.

Treatment Plan

The following information was provided on the CMS treatment plan form. Note that the clinician included the reason for referral, Mrs. Doe's level of functioning, and data that suggest Mrs. Doe has the potential to improve.

Mrs. Jane Doe is a 77-year-old female who has resided in the care facility for 6 months.

REASON FOR REFERRAL: Staff report that patient has a hard-to-hear voice, rarely expresses needs

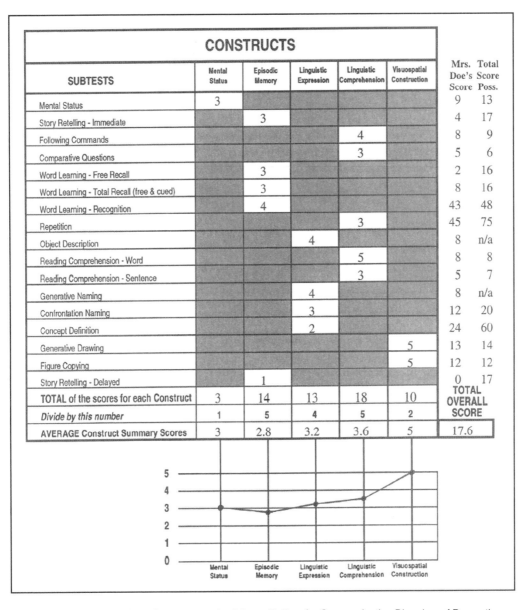

CONSTRUCTS

SUBTESTS	Mental Status	Episodic Memory	Linguistic Expression	Linguistic Comprehension	Visuospatial Construction	Mrs. Doe's Score	Total Score Poss.
Mental Status	3					9	13
Story Retelling - Immediate		3				4	17
Following Commands				4		8	9
Comparative Questions				3		5	6
Word Learning - Free Recall		3				2	16
Word Learning - Total Recall (free & cued)		3				8	16
Word Learning - Recognition		4				43	48
Repetition				3		45	75
Object Description			4			8	n/a
Reading Comprehension - Word				5		8	8
Reading Comprehension - Sentence				3		5	7
Generative Naming			4			8	n/a
Confrontation Naming			3			12	20
Concept Definition			2			24	60
Generative Drawing					5	13	14
Figure Copying					5	12	12
Story Retelling - Delayed		1				0	17
TOTAL of the scores for each Construct	3	14	13	18	10	TOTAL OVERALL SCORE	
Divide by this number	1	5	4	5	2		
AVERAGE Construct Summary Scores	3	2.8	3.2	3.6	5	17.6	

Figure V–1. Mrs. Doe's performance on the Arizona Battery for Communication Disorders of Dementia.

or communicates with other residents, and is socially isolated. Physician reports absence of vocal pathology.

LEVEL OF FUNCTION: The standardized Arizona Battery for Communication Disorders was administered as well as a speech and voice examination.

Cognition: Patient's test performance was typical of an individual with mild dementia. She was disoriented for time, could recount only 24% of a story immediately after hearing it, and remembered nothing 15 min later.

Comprehension: Patient could read and comprehend sentences with 71% accuracy, name objects and repeat with 60% accuracy, follow two-stage commands, and answer questions with 83% accuracy.

Expression: Patient could generate items in a category and define words with 40% accuracy. She has good grammar and pragmatics.

Table V–4. Relating Mrs. Doe's Arizona Battery for Communication Disorders (*ABCD*) Performance to Minimum Data Set (MDS) Items

MDS Functions	Information Provided by Analyzing ABCD Performance
Ability to recall	■ Disoriented for time but not for person
	■ Could recount only 24% of a short story immediately after hearing it; 20 min later, the story was forgotten
	■ Good recognition memory (83% accuracy)
	■ Performance improves with cues
Ability to Understand Communication/ Hearing Patterns	■ Read and comprehended single words with 88% accuracy
	■ Read and comprehended sentences with 71% accuracy
	■ Recognized and named objects with 60% accuracy repeated with 60% accuracy
	■ Followed two-stage commands
	■ Answered comparative questions with 83% accuracy
Making Self Understood	■ Generated items in a category
	■ Defined words with 40% accuracy
	■ Drew simple items with 50% accuracy
Skills for Daily Decision Making	■ Patient was oriented for self
	■ Could answer simple questions
	■ Followed one- and two-step commands
Indicators of Disoriented Thinking	■ Disoriented for time

Speech: Normal, no dysarthria.

Hearing: Able to discriminate speech with 90% accuracy.

Voice: Physician reports normal larynges and no pathology. Patient spoke in a barely audible voice 100% of the time but could increase loudness with cues.

OVERALL IMPRESSION: Mild cognitive-communication deficit secondary to dementia. Voice is soft and hard to hear. Likely patient has withdrawn because others fail to hear her.

POTENTIAL: Excellent for stated goals because of good recognition memory, ability to follow two-stage commands, reads with 71% accuracy, names with 60% accuracy, and answers questions with 83% accuracy. Patient could increase vocal loudness when stimulated to do so.

A Case-Based Example of a Maintenance Program

As was the case with Mrs. Doe's restorative care plan, the maintenance program (MP) must be based on comprehensive evaluation of the patient. Whereas Mrs. Doe presented with a mild dementia for which the ABCD was appropriate, Mr. John Doe's dementia is more severe. Both the Functional Linguistic Communication Inventory (Bayles & Tomoeda, 1994) and the Severe Impairment Battery (Saxton et al., 2005; Saxton & Swihart, 1989) were used to evaluate his mental status and level of communicative functioning. Mr. Doe's performance on the Functional Linguistic Communication Inventory is shown in Figure V–2. Mr. Doe is both nonambulatory and incontinent; however, he is not bedridden. He is unable to control his wheelchair and therefore is often isolated from activities. Mr. Doe is docile and accepting of care and was an avid football fan before his illness. When developing the MP, the clinician noted Mr. Doe's strengths and weaknesses. His deficits are suf-

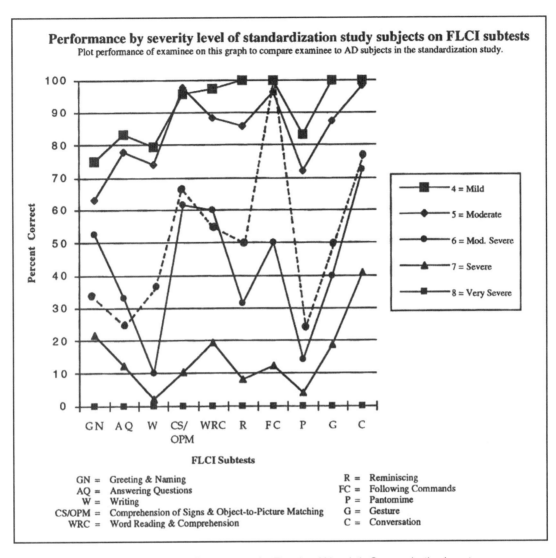

Figure V-2. Mr. Doe's performance on the Functional Linguistic Communication Inventory.

ficiently severe, thus restorative therapy is not justifiable. But he has many retained abilities that can be used to provide quality care. They are:

- Can give an appropriate verbal response
- Able to shake hands
- Can state own name
- Recognizes the written and spoken forms of his name

- Can answer some yes/no questions
- Able to write some words to dictation
- Recognizes some signs
- Can do some object-to-picture matching
- Can read single words
- Able to follow simple one-step commands
- Can give an appropriate response to a compliment
- Can correct misinformation given by the examiner

- Can make an appropriate verbal response to examiner's closing remarks.

Thus, the examiner formulated the following long-term goal and short-term steps for maintaining his function and quality of life.

Long-Term Goal

- Establish a routine of care that enables Mr. Doe to participate in activities daily that he enjoys through which he can have social interchange with caregivers and other residents.

Maintenance Program

- Address Mr. Doe by name when providing care
- Shake hands when greeting Mr. Doe
- Move from the handshake to a gentle massage of hands and arms
- Talk to Mr. Doe in a nurturing voice about a tangible object (e.g., picture, ball) for at least 5 min daily
- Encourage him to talk about the object
- Place pictures related to patient's favorite football team in patient's immediate environment
- Write single positive words on cards that relate to the pictures and place them where Mr. Doe can see them
- Incorporate throwing and catching a small football in his daily activity schedule
- Move Mr. Doe to at least three different locations in the facility daily where he can be near other people and activities
- Provide videos of football games on a trial basis to see if he enjoys watching them. Note the frequency and duration of his viewing and any affect changes
- Avoid asking patient questions that demand the free recall of information
- Use recognition and yes/no questions.

Documentation Is Critical

Documenting what you do is as important as providing the service. Without proper documentation, reimbursement claims will be denied. The documentation requirements for CMS can be found in their Benefit Policy Manual and are outlined below.

Evaluation and Plan of Care

The evaluation and plan of care are as follows:

- A diagnosis and description of the problem
- Specification of objective measures, preferably standardized measures or functional outcome measurement tools (e.g., ABCD-2 or FLCI)
- A clinical judgment of the patient's condition
- The need for treatment
- Certification that the client is under a physician's care.

Progress Notes

When treatment exceeds 10 treatment days or 30 calendar treatment days, whichever is less, progress notes must include:

- Date of the beginning of the treatment interval
- Date the report was written
- Signature of the qualified professional
- Objective reports of the patient's progress (both positive and negative clinical changes)
- Objective measurements of changes in status relative to current goals
- Plans for continuing treatment
- Changes to long- and short-term treatment goals.

Treatment Encounter Notes

With regard to treatment encounter notes,

- documentation is required for every treatment day and every therapy service;
- the note must contain the name of the treatment and intervention provided;
- total treatment time must be noted;
- the note must be signed by the professional providing the service; and
- when treatment is changed, or a new treatment added between the progress note

intervals, the change must be noted and justified.

Documentation Pitfalls

The necessary paperwork involved in gaining approval and reimbursement for services can be frustrating. Learn the rules early and adhere to them because it will reduce your frustration in the long run. The most common reason for denial of a claim is incomplete documentation, other reasons include:

- A skilled service is not being provided
- Therapy goals are not functional
- Requested services are not reasonable
- Requested services are not necessary
- The frequency and/or duration of therapy are inappropriate
- "Best practice" standards are not apparent in the treatment plan
- The therapy goal is to take the patient to a higher level than the patient was premorbidly

Synopsis

- The passage of OBRA and subsequent passage of IMPACT mandated that long-term-care facilities establish practices that maintain the highest level of function of long-term-care residents and promote quality of life.
- All long-term-care residents must be evaluated at admission and periodically thereafter using the MDS.

- Numerous MDS items are relevant to SLPs: cognitive patterns, communication and hearing patterns, oral/nutritional status, and special treatment and procedures.
- CAAs trigger the need for further evaluation of a long-term-care resident to identify problems that can be remediated.
- The CMS oversees the Medicare program and has established a process that must be followed for individuals admitted to long-term-care facilities.
- Speech-language pathology services are reimbursable by Medicare if the therapy requires the special skills of the SLP, is necessary and physician approved, and if the patient has the potential to improve in a reasonable amount of time.
- SLPs also can be reimbursed for creating a skilled maintenance program and overseeing its implementation.
- Medicare will pay for cognitive therapy by an SLP when documentation supports the therapy plan.
- Medicare has a cap on the amount of dollars that can be spent per individual for SLP and physical therapy services combined; however, CMS will make exceptions to the cap when additional services are medically necessary.
- CMS has standard forms for filing a treatment plan and reporting progress.
- Careful documentation and completion of forms according to CMS rules are necessary for Medicare approval of therapy and reimbursement.

References for Clinical Guide

Section I

Aarsland, D., Bronnick, K., Williams-Gray, C., Weintraub, D., Marder, K., Kulisevsky, J., . . . Emre, M. (2010). Mild cognitive impairment in Parkinson's disease. *Neurology, 75*, 1062–1069.

Aarsland, D., Litvan, I., Salmon, D., Galasko, D., Wentzel-Larsen, T., & Larsen, J. P. (2003). Performance on the dementia rating scale in Parkinson's disease with dementia and dementia with Lewy bodies: Comparison with progressive supranuclear palsy and Alzheimer's disease. *Journal of Neurology, Neurosurgery, and Psychiatry, 74*, 1215–1220.

Adlam, A. L. R., Patterson, K., Bozeat, S., & Hodges, J. R. (2010). The Cambridge Semantic Memory Test Battery: Detection of semantic deficits in semantic dementia and Alzheimer's disease. *Neurocase, 16*, 193–207.

Albert, M., DeKosky, S., Dickson, D., Dubois, B., Feldman, H., Fox, N., . . . Snyder, P. (2011). The diagnosis of mild cognitive impairment due to Alzheimer's disease: Recommendations from the National Institute on Aging-Alzheimer's Association workgroups on diagnostic guidelines for Alzheimer's disease. *Alzheimer's & Dementia, 7*, 270–279.

Alexopoulos, G. S. (2003). Depressive dementia. In V. O. B. Emery & T. E. Oxman (Eds.), *Dementia: Presentation, differential diagnosis, and nosology* (pp. 398–416). Baltimore: The Johns Hopkins University Press.

Alexopoulos, G., Young, R., & Meyers, B. (1993). Geriatric depression: Age of onset and dementia. *Biological Psychiatry, 34*, 141–145.

American Psychiatric Association. (2013). *Diagnostic and statistical manual of mental disorders, (5th ed.).* Arlington, VA: American Psychiatric Publishing.

American Psychiatric Association, Work Group on Delirium. (1999). Practice guideline for the treatment of patients with delirium. *The American Journal of Psychiatry, 156* (Suppl.), 1–20.

Armstrong, L., Borthwick, S. E., Bayles, K. A., & Tomoeda, C. K. (1996). Use of the Arizona Battery for Communication Disorders of Dementia in the UK. *European Journal of Disorders of Communication, 31*, 171–180.

Bayles, K. A., & Tomoeda, C. K. (1993). *Arizona Battery for Communication Disorders of Dementia.* Austin, TX: Pro-Ed.

Bayles, K. A., & Tomoeda, C. K. (1994). *Functional Linguistic Communication Inventory.* Austin, TX: Pro-Ed.

Bayles, K. A., Tomoeda, C. K., Montgomery, E. B., Cruz, R. F., & Azuma, T. (2000). The relationship of mental status to performance on lexical- semantic tasks in Parkinson's disease. *Advances in Speech-Language Pathology, 2*, 67–75.

Bayles, K. A., Tomoeda, C. K., Wood, J. A., Cruz, R. F., & McGeagh, A. (1996). Comparison of the sensitivity of the ABCD and other measures of Alzheimer 's dementia. *Journal of Medical Speech-Language Pathology, 4*, 183–194.

Bayles, K. A., Trosset, M. W., Tomoeda, C. K., Montgomery, E. B., & Wilson, J. (1993). Generative naming in Parkinson's disease patients. *Journal of Clinical and Experimental Neuropsychology, 15*, 547–562.

Benton, A. L. (1983). *Contributions to neuropsychological assessment.* New York: Oxford University Press.

Borson, S., Scanlan, J., Brush, M., Vitaliano, P., & Dokmak, A. (2000). The Mini-Cog: A cognitive 'vital signs' measure for dementia screening in multi-lingual elderly. *International Journal of Geriatric Psychiatry, 15*, 1021–1027.

Borson, S., Scanlan, J. M., Chen, P., & Ganguli, M. (2003). The Mini-Cog as a screen for dementia: Validation in a population-based sample. *Journal of the American Geriatrics Society, 51*, 1451–1454.

Borson, S., Scanlan, J., Watanabe, J., Tu, S. P., Lessig, M. (2005). Simplifying detection of cognitive impairment: Comparison of the Mini-Cog and Mini-Mental State Examination in a multiethnic sample. *Journal of the American Geriatrics Society, 53*, 871–874.

Bossers, W. J. R., van der Woude, L. H. V., Boersma, F., Scherder, E. J. A., & van Heuvelen, M. J. G. (2012). Recommended measures for the assessment of cognitive and physical performance in older patients with dementia: A systematic review. *Dementia and Geriatric Cognitive Disorders EXTRA, 2*, 589–609.

Bozeat, S., Gregory, C. A., Lambon Ralph, M. A., & Hodges, J. R. (2000). Which neuropsychiatric and behavioural features distinguish frontal and temporal variants of frontotemporal dementia from Alzheimer's disease? *Journal of Neurology, Neurosurgery, and Psychiatry, 69*, 178–186.

Brodaty, H., Low, L. F., Givson, L., & Burns, K. (2006). What is the best dementia screening instrument for general practitioners to use? *American Journal of Geriatric Psychiatry, 14*, 391–400.

Buschke, H., & Fuld, P. A. (1974). Evaluating storage, retention, and retrieval in disordered memory and learning. *Neurology, 24*, 1019–1025.

Buschke, H., Kuslansky, G., Katz, M., Stewart, W. F., Sliwinski, M. J., Eckholdt, H. M., & Lipton, R. B. (1999). Screening for dementia with the memory impairment screen. *Neurology, 52*, 231–238.

Chou, K. L., Amick, M. M., Brandt, J., Camicioli, R., Frei, K., Gitelman, D., . . . Uc, E.Y. (2010). A recommended scale for cognitive screening in clinical trials of Parkinson's disease. *Movement Disorders, 25*, 2501–2507.

Clark, L. J., Gatz, M., Zheng, L., Chen, Y. L., McCleary, C., & Mack W. J. (2009). Longitudinal verbal fluency in normal aging, preclinical, and prevalent Alzheimer's disease. *American Journal of Alzheimer's Disease & Other Dementias, 24*, 461–468.

Clark, J. H., Hobson, V. L., & O'Bryant, S. E. (2010). Diagnostic accuracy of percent retention scores on RBANS verbal memory subtests for the diagnosis of Alzheimer's disease and mild cognitive impairment. *Archives of Clinical Neuropsychology, 25*, 318–326.

Cole, M.G., McCusker, J., Voyer, P., Monette, J., Champoux, N., Ciampi, A., . . . Belzile, E. (2011). Subsyndromal delirium in older long-term care residents: Incidence, risk factors, and outcomes. *Journal of the American Geriatric Society, 59*, 1829–1836.

Collerton, D., Burn, D., McKeith, I., & O'Brien, J. (2003). Systematic review and meta-analysis show that dementia with Lewy bodies is a visual-perceptual and attentional-executive dementia. *Dementia and Geriatric Cognitive Disorders, 16*, 229–237.

Cruickshanks, K. (2009). Population-based epidemiologic studies of aging: The contributions of a Wisconsin community. *WMJ Wisconsin Medical Journal, 108*, 271–272.

Crum, R.M., Anthony, J. C., Bassett, S. S., & Folstein, M. F. (1993). Population-based norms for the Mini-Mental State Examination by age and educational level. *JAMA, 269*, 2386–2391.

Cummings, J. L. (1997). The Neuropsychiatric Inventory: Assessing psychopathology in dementia patients. *Neurology, 48* (Suppl. 6), S10–S16.

Cummings, J. L., Mega, M., Gray, K., Rosenberg-Thompson, S., Carusi, D. A., & Gornbein, J. (1994). The Neuropsychiatric Inventory: Comprehensive assessment of psychopathology in dementia. *Neurology, 44*, 2308–2314.

Delis, D. C., Kramer, J. H., Kaplan, E., & Ober, B. A. (2000). *California Verbal Learning Test®—Second Edition (CVLT®—II)*. San Antonio, TX: Harcourt Assessment.

Desmond, D. W. (2002). General approaches to neuropsychological assessment. In T. Erkin-Juntti & S. Gauther (Eds.), *Vascular cognitive impairment* (pp. 323–338). London: Martin Dunitz.

Dobie, D. J. (2002). Depression, dementia and pseudodementia. *Seminars in Clinical Neuropsychiatry, 7*, 170–186.

Donaghy, P. C., & McKeith, I. G. (2014). The clinical characteristics of dementia with Lewy bodies and a consideration of prodromal diagnosis. *Alzheimer's Research & Therapy, 6*, 46.

Doraiswamy, P. M., Kaiser, L., Beiber, F., & Garman, R. L. (2001). The Alzheimer's disease assessment scale: Evaluation of psychometric properties and patterns of cognitive decline in multicenter clinical trials of mild and moderate Alzheimer's disease. *Alzheimer Disease and Associated Disorders, 15*, 174–183.

Downing, L. J., Caprio, T. V., & Lyness, J. M. (2013). Geriatric psychiatry review: Differential diagnosis and treatment of the 3 D's – delirium, dementia, and depression. *Current Psychiatry Reports, 15*, 1–10.

Duff, K., Hobson, V. L., Beglinger, L. J., & O'Bryant, S. E. (2010). Diagnosic accuracy of the RBANS in mild cognitive impairment: Limitations on assessing milder impairments. *Archives of Clinical Neuropsychology, 25*, 429–441.

Emery, V. O. B., & Oxman, T. E. (2003). Depressive dementia. In V. O. B. Emery & T. E. Oxman (Eds.), *Dementia: Presentation, differential diagnosis, and nosology* (pp. 361–397). Baltimore, MD: The Johns Hopkins University Press.

Emre, M., Aarsland, D., Brown, R., Burn, D.J., Duyckaerts, C., Mizuno, Y., . . . Dubois, B. (2007). Clinical diagnostic criteria for dementia associated with Parkinson's disease. *Movement Disorders, 22*, 1689–1707.

Folstein, M. F., Folstein, S. E., & McHugh, P. R. (1975). "Mini-Mental State": A practical method for grading the mental state of patients for the clinician. *Journal of Psychiatric Research, 12*, 189–198.

Freilich, B. M., & Hyer, L. A. (2007). Relation of the Repeatable Battery for Assessment of Neuropsychological Status to measures of daily functioning in dementia. *Psychological Reports, 101*, 119–129.

Gorno-Tempini, M. L., Hillis, A. E., Weintraub, S., Kertesz, A., Mendez, M., Cappa, S. F., . . . Grossman, M. (2011). Classification of primary progressive aphasia and its variants. *Neurology, 76*, 1006–1014.

Graham, N., Emery, T., & Hodges, J. (2004). Distinctive cognitive profiles in Alzheimer's disease and subcortical vascular dementia. *Journal of Neurology, Neurosurgery, & Psychiatry, 75*, 61–71.

Grober, E., & Kawas, C. (1997). Learning and retention in preclinical and early Alzheimer's disease. *Psychology and Aging, 12*, 183–188.

Hachinski, V. C., Iliff, L. D., Zilhka, E., duBoulay, G. H. D., McAllister, V. L., Marshall, J., . . . Symon, L. (1975).

Cerebral blood flow in dementia. *Archives of Neurology,* 32, 632–637.

Hamilton, J. M., Salmon, D. P., Galasko, D., & Hansen, L. A. (2004). Distinct memory deficits in dementia with Lewy bodies and Alzheimer 's disease. *Journal of the International Neuropsychological Society,* 10, 689–697.

Hancock P., & Larner, A. J. (2008). Cambridge Behavioural Inventory for the diagnosis of dementia. *Progress in Neurology and Psychiatry,* 12, 23–25.

Hansen, L., Salmon, D., Galasko, D., Masliah, E., Katzman, R., DeTeresa, R., . . . Alford, M. (1990). The Lewy body variant of Alzheimer 's disease: A clinical and pathological entity. *Neurology,* 40, 1–8.

Hart, R. P., Kwentus, J. A., Wade, J. B., & Taylor, J. R. (1988). Modified Wisconsin Card Sorting Test in elderly normal, depressed, and demented patients. *Clinical Neuropsychologist,* 2, 49–52.

Helm-Estabrooks, N. (2001). Cognitive Linguistic Quick Test (CLQT): Examiner's manual. San Antonio, TX: The Psychological Corporation.

Hines, L. E., & Murphy, J. E. (2011). Potentially harmful drug-drug interactions in the elderly: A review. *American Journal of Geriatric Pharmacotherapy,* 9, 364–377.

Hoffman, H. J., Dobie, R. A., Losonczy, K. G., Themann, C. L., & Flamme, G. A. (2017). Declining prevalence of hearing loss in US adults aged 20 to 69 years. *JAMA Otolaryngology Head Neck Surgery,* 143, 274–285.

Humphreys, J. D., Dempsey, J. P., O'Bryant, S. E., & Sutker, P. B. (2006). Convergent validity of the Repeatable Battery for the Assessment of Neuropsychological Status in a memory disorder clinic sample. *Archives of Clinical Neuropsychology,* 21, 557–558.

Ijuin, M., Homma, A., Mimura, M., Kitamura, S., Kawai, Y., Imai, Y., & Gondo, Y. (2008). Validation of the 7-Minute Screen for the detection of early-stage AD. *Dementia and Geriatric Cognitive Disorders,* 25, 248–255.

Inouye, S. K., Van Dyck, C. H., Alessi, C. A., Balkin, S., Siegal, A. P., & Horwitz, R.I. (1990). Clarifying confusion: The Confusion Assessment Method. A new method for detection of delirium. *Annals of Internal Medicine,* 113, 941–948.

Ismail, Z., Rajji, T.K., & Shulman, K.I. (2010). Brief cognitive screening instruments: An update. *International Journal of Geriatric Psychiatry,* 25, 111–120.

Jenkins, R. L., & Parsons, O. A. (1978). Cognitive deficits in male alcoholics as measured by a modified Wisconsin Card Sorting Test. *Alcohol Technical Reports,* 7, 76–83.

Johnson, D. K., Morris, J. C., & Galvin, J. E. (2005). Verbal and visuospatial deficits in dementia with Lewy bodies. *Neurology,* 65, 1232–1238.

Karantzoulis, S., Novitski, J., Gold, M., & Randolph, C. (2013). The Repeatable Battery for the Assessment of Neuropsychological Status (RBANS): Utility in detection and characterization of mild cognitive impairment due to Alzheimer's disease. *Archives of Clinical Neuropsychology,* 28, 837–844.

Kaufer, D. I., Cummings, J. L., Ketchel, P., Smith, V., MacMillan, A., Shelley, T., . . . DeKosky, S. T. (2000). Validation of the NPI-Q, a brief clinical form of the neuropsychiatric inventory. *Journal of Neuropsychiatry and Clinical Neurosciences,* 12, 233–239.

Kehagia, A. A., Barker, R. A., & Robbins, T. W. (2010). Neuropsychological and clinical heterogeneity of cognitive impairment and dementia in patients with Parkinson's disease. *Lancet Neurology,* 9, 1200–1213.

Kemp, J., Philippi, N., Phillipps, C., Demuynck, C., Albasser, T., Martin-Hunyadi, C., . . . Blanc, F. (2017). Cognitive profile prodromal dementia with Lewy bodies. *Alzheimer's Research & Therapy,* 91, 1–10.

Kertesz, A., Davidson, W., & Fox, H. (1997). Frontal behavioral inventory: Diagnostic criteria for frontal lobe dementia. *Canadian Journal of Neurological Sciences,* 24, 29–36.

Kertesz, A., Davidson, W., McCabe, P., & Munoz, D. (2003). Behavioral quantitation is more sensitive than cognitive testing in frontotemporal dementia. *Alzheimer Disease and Associated Disorders,* 17, 223–229.

Kertesz, A., Nadkarni, N., Davidson, W., & Thomas, A. W. (2000). The Frontal Behavioral Inventory in the differential diagnosis of frontotemporal dementia. *Journal of the International Neuropsychological Society,* 6, 460–468.

Kiloh, L.G. (1961). Pseudo-dementia. *Acta Psychiatrica Scandinavica,* 37, 336–351.

Konstantinopoulou, E., Aretouli, E., Ioannidis, P., Karacostas, D., & Kosmidis, M. H. (2013). Behavioral disturbances differentiate frontotemporal lobar degeneration subtypes and Alzheimer's disease: Evidence from the Frontal Behavioral Inventory. *International Journal of Geriatric Psychiatry,* 28, 939–946.

Kral, V. A., & Emery, O. B. (1989). Long-term follow up of depressive pseudodementia of the aged. *Canadian Journal of Psychiatry,* 34, 445–446.

Lamy, P. P. (1986). The elderly and drug interactions. *Journal of the American Geriatric Society,* 34, 586–592.

Larner, A. J. (2007). Addenbrooke's Cognitive Examination (ACE) for the diagnosis and differential diagnosis of dementia. *Clinical Neurology and Neurosurgery,* 109, 491–494.

Larson, E. B., Kukull, W. A., Buchner, D., & Reifler, B. V. (1987). Adverse drug reactions associated with global cognitive impairment in elderly persons. *Annals of Internal Medicine,* 107, 169–173.

Le Rhun, E., Richard, F., & Pasquier, F. (2006). Different patterns of Mini Mental Status Examination responses in primary progressive aphasia and Alzheimer 's disease. *European Journal of Neurology,* 13, 1124–1127.

Levy, M. L., Miller, B. L., Cummings, J. L., Fairbanks, L. A., & Craig, A. (1996). Alzheimer disease and frontotemporal dementias: Behavioral distinctions. *Archives of Neurology,* 53, 687–690.

Lezak, M. D., Howieson, D. B., Loring, D. W., Hannay, H. J., & Fischer, J. S. (2004). *Neuropsychological assessment* (4th ed.). New York, NY: Oxford University Press.

Locascio, J. J., Growden, J. H., & Corkin, S. (1995). Cognitive test performance in detecting, staging and tracking Alzheimer 's disease. *Archives of Neurology,* 52, 1087–1099.

Maguire, E. A., Kumaran, D., Hassabis, D., & Kopelman, M. D. (2010). Autobiographical memory in semantic dementia: A longitudinal fMRI study. *Neuropsychologia, 48*, 123–136.

Malloy, P., & Grace, J. (2005). A review of rating scales for measuring behavior change due to frontal systems damage. *Cognitive and Behavioral Neurology, 18*, 18–27.

Massey, A. J. (2005). Medication-related issues associated with the management of dementia. *The ASHA Leader, 10*, 12–13.

Mathias, J. L., & Morphett, K. (2010). Neurobehavioral differences between Alzheimer's disease and frontotemporal dementia: A meta-analysis. *Journal of Clinical and Experimental Neuropsychology, 32*, 682–698.

Mathuranath, P. S., Nestor, P. J., Berrios, G. E., Rakowicz, W., & Hodges, J. R. (2000). A brief cognitive test battery to differentiate Alzheimer's disease and frontotemporal dementia. *Neurology, 55*, 1613–1620.

Mattis, S. (1976). Mental status examination for organic mental syndrome in the elderly patient. In L. Bellak & T. B. Karasu (Eds.), *Geriatric psychiatry* (pp. 77–121). New York, NY: Grune & Stratton.

McKhann, G., Knopman, D., Chertkow, H., Hyman Jr., B. T., Jack Jr., C. R., Kawas, C. H., . . . Phelps, C.H. (2011). The diagnosis of dementia due to Alzheimer's disease: Recommendations from the National Institute on Aging-Alzheimer's Association workgroups on diagnostic guidelines for Alzheimer's disease. *Alzheimer's and Dementia: The Journal of the Alzheimer's Association, 7*, 263–269.

Milne, A., Culverwell, A., Guss, R., Tuppen, J., & Whelton, R. (2008). Screening for dementia in primary care: A review of the use, efficacy and quality of measures. *International Psychogeriatrics, 20*, 911–926.

Mioshi, E., Dawson, K., Mitchell, J., Arnold, R., & Hodges, J. R. (2006). The Addenbrooke's Cognitive Examination Revised (ACE-R): A brief cognitive test battery for dementia screening. *International Journal of Geriatric Psychiatry, 21*, 1078–1085.

Mitchell, A. J. (2009). A meta-analysis of the accuracy of the Mini-Mental State Examination in the detection of dementia and mild cognitive impairment. *Journal of Psychiatric Research, 43*, 411–431.

Monsch, A. U., Foldi, N. S., Ermini-Fünfschillin, D. E., Berres, M., Taylor, K. I., Seifritz, E., . . . Spiegel, R. (1995). Improving the diagnostic accuracy of the Mini-Mental State Examination. *Acta Neurologica Scandinavica, 92*(2), 145–150.

Moorhouse, B., Douglas, J., Panaccio, J., & Steel, G. (1999). Use of the Arizona Battery for Communication Disorders of Dementia in an Australian context. *Asia Pacific Journal of Speech, Language and Hearing, 4*, 93–107.

Moroney, J. T., Bagiella, E., Desmond, D. W., Hachinski, V. C., Molsa, P. K., Gustafson, L., . . . Tatemichi, T. K. (1997). Meta-analysis of the Hachinski Ischemic Score in pathologically verified dementias. *Neurology, 49*, 1096–1105.

Moss, S. E., Tomoeda, C. K., & Bayles, K.A. (2000). Comparison of the cognitive-linguistic profiles of Down syndrome adults with and without dementia to individuals with Alzheimer's disease. *Journal of Medical Speech-Language Pathology, 8*, 69–81.

Mueller, K. D., Koscik, R. L., LaRue, A., Clark, L. R., Hermann, B., Johnson, S. C., & Sager, M. A. (2015). Verbal fluency and early memory decline: Results from the Wisconsin Registry for Alzheimer's Prevention. *Archives of Clinical Neuropsychology, 30*, 448–457.

Nagahama, Y., Okina, T., Suzuki, N., & Matsuda, M. (2006). The Cambridge Behavioral Inventory: Validation and application in a memory clinic. *Journal of Geriatric Psychiatry and Neurology, 19*, 220–225.

Nasreddine, Z. (2011). Montreal Cognitive Assessment (MoCA) Version 3. Retrieved December 6, 2017, from www.mocatest.org.

Nasreddine, Z., Phillips, N. A., Bédirian, V., Charbonneau, S., Whitehead, V., Collin, I., . . . Chertkow, H. (2005). The Montreal Cognitive Assessment, MoCA: A brief screening tool for mild cognitive impairment. *Journal of the American Geriatric Society, 53*, 695–699.

National Institute on Aging. (2017).What are Frontotemporal dementias. Retrieved from https://www.nia.nih .gov/health/what-are-frontotemporal-disorders.

National Institute on Deafness and Other Communication Disorders (NIDCD). (2017). *Age-related hearing loss*. National Institutes of Health. Retrieved December 6, 2017, from https://www.nidcd.nih.gov/health/age-related -hearing-loss.

Noe, E., Marder, K., Bell, K. L., Jacobs, D. M., Manly, J. J., & Stern, Y. (2004). Comparison of dementia with Lewy bodies to Alzheimer's disease and Parkinson's disease with dementia. *Movement Disorders, 19*, 60–67.

Orange, J. B. (2001). Family caregivers, communication, and Alzheimer 's disease. In M. L. Hummert & J. F. Nussbaum (Eds.), *Aging, communication, and health: Linking research and practice for successful aging* (pp. 225–248). Mahwah, NJ: Lawrence Earlbaum Associates.

Parashos, S. A., Johnson, M. L., Erickson-Davis, C., & Wielinski, C.L. (2009). Assessing cognition in Parkinson disease: Use of the Cognitive Linguistic Quick Test. *Journal of Geriatric Psychiatry & Neurology, 22*, 228–234.

Popplewell, P., & Phillips, R. (2002). Is it dementia?— Which one? *Australian Family Physician, 31*, 319–322.

Randolph, C., Tierney, M. C., Mohr, E., & Chase T. N. (1998). The Repeatable Battery for the Assessment of Neuropsychological Status (RBANS): Preliminary clinical validity. *Journal of Clinical and Experimental Neuropsychology, 20*, 310–319.

Reisberg, B., Ferris, S. H., de Leon, M. J., & Crook, T. (1982). The Global Deterioration Scale (GDS): An instrument for the assessment of primary degenerative dementia (PDD). *American Journal of Psychiatry, 139*, 1136–1139.

Reisberg, B., Ferris, S. H., & Franssen, E. (1985). An ordinal functional assessment tool for Alzheimer's type dementia. *Hospital and Community Psychiatry, 36*, 593–595.

Rentz, D. M., & Weintraub, S. (2000). Neuropsychological detection of early probable Alzheimer's disease. In L. F. M. Scinto & K. R. Daffner (Eds.), *Early diagnosis of Alzheimer's disease* (pp. 169–189). Totowa, NJ: Humana Press.

Robinson-Whelen, S., & Storandt, M. (1992). Immediate and delayed prose recall among normal and demented adults. *Archives of Neurology, 49*, 32–34.

Rosen, W. G., Mohs, R. C., & Davis, K. L. (1984). A new rating scale for Alzheimer's disease. *American Journal of Psychiatry, 141*, 1356–1364.

Rosen, W. G., Mohs, R. C., & Davis, K. L. (1986). Longitudinal changes: Cognitive, behavioral, and affective patterns in Alzheimer's disease. In L. W. Poon (Ed.), *Handbook for clinical memory assessment of older adults* (pp. 294–301). Washington, DC: American Psychological Association.

Rossetti, H. C., Lacritz, L. H., Cullum, C. M., & Weiner, M. F. (2011). Normative data for the Montreal Cognitive Assessment (MoCA) in a population-based sample. *Neurology, 77*, 1272–1275.

Rubin, E. H., Storandt, M., Miller, J. P., Kinscherf, D. A., Grant, E. A., Morris, J. C., & Berg, L. (1998). A prospective study of cognitive function and onset of dementia in cognitively healthy elders. *Archives of Neurology, 55*, 395–401.

Sachdev, P. S., & Looi, J. C. L. (2003). Neuropsychological differentiation of Alzheimer's disease and vascular dementia. In J. V. Bowler & V. Hachinski (Eds.), *Vascular cognitive impairment* (pp. 153–175). New York, NY: Oxford University Press.

Saczynski, J. S., Beiser, A., Seshadri, S., Auerbach, S., Wolf, P. A., & Au, R. (2010). Depressive symptoms and risk of dementia. *Neurology, 75*, 35–41.

Sevigny, J. J., Peng, Y., Liu, L., & Lines, C. R. (2010). Item analysis of ADAS-Cog: Effect of baseline cognitive impairment in a clinical AD trial. *American Journal of Alzheimer Disease and Other Dementias, 25*, 119–124.

Seymour, R., & Routledge, P. (1998). Important drug-drug interactions in the elderly. *Drugs & Aging, 12*, 485–494.

Shulman, K. I., Herrmann, N., Brodaty, H., Chiu, H., Lawlor, B., Ritchie, K., & Scanlan, J. M. (2006). IPA survey of brief cognitive screening instruments. *International Psychogeriatrics, 18*, 281–294.

Silva, J. D., Humphreys, J. D., Dempsey, J. P., O'Bryant, S. E., & Sutker, P. B. (2006) Test-retest reliability of the Repeatable Battery for the Assessment of Neuropsychological Status in a memory disorder clinic sample. *Archives of Clinical Neuropsychology, 21*, 560–561.

Sloan, R. W. (1983). Drug interactions. *American Family Physician, 27*, 229–238.

Snowden, J. S. (2005). Semantic dementia. In A. Burns, J. O'Brien, & D. Ames (Eds.), *Dementia* (3rd, ed., pp. 702–712). London: Hodder Arnold.

Solomon, P. R., Hirschoff, A., Kelly, B., Relin, M., Brush, M., DeVeaux, R. D., & Pendlebury, W. W. (1998). A 7 minute neurocognitive screening battery highly sensitive to Alzheimer's disease. *Archives of Neurology, 55*, 349–355.

Sperling, R. A., Aisen, P. S., Beckett, L. A., Bennett, D. A., Craft, S., Fagan, A. M., . . . Phelps, C. H. (2011). Toward defining the preclinical stages of Alzheimer's disease: Recommendations from the National Institute on Aging-Alzheimer's Association work groups on diagnostic guidelines for Alzheimer's disease. *Alzheimer's and Dementia: The Journal of the Alzheimer's Association, 7*, 280–292.

Taler, V., & Phillips, N.A. (2008). Language performance in Alzheimer's disease and mild cognitive impairment: A comparative review. *Journal of Clinical and Experimental Neuropsychology, 30*, 501–556.

Taylor, W. D. (2014). Depression in the elderly. *New England Journal of Medicine, 371*, 1228–1236.

Tiraboschi, P., Salmon, D. P., Hansen, L. A., Hostetter, R. C., Thal, L. J., & Corey-Bloom J. (2006). What best differentiates Lewy body from Alzheimer's disease in early-stage dementia. *Brain, 129*, 729–735.

Tombaugh, T., & McIntyre, N. (1992). The Mini-Mental State Examination: A comprehensive review. *Journal of the American Geriatrics Society, 40*, 922–935.

Tomoeda, C. K., & Bayles, K. A. (1993). Longitudinal effects of Alzheimer's disease on discourse production. *Alzheimer's Disease and Associated Disorders, 7*, 223–236.

Tröster, A.I. (2008). Neuropsychological characteristics of dementia with Lewy bodies and Parkinson's disease with dementia: Differentiation, early detection, and implications for "mild cognitive impairment" and biomarkers. *Neuropsychology Review, 18*, 103–119.

Verhey, F. R., Houx, P., van Lang, N., Huppert, F., Stoppe, G., Saerens, J., . . . Jolles, J. (2004). Cross-national comparison and validation of the Alzheimer's Disease Assessment Scale: Results from the European Harmonization Project for Instruments in Dementia (EURO-HARPID). *International Journal of Geriatric Psychiatry, 19*, 41–50.

Wallace, G. L., & Holmes, S. (1993). Cognitive-linguistic assessment of individuals with multiple sclerosis. *Archives of Physical Medical Rehabilitation, 74*, 637–643.

Warren, J. D., Harvey, R. J., & Rossor, M. N. (2005). Progressive aphasia and other focal syndromes. In A. Burns, J. O'Brien, & D. Ames (Eds.), *Dementia* (3rd ed., pp. 720–728). London, England: Hodder Arnold.

Warrington, E.K., & James, M. (1991). *The visual object and space perception battery*. Bury St. Edmunds, England: Thames Valley Test Company.

Wear, H. J., Wedderburn, C. J., Mioshi, E., Williams-Gray, C. H., Mason, S. L., Barker, R. A., & Hodges, J. R. (2008). The Cambridge Behavioural Inventory revised. *Dementia & Neuropsychologia, 2*, 102–107.

Wechsler, D. (1981). *Wechsler Adult Intelligence Scale—Revised manual*. New York: Harcourt Brace & Jovanovich.

Wechsler, D. (1987). *Wechsler Memory Scale—Revised*. New York: The Psychological Corporation.

Wechsler, D. (2009). *Wechsler Memory Scale—Fourth Edition*. San Antonio, TX: Pearson.

Wedderburn, C., Wear, H., Brown, J., Mason, S. J., Barker, R. A., Hodges, J., & Williams-Gray, C. (2008). The utility of the Cambridge Behavioural Inventory in neurodegenerative disease. *Journal of Neurology, Neurosurgery & Psychiatry, 79*, 500–503.

Wei, L. A., Fearing, M. A., Sternberg, E. J., & Inouye, S. K. (2008). The Confusion Assessment Methods (CAM): A systematic review of current usage. *Journal of the American Geriatric Society, 56*, 823–830.

Weiner, M. F. (2003). Clinical diagnosis of cognitive dysfunction and dementing illness. In M. F. Weiner & A. M. Lipton (Eds.), *The dementias: Diagnosis, treatment, and research* (pp. 1–48). Washington, DC: American Psychiatric Publishing.

Welsh, K., Butters, N., Hughes, J., Mohs, R., & Heyman, A. (1991). Detection of abnormal memory decline in mild cases of Alzheimer's disease using CERAD neuropsychological measures. *Archives of Neurology, 48*, 278–281.

Weytingh, M. D., Bossuyt, P. M. M., & van Crevel, H. (1995). Reversible dementia: More than 10% or less an 1%? A quantitative review. *Journal of Neurology, 242*, 466–471.

Williams-Gray, C. H., Evans, J. R., Goris, A., Foltynie, T., Ban, M., Robbins, T. W., . . . Barker, R.A. (2009). The distinct cognitive syndromes of Parkinson's disease: 5 year follow-up of the CamPaIGN cohort. *Brain, 132*, 2958–2969.

Williams-Gray, C. H., Foltynie, T., Brayne, C. E. G., Robbins, T. W., & Barker, R. A. (2007). Evolution of cognitive dysfunction in an incident Parkinson's disease cohort. *Brain, 130*, 1787–1798.

Wilson, B., Cockburn, J., & Baddeley, A. (1991). *Rivermeade Behavioral Memory Test* (2nd ed.). Reading, England: Thames Valley Test Co.

Yokomizo, J. E., Simon, S. S., & Bottino, C. M. (2014). Cognitive screening for dementia in primary care: A systematic review. *International Psychogeriatrics, 26*, 1783–1804.

Section II

Arriagada, P. V., Growdon, J. H., Hedley-Whyte, E. T., & Hyman, B. T. (1992). Neurofibrillary tangles but not senile plaques parallel duration and severity of Alzheimer's disease. *Neurology, 42*(3), 631–631.

Barnes, D. E., Yaffe, K., Belfor, N., Jagust, W. J., Decarli, C., Reed, B. R., & Kramer, J. H. (2009). Computer-based cognitive training for mild cognitive impairment: Results from a pilot randomized, controlled trial. *Alzheimer Disease and Associated Disorders, 23*, 205–210. doi:10.1097/ WAd.0b013e31819c6137

Basak, C., Boot, W. R., Voss, M. W., & Kramer, A.F. (2008). Can training in a real-time strategy video game attenuate cognitive decline in older adults? *Psychology and Aging, 23*, 765–777.

Belleville, S., & Bherer, L. (2012). Biomarkers of cognitive training effects in aging. *Current Translational Geriatrics and Gerontology Reports, 1*, 104–110.

Belleville, S., Clément, F., Mellah, S., Gilbert, B., Fontaine, F., & Gauthier, S. (2011). Training-related brain plasticity in subjects at risk of developing Alzheimer's disease. *Brain, 134*(6), 1623–1634.

Belleville, S., Gilbert, B., Fontaine, F., Gagnon, L., Ménard, E., & Gauthier, S. (2006). Improvement of episodic memory in persons with mild cognitive impairment and healthy older adults: Evidence from a cognitive intervention program. *Dementia and Geriatric Cognitive Disorders, 22*, 486–499.

Belleville, S., Hudon, C., Bier, N., Brodeur, C., Gilbert, B., Grenier, S., . . . Gauthier, S. (2018). MEMO+: Efficacy, durability and effect of cognitive training and psychosocial intervention in individuals with mild cognitive impairment. *Journal of the American Geriatrics Society*, 1–9. doi:10.1111/jgs.15192

Bennett, D. A., Schneider, J. A., Arvanitakis, Z., Kelly, J. F., Aggarwal, N. T., Shah, R. C., & Wilson, R. S. (2006). Neuropathology of older persons without cognitive impairment from two community-based studies. *Neurology, 66*(12), 1837–1844.

Brehmer, Y., Westerberg, H., & Bäckman, L. (2012). Working-memory training in younger and older adults: Training gains, transfer, and maintenance. *Frontiers in Human Neuroscience, 6*, 63.

Caeyenberghs, K., Clemente, A., Imms, P., Egan, G., Hocking, D. R., Leemans, A., . . . Wilson, P. H. (2018). Evidence for training-dependent structural neuroplasticity in brain-injured patients: A critical review. *Neurorehabilitation and Neural Repair*, 1–16.

Cipriani, G., Bianchetti, A., & Trabucchi, M. (2006). Outcomes of a computer-based cognitive rehabilitation program on Alzheimer's disease patients compared with those on patients affected by mild cognitive impairment. *Archives of Gerontology and Geriatrics, 43*, 327–335.

Clare, L., Evans, S., Parkinson, C., Woods, R. T., & Linden, D. (2011). Goal-setting in cognitive rehabilitation for people with early-stage Alzheimer's disease. *Clinical Gerontologist, 34*(3), 220–236.

Clare, L., van Paasschen, J., Evans, S. J., Parkinson, C., Woods, R. T., & Linden, D. E. J. (2009). Goal-oriented cognitive rehabilitation for an individual with mild cognitive impairment: Behavioural and neuroimaging outcomes. *Neurocase, 15*(4), 318–331.

Clare, L., & Woods, R. T. (2004). Cognitive training and cognitive rehabilitation for people with early-stage Alzheimer's disease: A review. *Neuropsychological Rehabilitation, 14*, 385–401.

Devanand, D. P., Liu, X., & Brown, P. J. (2017). Impact of functional deficits in instrumental activities of daily living in mild cognitive impairment: A clinical algorithm to predict progression to dementia. *Alzheimer Disease and Associated Disorders*, 31(1), 55–61. http://doi.org/10.1097/WAD.0000000000000160

Driscoll, I., & Troncoso, J. (2011). Asymptomatic Alzheimer's disease: A prodrome or a state of resilience? *Current Alzheimer Research*, 8(4), 330–335.

Engvig, A., Fjell, A. M., Westlye, L. T., Moberget, T., Sundseth, Ø., Larsen, V. A., & Walhovd, K. B. (2010). Effects of memory training on cortical thickness in the elderly. *NeuroImage*, 52(4), 1667–1676.

Epstein, R. M., Fiscella, K., Lesser, C. S., & Stange, K. C. (2010). Why the nation needs a policy push on patient-centered health care. *Health Affairs*, 29(8), 1489–1495.

Hampstead, B. M., Stringer, A. Y., Stilla, R. F., Deshpande, G., Hu, X., Moore, A. B., & Sathian, K. (2011). Activation and effective connectivity changes following explicit-memory training for face-name pairs in patients with mild cognitive impairments: A pilot study. *Neurorehabilitation and Neural Repair*, 25, 210–222.

Hampstead, B. M., Stringer, A. Y., Stilla, R. F., Giddens, M., & Sathian, K. (2012). Mnemonic strategy training partially restores hippocampal activity in patients with mild cognitive impairment. *Hippocampus*, 22, 1652–1658.

Hampstead, B. M., Towler, S., Stringer, A. Y., & Sathian, K. (2018). Continuous measurement of object location memory is sensitive to effects of age and mild cognitive impairment and related to medial temporal lobe volume. *Alzheimer's & Dementia: Diagnosis, Assessment & Disease Monitoring*, 10, 76–85.

Ince, P. (2001). Pathological correlates of late-onset dementia in a multicenter community-based population in England and Wales. *Lancet*, 357, 169–175.

Institute of Medicine. (2001). *Crossing the quality chasm: A new health system for the 21st century*. Washington, DC: National Academies Press.

Jak, A. J., Seelye, A. M., & Jurick, S. M. (2013). Crosswords to computers: A critical review of popular approaches to cognitive enhancement. *Neuropsychology Rreview*, 23(1), 13–26.

Jean, L., Bergeron, M. È., Thivierge, S., & Simard, M. (2010). Cognitive intervention programs for individuals with mild cognitive impairment: Systematic review of the literature. *American Journal of Geriatric Psychiatry*, 18, 281–296.

Jelcic, N., Cagnin, A., Meneghello, F., Turolla, A., Ermani, M., & Dam, M. (2012). Effects of lexical–semantic treatment on memory in early Alzheimer disease: An observer-blinded randomized controlled trial. *Neurorehabilitation and Neural Repair*, 26(8), 949–956.

Karow, C. M., Harvey, J., Helm-Estabrooks, N., Bloom, C., & Cuellar, M. (2011). *Cognitive decline in normal aging and mild cognitive impairment*. Presented at ASHA, San Diego, C.A.

Katzman, R., Terry, R., DeTeresa, R., Brown, T., Davies, P., Fuld, P., . . . Peck, A. (1988). Clinical, pathological, and neurochemical changes in dementia: A subgroup with preserved mental status and numerous neocortical plaques. *Annals of Neurology*, 23(2), 138–144.

Kaye, J. A., Maxwell, S. A., Mattek, N., Hayes, T. L., Dodge, H., Pavel, M., . . . Zitzelberger, T. A. (2011). Intelligent systems for assessing aging changes: Home-based, unobtrusive, and continuous assessment of aging. *Journals of Gerontology Series B: Psychological Sciences and Social Sciences*, 66(Suppl. 1), i180–i190.

Kinsella, G. J., Mullaly, E., Rand, E., Ong, B., Burton, C., Price, S., . . . Storey, E. (2009). Early intervention for mild cognitive impairment: A randomised controlled trial. *Journal of Neurology, Neurosurgery and Psychiatry*, 80(7), 730–736.

Kleim, J. A., & Jones, T. A. (2008). Principles of experience-dependent neural plasticity: implications for rehabilitation after brain damage. *Journal of Speech, Language, and Hearing Research*, 51, 225–239.

Kueider, A. M., Parisi, J. M., Gross, A. L., & Rebok, G. W. (2012). Computerized cognitive training with older adults: A systematic review. *PLoS One*, 7(7), e40588. doi:10.1371/journal.pone.0040588

Kurz, A., Pohl, C., Ramsenthaler, M., & Sorg, C. (2009). Cognitive rehabilitation in patients with mild cognitive impairment. *International Journal of Geriatric Psychiatry*, 24, 163–168.

Li, H., Li, J., Li, N., Li, B., Wang, P., & Zhou, T. (2011). Cognitive intervention for persons with mild cognitive impairment: A meta-analysis. *Ageing Research Reviews*, 10(2), 285–296.

Lin, F., Yaffe, K., Xia, J., Xue, Q., Harris, T., & Simonsick, A. M. (2013) Hearing loss and cognitive decline in older adults. *Journal of the American Medical Association Internal Medicine*, 173, 293–299.

Mavandadi, S., Rook, K. S., & Newsom, J. T. (2007). Positive and negative social exchanges and disability in later life: An investigation of trajectories of change. *Journal of Gerontology Social Sciences*, 62, 361–370.

Mendes de Leon, C. F., Glass, T. A., & Berkman, L. F. (2003). Social engagement and disability in a community population of older adults: The New Haven EPESE. *American Journal of Epidemiology*, 157(7), 633–642.

Moebs, I., Gee, S., Miyahara, M., Paton, H., & Croucher, M. (2017). Perceptions of a cognitive rehabilitation group by older people living with cognitive impairment and their caregivers: A qualitative interview study. *Dementia*, 16(4), 513–522.

Mufson, E. J., Mahady, L., Waters, D., Counts, S. E., Perez, S. E., DeKosky, S. T., . . . Binder, L. I. (2015). Hippocampal plasticity during the progression of Alzheimer's disease. *Neuroscience*, 309, 51–67. https://doi.org/10.1016/j.neuroscience.2015.03.006

Mufson, E. J., Malek-Ahmadi, M., Perez, S. E., & Chen, K. (2016). Braak staging, plaque pathology, and APOE status in elderly persons without cognitive impairment. *Neurobiology of Aging*, 37, 147–153.

National Academies of Sciences, Engineering, and Medicine. (2017). *Preventing cognitive decline and dementia: A way forward*. Washington, DC: The National Academies Press. https://doi.org/10.17226/24782.

Ngandu, T., Lehtisalo, J., Solomon, A., Levälahti, E., Ahtiluoto, S., Antikainen, R., . . . Lindström, J. (2015). A 2 year multidomain intervention of diet, exercise, cognitive training, and vascular risk monitoring versus control to prevent cognitive decline in at-risk elderly people (FINGER): A randomised controlled trial. *The Lancet, 385*(9984), 2255–2263.

Nudo, R. J., & Bury, S. (2011). Motor and sensory reorganization in primates. In S. Raskin (Ed.), *Neuroplasticity and rehabilitation* (pp. 65–88). New York, NY: Guilford Press.

Petersen, R. C., Lopez, O., Armstrong, M. J., Getchius, T. S., Ganguli, M., Gloss, D., . . . Sager, M. (2018). Practice guideline update summary: Mild cognitive impairment: Report of the guideline development, dissemination, and implementation subcommittee of the American Academy of Neurology. *Neurology, 90*(3), 126–135.

Pistacchi, M., Gioulis, M., Contin, F., Sanson, F., & Marsala, S. Z. (2015). Cognitive profiles in mild cognitive impairment (MCI) patients associated with Parkinson's disease and cognitive disorders. *Annals of Indian Academy of Neurology, 18*(2), 200–205. http://doi.org/10.4103/0972-2327.150611

Rebok, G. W., Ball, K., Guey, L. T., Jones, R. N., Kim, H. Y., King, J. W., . . . Willis, S. L. (2014). Ten-year effects of the ACTIVE cognitive training trial on cognition and everyday functioning in older adults. *Journal of the American Geriatrics Society, 62*(1), 16–24. http://doi.org/10.1111/jgs.12607

Rosen, A. C., Sugiura, L., Kramer, J. H., Whitfield-Gabrieli, S., & Gabrieli, J. D. (2011). Cognitive training changes hippocampal function in mild cognitive impairment: A pilot study. *Journal of Alzheimer's Disease, 26*(s3), 349–357.

Rosenberg, A., Ngandu, T., Rusanen, M., Antikainen, R., Bäckman, L., Havulinna, S., . . . Lindström, J. (2017). Multidomain lifestyle intervention benefits a large elderly population at risk for cognitive decline and dementia regardless of baseline characteristics: The FINGER trial. *Alzheimer's & Dementia, 1–8.*

Rouillard, M., Audiffren, M., Albinet, C., Ali Bahri, M., Garraux, G., & Collette, F. (2017). Contribution of four lifelong factors of cognitive reserve on late cognition in normal aging and Parkinson's disease. *Journal of Clinical and Experimental Neuropsychology, 39*(2), 142–162.

Rowland, C. A., & DeLosh, E. L. (2015). Mnemonic benefits of retrieval practice at short retention intervals. *Memory, 23* (3), 403–419.

Rozzini, L., Costardi, D., Chilovi, B. V., Franzoni, S., Trabucchi, M., & Padovani, A. (2007). Efficacy of cognitive rehabilitation in patients with mild cognitive impairment treated with cholinesterase inhibitors. *International Journal of Geriatric Psychiatry, 22*(4), 356–360.

Shankar, A., McMunn, A., Demakakos, P., Hamer, M., & Steptoe, A. (2017). Social isolation and loneliness: Prospective associations with functional status in older adults. *Health Psychology, 36*(2), 179–187. http://dx.doi.org/10.1037/hea0000437

Sherman, D. S., Mauser, J., Nuno, M., & Sherzai, D. (2017). The efficacy of cognitive intervention in mild cognitive impairment (MCI): A meta-analysis of outcomes on neuropsychological measures. *Neuropsychology Review, 27*(4), 440–484. doi: 10.1007/s11065-017-9363-3

SharpBrains.com. (2013). The Digital Brain Health Market 2012–2020: Web-based, mobile and biometrics-based technology to assess, monitor and enhance cognition and brain functioning 2013. Retrieved May 10, 2013, from http://www.sharpbrains.com/market-report/

Simon, S. S., Hampstead, B. M., de Campos Bottino, C. M., de Gobbi Porto, F. H., Duran, F. L., Brucki, S. M. D., . . . Fonseca, L. M. (2017). Transfer effect after mnemonic strategy training in amnestic mild cognitive impairment: evidence from a randomized, single-blind study. *Alzheimer's & Dementia: The Journal of the Alzheimer's Association, 13*(7), P900.

Simon, S. S., Yokomizo, J. E., & Bottino, C. M. C. (2012). Cognitive intervention in amnestic mild cognitive impairment: A systematic review. *Neuroscience and Biobehavioral Reviews, 36*, 1163–1178.

Smith, M. A., & Karpicke, J. D. (2014). Retrieval practice with short-answer, multiple-choice, and hybrid tests. *Memory, 22* (7), 784–802.

Stott, J., & Spector, A. (2011). A review of the effectiveness of memory interventions in mild cognitive impairment (MCI). *International Psychogeriatrics, 23*, 526–538.

Tesky, V. A., Köbe, T., Witte, A. V., Flöel, A., Schuchardt, J. P., Hahn, A., & Pantel, J. (2017). Feasibility and first results of a group program to increase the frequency of cognitively stimulating leisure activities in people with mild cognitive impairment (AKTIVA-MCI). *Clinical Interventions in Aging, 12*, 1459–1469. http://doi.org/10.2147/CIA.S139146

Tripodis, Y., Coleman, B., Martin, B. M., Chaisson, C. E., Steinberg, E., Kowall, N. W., . . . Stern, R. A. (2017). Significant subjective memory and language complaints predict conversion to MCI and Alzheimer's disease dementia. *Alzheimer's & Dementia: The Journal of the Alzheimer's Association, 13*(7), P743.

Troyer, A. K., Murphy, K. J., Anderson, N. D., Moscovitch, M., & Craik, F. I. (2008). Changing everyday memory behaviour in amnestic mild cognitive impairment: A randomised controlled trial. *Neuropsychological Rehabilitation, 18*(1), 65–88.

van Paasschen, J., Clare, L., Yuen, K. S., Woods, R. T., Evans, S. J., Parkinson, C. H., . . . Linden, D. E. (2013). Cognitive rehabilitation changes memory-related brain activity in people with Alzheimer disease. *Neurorehabilitation and Neural Repair, 27*(5), 448–459.

Wolinsky, F. D., Vander Weg, M. W., Martin, R., Unverzagt, F. W., Willis, S. L., Marsiske, M., . . . Tennstedt, S. L. (2009). Does cognitive training improve internal locus of control among older adults? *Journals of Gerontology*

Series B: Psychological Sciences and Social Sciences, 65(5), 591–598.

Woods, B., Aguirre, E., Spector, A. E., & Orrell, M. (2012). Cognitive stimulation to improve cognitive functioning in people with dementia. *The Cochrane Library.*

World Health Organization. (2001). International classification of functioning, disability and health (ICF). *Fifty-Fourth World Health Assembly Health Assembly, WHA54.21,* 13.9. Retrieved from http://www.who.int/classifications/icf/wha-en.pdf.

World Health Organization. (2017). Global action plan on the public health response to dementia 2017–2025. In *Global action plan on the public health response to dementia 2017–2025.*

Yang, Y. C., Boen, C., Gerken, K., Li, T., Schorpp, K., & Harris, K. M. (2016). Social relationships and physiological determinants of longevity across the human life span. *Proceedings of the National Academy of Sciences, 113*(3), 578–583.

Section III

Abrahams, J. P., & Camp, C. J. (1993). Maintenance and generalization of object naming training in anomia associated with degenerative dementia. *Clinical Gerontology, 12,* 57–72.

Anderson, J. R., & Bower, G. H. (1972). Recognition and retrieval processes in free recall. *Psychological Review, 79*(2), 97.

Arbuthnott, K. D., & Kratzig, G. P. (2015). Effective teaching: Sensory learning styles versus general memory processes. *Comprehensive Psychology, 4,* Article 2, 2165–2228.

Arkin, S. M., Rose, C., & Hopper, T. (2000). Implicit and explicit learning gains in Alzheimer's patients: Effects of naming and information retrieval training. *Aphasiology, 14,* 723–742.

Baddeley, A. D., & Wilson, B. A. (1994). When implicit learning fails: Amnesia and the problem of error elimination. *Neuropsychologia, 32,* 53–68.

Bayles, K. A., Tomoeda, C. K., Kaszniak, A. W., & Trosset, M. W. (1991). Alzheimer's disease effects on semantic memory: Loss of structure or function. *Journal of Cognitive Neuroscience, 3,* 166–182.

Belleville, S., Peretz, I., & Malenfant, D. (1996). Examination of the working memory components in normal aging and in dementia of the Alzheimer type. *Neuropsychologia, 34,* 195–207.

Bettcher, B. M., Giovannetti, T., Libon, D. J., Eppig, J., Wambach, D., & Klobusicky, E. (2011). Improving everyday error detection, one picture at a time: A performance-based study of everyday task training. *Neuropsychology, 25*(6), 771–783.

Bier, N., Van Der Linden, M., Gagnon, L., Desrosiers, J., Adam, S., Louveaux, S., & Saint-Mleux, J. (2008). Face–name association learning in early Alzheimer's disease: A comparison of learning methods and their underlying mechanisms. *Neuropsychological Rehabilitation, 18*(3), 343–371.

Bird, M. J. (2000). Psychosocial rehabilitation for problems arising from cognitive deficits in dementia. In R. D. Hill, L. Bäckman, & A. Stigsdotter-Neely (Eds.), *Cognitive rehabilitation in old age* (pp. 249–267). New York, NY: Oxford University Press.

Blunt, J. R. & Karpicke, J. D. (2014). Learning with retrieval-based concept mapping. *Journal of Educational Psychology, 106* (3), 849–858.

Boczko, F. (1994). The Breakfast Club: A multimodal language stimulation program for nursing home residents with Alzheimer's disease. *American Journal of Alzheimer's Disease and Other Dementias, 9,* 35–38.

Bourgeois, M. S. (1990). Enhancing conversation skills in patients with Alzheimer's disease using a prosthetic memory aid. *Journal of Applied Behavior Analysis, 23,* 29–42.

Bourgeois, M. S. (1991). Communication treatment for adults with dementia. *Journal of Speech and Hearing Research, 34,* 831–844.

Bourgeois, M. S. (1992). Evaluating memory wallets in conversations with persons with dementia. *Journal of Speech and Hearing Research, 35,* 1344–1357.

Bourgeois, M.S. (2007). *Memory books and other graphic cuing systems: Practical communication and memory aids for adults with dementia.* Baltimore, MD: Health Professions Press.

Bourgeois, M. S., Camp, C. J., Antenucci, V., & Fox, K. (2016). VoiceMyChoice™: Facilitating Understanding of Preferences of Residents with Dementia. *Advances in Aging Research, 5*(6), 131.

Brush, J. A., & Camp, C. J. (1998a). *A therapy technique for improving memory: Spaced retrieval.* Beachwood, OH: Authors.

Brush, J. A., & Camp, C. J. (1998b). Using spaced-retrieval as an intervention during speech-language therapy. *Clinical Gerontologist, 19,* 51–64.

Budde, H., Wegner, M., Soya, H., Voelcker-Rehage, C., & McMorris, T. (2016). Neuroscience of exercise: Neuroplasticity and its behavioral consequences. *Neural Plasticity, 2016.* doi: doi.org/10.1155/2016/3643879

Camicioli, R., Howieson, D., Lehman, S., & Kaye, J. (1997). Talking while walking: The effect of a dual task in aging and Alzheimer's disease. *Neurology, 48*(4), 955–958.

Camp, C. J. (1989). Facilitation of new learning in Alzheimer's disease. In G. C. Gilmore, P. J. Whitehouse, & M. L. Wykle (Eds.), *Memory, aging and dementia* (pp. 212–225). New York, NY: Springer.

Camp, C. J., Bird, M. J, & Cherry, K. E. (2000). Retrieval strategies as a rehabilitation aid for cognitive loss in pathological aging. In R.D. Hill, L. Bäckman, & A. Stigsdotter-Neely (Eds.), *Cognitive rehabilitation in old age* (pp. 224–248). New York, NY: Oxford University Press.

Camp, C. J., & Schaller, J. R. (1989). Epilogue: Spaced-retrieval memory training in an adult day-care center. *Educational Gerontology, 15*(6), 641–648.

Cherry, B. J., Buckwalter, J. G., & Henderson, V. W. (1996). Memory span procedures in Alzheimer's disease. *Neuropsychology, 10*, 286–293.

Christie, M. E. (1992). Music therapy applications in a skilled and intermediate care nursing home facility: A clinical study. *Activities, Adaptation and Aging, 16*, 69–87.

Clare, L., & Jones, R. S. P. (2008). Errorless learning in the rehabilitation of memory impairment: A critical review. *Neuropsychological Review, 18*, 1–23.

Clare, L., Wilson, B. A., Carter, G., Breen, K., Gosses, A., & Hodges, J. R. (2000). Intervening with everyday memory problems in dementia of Alzheimer type: An errorless learning approach. *Journal of Clinical and Experimental Neuropsychology, 22*(1), 132–146.

Cofer, C. N. (1960). Experimental studies of the role of verbal processes in concept formation and problem solving. *Annals of the New York Academy of Sciences, 91*, 94–107.

Comblain, C., D'Argembeau, A., & Van der Linden, M. (2005). Phenomenal characteristics of autobiographical memories for emotional and neutral events in older and younger adults. *Experimental Aging Research, 31*, 173–189.

Cotman, C. W., Berchtold, N. C., & Christie, L. A. (2007). Exercise builds brain health: Key roles of growth factor cascades and inflammation. *Trends in Neurosciences, 30*(9), 464–472.

Cuddy, L. L., & Duffin, J. (2005). Music, memory, and Alzheimer's disease: Is music recognition spared in dementia, and how can it be assessed? *Medical Hypotheses, 645*, 229–235.

Cuddy, L. L., Duffin, J. M., Gill, S. S., Brown, C. L., Sikka, R., & Vanstone, A. D. (2012). Memory for melodies and lyrics in Alzheimer's disease. *Music Perception, 29*, 479–491.

Cuddy, L. L., Sikka, R., Silveira, K., Bai, S., & Vanstone, A. (2017). Music-evoked autobiographical memories (MEAMs) in Alzheimer disease: Evidence for a positivity effect. *Cogent Psychology, 4*(1), 1277578 https://doi.org/10.1080/23311908.2016.1277578

Damasio, A. R. (1999). *The feeling of what happens: Body and emotion in the making of consciousness*. New York, NY: Harcourt, Brace.

Danckert, S. L., & Craik, F. I. (2013). Does aging affect recall more than recognition memory?. *Psychology and Aging, 28*(4), 902.

Daneman, M., & Carpenter, P. A. (1980). Individual differences in working memory and reading. *Journal of Verbal Learning and Verbal Behavior, 19*, 450–466.

Darwin, C. (1872). The *expression of the emotions in man and animals*. London, UK: Murray.

Davis, R. N., Massman, P. J., & Doody, R. S. (2001). Cognitive intervention in Alzheimer's disease: A randomized placebo-controlled study. *Alzheimer Disease and Associated Disorders, 15*, 1–9.

Diesfeldt, H. F. A. (1984). The importance of encoding instructions and retrieval cues in the assessment of memory in senile dementia. *Archives of Gerontology and Geriatrics, 3*, 51–57.

Duchek, J. M., Hunt, L., Ball, K., Buckles, V., & Morris, J. C. (1997). The role of selective attention in driving and dementia of the Alzheimer type. *Alzheimer Disease and Associated Disorders, 11*(1), 48–56.

Ehlhardt, L. A., Sohlberg, M. M., Kennedy, M., Coehlo, C., Turkstra, L., Ylvisaker, M., . . . Yorkston, K. (2008). Evidence-based practice guidelines for instructing individuals with acquired memory impairments: What have we learned in the past 20 years? *Neuropsychological Rehabilitation, 18*, 300–342.

Ellenbogen, J. M., Payne, J. D., & Stickgold, R. (2006). The role of sleep in declarative memory consolidation: Passive, permissive, active or none?. *Current Opinion in Neurobiology, 16*(6), 716–722.

Ellis, Y., Daniels, B., & Jauregui, A. (2010). The effect of multitasking on the grade performance of business students. *Research in Higher Education Journal, 8*, 1–10.

Emery, V. O. B. (2003). Retrophylogenesis. In V. O. B. Emery & T. E. Oxman (Eds.), *Dementia* (pp. 177–236). Baltimore, MD: Johns Hopkins University Press.

Erkes, J., Raffard, S., & Meulemans, T. (2009). Spaced-retrieval in patients with Alzheimer's disease: Critical review and clinical applications. *Psychologie Neuropsychiatrie du Vieillissement, 7*(4), 275–286.

Filoteo, J. V., Delis, D. C., Massman, P. J., Demadura, T., Butters, N., & Salmon, D. P. (1992). Directed and divided attention in Alzheimer's disease: Impairment in shifting of attention to global and local stimuli. *Journal of Clinical and Experimental Neuropsychology, 14*(6), 871–883.

Fish, J. E., Manly, T., Kopelman, M. D., & Morris, R. G. (2015). Errorless learning of prospective memory tasks: An experimental investigation in people with memory disorders. *Neuropsychological Rehabilitation, 25*(2), 159–188.

Fontaine, F. (1995). *Apprentissage de nouvelles connaissances chez les patients Alzheimer* [Acquisition of new knowledge in Alzheimer patients]. Unpublished doctoral dissertation, Université de Montreal, Quebec, Canada.

Foster, N. A., & Valentine, E. R. (2001). The effect of auditory stimulation on autobiographical recall in dementia. *Experimental Aging Research, 27*, 215–228.

Franck, L., Molyneux, N., & Parkinson, L. (2016). Systematic review of interventions addressing social isolation and depression in aged care clients. *Quality of Life Research, 25*(6), 1395–1407.

Gerdner, L., & Swanson, E. (1993). Effects of individualized music on confused and agitated elderly patients. *Archives of Psychiatric Nursing, 7*, 284–291.

Gillies, C., & James, A. (1994). *Reminiscence work with old people*. London, UK: Chapman & Hall.

Glisky, E. L. (1997). Rehabilitation and memory disorders: Tapping into preserved mechanisms. *Brain and Cognition, 35*, 291–292.

Glisky, E. L., Schacter, D. L., & Tulving, E. (1986). Learning and retention of computer-related vocabulary in memory-impaired patients: Method of vanishing cues. *Journal of Clinical and Experimental Neuropsychology, 8*, 292–312.

Gordon, B. A., Zacks, J. M., Blazey, T., Benzinger, T. L., Morris, J. C., Fagan, A. M., . . . Balota, D. A. (2015). Task-evoked fMRI changes in attention networks are associated with preclinical Alzheimer's disease biomarkers. *Neurobiology of Aging, 36*(5), 1771–1779. http://doi.org/10.1016/j.neurobiolaging.2015.01.019

Gorgoni, M., D'Atri, A., Lauri, G., Rossini, P. M., Ferlazzo, F., & De Gennaro, L. (2013). Is sleep essential for neural plasticity in humans, and how does it affect motor and cognitive recovery?. *Neural Plasticity, 2013*, 1–13.

Green, R. L. (1992). *Human memory: Paradigms and paradoxes*. Hillsdale, NJ: Lawrence Erlbaum Associates.

Haj, M. E., Postal, V., & Allain, P. (2012). Music enhances autobiographical memory in mild Alzheimer's disease. *Educational Gerontology, 38*, 30–41.

Halle, J. W., & Spradlin, J. E. (1993). Identifying stimulus control of challenging behavior. In J. Reichle & D. W. Wacker (Eds.), *Communicative alternatives to challenging behavior: Integrating functional assessment and intervention strategies* (pp. 83–109). Baltimore, MD: Paul H. Brookes.

Hasher, L., & Zacks, R. T. (1979). Automatic and effortful processes in memory. *Journal of Experimental Psychology: General, 108*(3), 356.

Haslam, C., Hodder, K. I., & Yates, P. J. (2011). Errorless learning and spaced retrieval: How do these methods fare in healthy and clinical populations?. *Journal of Clinical and Experimental Neuropsychology, 33*(4), 432–447.

Haslam, C., Moss, Z., & Hodder, K. (2010). Are two methods better than one? Evaluating the effectiveness of combining errorless learning with vanishing cues. *Journal of Clinical and Experimental Neuropsychology, 32*(9), 973–985.

Hattie, J. A. C., & Donoghue, G. M. (2016). Learning strategies: A synthesis and conceptual model. *Science of Learning, 1*, Article number 16013.

Hellen, C. R. (1992). *Alzheimer's disease: Activity-focused care*. Newton, MA: Butterworth-Heinemann.

Helmes, E., & Wiancko, D. (2006). *Effects of music in reducing disruptive behavior in a general hospital*. Paper presented at the 16th congress of the International Association of Gerontology, Adelaide, Australia.

Herlitz, A., & Viitanen, M. (1991). Semantic organization and verbal episodic memory in patients with mild and moderate Alzheimer's disease. *Journal of Clinical and Experimental Neuropsychology, 13*, 559–574.

Heun, R., Burkart, M., & Benkert, O. (1997). Improvement of picture recall by repetition in patients with dementia of the Alzheimer type. *International Journal of Geriatric Psychiatry, 12*, 85–92.

Hopper, T., Bayles, K. A., & Tomoeda, C. K. (1998). Using toys to stimulate communicative function in individuals with Alzheimer's disease. *Journal of Medical Speech-Language Pathology, 6*, 73–80.

Hopper, T., Drefs, S. J., Bayles, K. A., Tomoeda, C. K., & Dinu, I. (2010). The effects of modified spaced-retrieval training on learning and retention of face-name associations by individuals with dementia. *Neuropsychological Rehabilitation, 20*, 81–102.

Hopper, T., Mahendra, N., Kim, E., Azuma, T., Bayles, K. A., Cleary, S. J., & Tomoeda, C. K. (2005). Evidence-based practice recommendations for working with individuals with dementia: Spaced-retrieval training. *Journal of Medical Speech-Language Pathology, 13*(4), xxvii–xxxiv.

Hotting, K., & Roder, B. (2013). Beneficial effects of physical exercise on neuroplasticity and cognition. *Neuroscience and Biobehavioral Reviews, 37*(9), 2243–2257.

Irish, M., Cunningham, C. J., Walsh, J. B., Coakly, D., Lawlor, A.B., Robertson, I. H., & Coen, R. F. (2006). Investigating the enhancing effect of music on autobiographical memory in mild Alzheimer's disease. *Dementia and Geriatric Cognitive Disorders, 22*, 108–120.

Jacquemin, A., Van der Linden, M., & Feyereisen, P. (1993). Thérapie du manque du mot chez un patient bilingue présentant une maladie d'Alzheimer probable. *Questions de Logopédie, 27*, 91–96.

Just, M. A., Carpenter, P. A., Keller, T. A., Emery, L., Zajac, H., & Thulborn, K. R. (2001). Interdependence of nonoverlapping cortical systems in dual cognitive tasks. *NeuroImage, 14*, 417–426.

Karlsson, T., Bäckman, L., Herlitz, A., Nilsson, L. G., Winblad, B., & Österlind, P. O. (1989). Memory improvement at different stages of Alzheimer's disease. *Neuropsychologia, 27*, 737–742.

Karpicke, J. D. (2012). Retrieval-based learning: active retrieval promotes meaningful learning. *Current Directions in Psychology, 21* (3), 157–163.

Karpicke, J. D. (2017). Retrieval-based learning: A decade of progress. In J. T. Wixted & J. H. Byrne (Eds.), *Learning & memory: a comprehensive reference (Vol. 2: Cognitive Psychology of Memory)*. Academic Press.

Kelley, P., & Whatson, T. (2013). Making long-term memories in minutes: A spaced learning pattern from memory research in education. *Frontiers in Human Neuroscience, 7*, 589.

Kintsch, W. (1970). Models for free recall and recognition. In D. A. Norman (Ed.), *Models of human memory* (pp. 333–374). New York, NY: Academic Press.

Kiran, S. (2007). Complexity in the treatment of naming deficits. *American Journal of Speech-Language Pathology, 16*(1), 18–29.

Kirk, M., & Berntsen, D. (2017). A short cut to the past: Cueing via concrete objects improves autobiographical memory retrieval in Alzheimer's disease patients. *Neuropschologia, 111*. https://doi.org/10.1016/j.neuropsy chologia.2017.06.034

Kolb, B., & Gibb, R. (2017). *The Neurobiology of brain and behavioral development*. Academic Press.

Kolb, B., Teskey, G. C., & Gibb, R. (2010). Factors influencing cerebral plasticity in the normal and injured brain. *Frontiers in Human Neuroscience, 4*, 204.

Kuhn, M., Wolf, E., Maier, J. G., Mainberger, F., Feige, B., Schmid, H., . . . Reis, J. (2016). Sleep recalibrates homeostatic and associative synaptic plasticity in the human cortex. *Nature Communications, 7*, 12455.

LaBar, K. S., Mesulam, M. M., Gitelman, D. R., & Weintraub, S. (2000). Emotional curiosity: Modulation of visuospatial attention by arousal is preserved in aging and early-stage Alzheimer's disease. *Neuropsychologia, 38*, 1734–1740.

Landauer, T. K., & Bjork, R. A. (1978). Optimum rehearsal patterns and name learning. In M. M. Gruneberg, P. E. Morris, & R. N. Sykes (Eds.), *Practical aspects of memory* (pp. 625–632). New York, NY: Academic Press.

Landmann, N., Kuhn, M., Maier, J. G., Feige, B., Spiegelhalder, K., Riemann, D., & Nissen, C. (2016). Sleep strengthens but does not reorganize memory traces in a verbal creativity task. *Sleep, 39*(3), 705–713.

Leng, N. R. C., Copello, A. G., & Sayegh, A. (1991). Learning after brain injury by the method of vanishing cues: A case study. *Behavioural Psychotherapy, 19*, 173–181.

Levin, J. R. (1988). Elaboration-based learning strategies: Powerful theory = powerful application. *Contemporary Educational Psychology, 13* (3), 191–205.

Lipinska, B., Bäckman, L., Mäntylä, T., & Viitanen, M. (1994). Effectiveness of self-generated cues in early Alzheimer's disease. *Journal of Clinical and Experimental Neuropsychology, 16*(6), 809–819.

Little, A. G., Volans, P. J., Hemsley, D. R., & Levy, R. (1986). The retention of new information in senile dementia. *British Journal of Clinical Psychology, 25*, 71–72.

Mahendra, N. (1999, November). Manipulation of working memory through sensory stimulation. In Bayles, K. A., Hopper, T, Mahendra, N., Cleary, S., & Tomoeda, C. K., *What works with dementia patients and why*. Short course presented at the American Speech-Language-Hearing Association convention, San Francisco, CA.

Mahendra, N. (2001). Direct interventions for improving the performance of individuals with Alzheimer's disease. *Seminars in Speech and Language, 22*, 291–304.

Mahendra, N., Bayles, K., & Harris, F. (2005). Effect of presentation modality on immediate and delayed recall in individuals with Alzheimer's disease. *American Journal of Speech-Language Pathology, 14*, 144–155.

Martin, G., & Pear, J. (1996). *Behavior modification. What it is and how to do it*. Upper Saddle River, NJ: Prentice-Hall.

Materne, C. J., Luszcz, M. A., & Bond, M. J. (2014). Once-weekly spaced retrieval training is effective in supporting everyday memory activities in community dwelling older people with dementia. *Clinical Gerontologist, 37*(5), 475–492.

McGuinness, B., Barrett, S. L., Craig, D., Lawson, J., & Passmore, A. P. (2010). Attention deficits in Alzheimer's disease and vascular dementia. *Journal of Neurology, Neurosurgery & Psychiatry, 81*(2), 157–159.

McKitrick, L. A., & Camp, C. J. (1993). Relearning the names of things: The spaced retrieval intervention implemented by caregivers. *Clinical Gerontology, 14*, 60–62.

Merzenich, M. M., Van Vleet, T. M., & Nahum, M. (2014). Brain plasticity-based therapeutics. *Frontiers in Human Neuroscience, 8*, 385.

Millet, X., Le Goff, M., Bouisson, J., Dartigues, J. F., & Amieva, H. (2010). Encoding processes influence

word-stem completion priming in Alzheimer's disease: A meta-analysis. *Journal of Clinical and Experimental Neuropsychology, 32*(5), 494–504.

Mitchell, D. B., Hunt, R. R., & Schmitt, F. A. (1986). The generation effect and reality monitoring: Evidence from dementia and normal aging. *Journal of Gerontology, 41*(1), 79–84.

Moayeri, S. E., Cahill, L., Jin, Y., & Potkin, S. G. (2000). Relative sparing of emotionally influenced memory in Alzheimer's disease. *NeuroReport, 11*, 643–645.

Moffat, N. J. (1989). Home-based cognitive rehabilitation with the elderly. In L. Poon, D. C. Rubin, & B. A. Wilson (Eds.), *Everyday cognition in adulthood and late life* (pp. 659–690). Cambridge, UK: Cambridge University Press.

National Institute on Aging. (2017).Healthy eating. Retrieved from https://www.nia.nih.gov/health/healthy-eating.

Newman, S. D., Keller, T. A., & Just, M. A. (2007). Volitional control of attention and brain activation in dual task performance. *Human Brain Mapping, 28*(2), 109–117.

Ochsner, K. N, Chiu, C. Y. P., & Schacter, D. L. (1994). Varieties of priming. *Current Biology, 4*, 189–194.

Omar, R., Hailstone, J. C., & Warren, J. D. (2012). Semantic memory for music in dementia. *Music Perception: An Interdisciplinary Journal, 29*(5), 467–477.

Ophir, E., Nass, C., & Wagner, A. D. (2009). Cognitive control in media multitaskers. *Proceedings of the National Academy of Sciences, 106*(37), 15583–15587.

Oren, S., Willerton, C., & Small, J. (2014). Effects of spaced retrieval training on semantic memory in Alzheimer's disease: A systematic review. *Journal of Speech, Language, and Hearing Research, 57*(1), 247–270.

Perlmuter, L. C., & Monty, R. A. (1989). Motivation and aging. In L. Poon, D. C. Rubin, & B.A. Wilson (Eds.), *Everyday cognition in adulthood and late life* (pp. 373–393). Cambridge, UK: Cambridge University Press.

Perry, R. J., Watson, P., & Hodges, J. R. (2000). The nature and staging of attention dysfunction in early (minimal and mild) Alzheimer's disease: Relationship to episodic and semantic memory impairment. *Neuropsychologia, 38*(3), 252–271.

Pessoa, L. (2009). How do emotion and motivation direct executive function? *Trends in Cognitive Sciences, 13*, 160–166.

Potkin, K. T., & Bunney Jr, W. E. (2012). Sleep improves memory: The effect of sleep on long term memory in early adolescence. *PLoS One, 7*(8), e42191.

Rasch, B., & Born, J. (2013). About sleep's role in memory. *Physiological Reviews, 93*(2), 681–766.

Rees, G., Frith, C. D., & Lavie, N. (1997). Modulating irrelevant motion perception by varying attentional load in an unrelated task. *Science, 278*(5343), 1616–1619.

Ridder, H. M. O., Stige, B., Qvale, L. G., & Gold, C. (2013). Individual music therapy for agitation in dementia: An exploratory randomized controlled trial. *Aging & Mental Health, 17*(6), 667–678.

Schacter, D. L., Rich, S. A., & Stampp, M. S. (1985). Remediation of memory disorders: An experimental evaluation of the spaced retrieval technique. *Journal of Clinical and Experimental Neuropsychology, 7,* 79–96.

Schaefer, A., & Philippot, P. (2005). Selective effects of emotion on the phenomenal characteristics of autobiographical memories. *Memory, 13,* 148–160.

Shebilske, W. L., Goettl, B. P., Corrington, K., & Day, E. A. (1999). Interlesson spacing and task-related processing during complex skill acquisition. *Journal of Experimental Psychology: Applied, 5*(4), 413.

Sheridan, C. (1995). Reminiscence. In Alzheimer's Association (Ed.), *Activity programming for persons with dementia: A sourcebook.* Chicago, IL: Alzheimer's Association.

Sherratt, K., Thornton, A., & Hatton, C. (2004). Music interventions for people with dementia: A review of the literature. *Aging & Mental Health, 8*(1), 3–12.

Skaugset, L. M., Farrell, S., Carney, M., Wolff, M., Santen, S. A., Perry, M., & Cico, S. J. (2016). Can you multitask? Evidence and limitations of task switching and multitasking in emergency medicine. *Annals of Emergency Medicine, 68*(2), 189–195.

Slamecka, N. J., & Graf, P. (1978). The generation effect: Delineation of a phenomenon. *Journal of Experimental Psychology: Human Learning and Memory, 4*(6), 592–604.

Small, J. A., Kemper, S., & Lyons, K. (1997). Sentence comprehension in Alzheimer's disease: Effects of grammatical complexity, speech rate, and repetition. *Psychology and Aging, 12,* 3–11.

Storms, L. H. (1958). Apparent backward association: A situational effect. *Journal of Experimental Psychology, 55,* 390–395.

Summer, L. (1981). Guided imagery and music with the elderly. *Music Therapy, 1,* 39–42.

Svansdottir, H. B., & Snædal, J. (2006). Music therapy in moderate and severe dementia of Alzheimer's type: A case–control study. *International Psychogeriatrics, 18*(4), 613–621.

Talarico, J. M., LaBar, K. S., & Rubin, D. C. (2004). Emotional intensity predicts autobiographical memory experience. *Memory and Cognition, 32,* 1118–1132.

Thivierge, S., Simard, M., Jean, L., & Grandmaison, É. (2008). Errorless learning and spaced retrieval techniques to relearn instrumental activities of daily living in mild Alzheimer's disease: A case report study. *Neuropsychiatric Disease and Treatment, 4*(5), 987.

Thornton, S., & Brotchie, J. (1987). Reminiscence: A critical review of the empirical literature. *British Journal of Clinical Psychology, 26,* 93–111.

Tulving, E., & Schacter, D. L. (1990). Priming and human memory systems. *Science, 247,* 301–306.

Tulving, E., & Thomson, D. M. (1973). Encoding specificity and retrieval processes in episodic memory. *Psychological Review, 80,* 352–373.

U.S. Department of Health and Human Services. (2008). *2008 Physical Activity Guidelines for Americans.* ODPHP Publication No. U0036. Retrieved from http://www.health.gov/paguidelines.

Vandenberghe, R., Duncan, J., Dupont, P., Ward, R., Poline, J. B., Bormans, G., . . . Orban, G. A. (1997). Attention to one or two features in left or right visual field: A positron emission tomography study. *Journal of Neuroscience, 17*(10), 3739–3750.

Van der Linden, M., & Coyette. F. (1995). Acquisition of word processing knowledge in an amnesic patient: Implications for theory and rehabilitation. In R. Campbell & M. Conway (Eds.), *Broken memories: Neuropsychological case studies* (pp. 54–80). Oxford, UK: Blackwell.

Vanhalle, C., Van der Linden, M., Belleville, S., & Gilbert, B. (1998). Putting names on faces: Use of spaced retrieval strategy in a patient with dementia of Alzheimer type. American Speech, Language & Hearing Association, Special interest division 2 newsletter. *Neurophysiology and Neurogenic Speech and Language Disorders, 8,* 17–21.

Vanstone, A. D., Cuddy, L. L., Duffin, J. M., & Alexander, E. (2009). Exceptional preservation for memory for tunes and lyrics: Case studies of amusia, profound deafness and Alzheimer's disease. *Annals of the New York Academy of Sciences, 1169,* 291–294.

Vuilleumier, P. (2005). How brains beware: Neural mechanisms of emotional attention. *Trends in Cognitive Sciences, 9,* 585–594.

Walker, M. P. (2009). The role of sleep in cognition and emotion. *Annals of the New York Academy of Sciences, 1156*(1), 168–197.

Wilson, B. A., Baddeley, A., Evans, J., & Shiel, A. (1994). Errorless learning in the rehabilitation of memory impaired people. *Neuropsychological Rehabilitation, 4,* 307–326.

Wilson, B. A., & Moffat, N. (1992). The development of group memory therapy. In B. A. Wilson & N. Moffat (Eds.), *Clinical management of memory problems* (2nd ed., pp. 243–273). London, UK: Chapman & Hall.

Winter, J., & Hunkin, N. M. (1999). Re-learning in Alzheimer's disease. *International Journal of Geriatric Psychiatry, 14,* 988–990.

Ylvisaker, M., & Feeney, T. (2002). Executive functions, self-regulation, and learned optimism in pediatric rehabilitation: A review and implications for intervention. *Pediatric Rehabilitation, 5,* 51–70.

Section IV

Abreu, J., & Almeida, P. (2012). A social TV application for senior citizens. *EuroITV 2012 Adjunct Proceedings* (pp. 11–12). Berlin, Germany: Fraunhofer institute for open communication Systems, FOKUS.

Acar, B., Yurekli, M. F., Babademez, M. A., Karabulut, H., & Karasen, R. M. (2011). Effects of hearing aids on cognitive functions and depressive signs in elderly people. *Archives of Gerontology and Geriatrics, 52*(3), 250–252.

Adelman, R. D., Tmanova, L. L., Delgado, D., Dion, S., & Lachs, M. S. (2014). Caregiver burden: A clinical review. *Journal of the American Medical Association, 311*(10), 1052–1060.

Allen, A. P., Curran, E. A., Duggan, Á., Cryan, J. F., Chorcoráin, A. N., Dinan, T. G., . . . Clarke, G. (2017). A systematic review of the psychobiological burden of informal caregiving for patients with dementia: Focus on cognitive and biological markers of chronic stress. *Neuroscience & Biobehavioral Reviews, 73*, 123–164.

Allen, N. H., Burns, A., Newton, V., Hickson, F., Ramsden, R., Rogers, J. . . . Morris, J. (2003). The effects of improving hearing in dementia. *Age and Aging, 32*, 189–193.

Almor, A., Kempler, D., MacDonald, M. C., Andersen, E. S., & Tyler, L. K. (1999). Why do Alzheimer patients have difficulty with pronouns? Working memory, semantics, and reference in comprehension and production in Alzheimer's disease. *Brain and Language, 67*(3), 202–227.

Alzheimer's Association. (2013). 2013 Alzheimer's disease facts and figures. *Alzheimer's & Dementia, 9*(2), 1–69.

Alzheimer's Association. (2014). 2014 Alzheimer's disease facts and figures. Retrieved from https://www.alz.org /downloads/Facts_Figures_2014.pdf.

Alzheimer's Association. (2015). 2015 Alzheimer's disease facts and figures. *Alzheimer's & Dementia, 11*, 332–384.

American Academy of Ophthalmology. (2017). What is presbyopia? Retrieved from https://www.aao.org/eye -health/diseases/what-is-presbyopia.

American Macular Degeneration Foundation. (n.d.). What is macular degeneration? Retrieved from https://www .macular.org/what-macular-degeneration.

Ancoli-Israel, S., Martin, J., Gehrman, P., Shochat, T., Corey-Bloom, J., Marler, M., . . . Levi, L. (2003). Effect of light on agitation in institutionalized patients with severe Alzheimer disease. *American Journal of Geriatric Psychiatry, 11*, 194–203.

Arévalo-Flechas, L. C., Acton, G., Escamilla, M. I., Bonner, P. N., & Lewis, S. L. (2014). Latino Alzheimer's caregivers: What is important to them?. *Journal of Managerial Psychology, 29*(6), 661–684.

Arthur, P. B., Gitlin, L. N., Kairalla, J. A., & Mann, W. C. (2017). Relationship between the number of behavioral symptoms in dementia and caregiver distress: What is the tipping point? *International Psychogeriatrics*, 1–9.

Baddeley, A. D., Baddeley, H. A., Bucks, R. S., & Wilcock, G. K. (2001). Attentional control in Alzheimer's disease. *Brain, 124*, 1492–1508.

Baumgarten, M., Battista, R. N., Infant-Rivard, C., Hanley, J. A., Becker, R., & Gauthier, S. (1992). The psychological and physical health of family members caring for an elderly person with dementia. *Journal of Clinical Epidemiology, 45*, 61–70.

Bayles, K. A., & Tomoeda, C. K. (1993). *Arizona Battery for Communication Disorders in Dementia*. Austin, TX: Pro-Ed.

Beeson, R. A. (2004). Loneliness and depression in caregivers. In R. W. Richter & B. Zoeller Richter (Eds.), *Alzheimer's disease: A physician's guide to practical management* (pp. 449–453). Totowa, NJ: Humana Press.

Belle, S. H., Czaja, S. J., Schulz, R., Zhang, S., Burgio, L. D., Gitlin, L. N., . . . Ory, M. G. REACH investigators.

(2003). Using a new taxonomy to combine the uncombinable: Integrating results across diverse caregiving interventions. *Psychology and Aging, 18*, 396–405.

Bemelmans, R., Gelderblom, J., Jonker, P., & de Witt, L. (2012). Socially assistive robots in elderly care: A systematic review into effects and effectiveness. *American Medical Directors Association, 13*, 114–120.

Bergman-Evans, B. (2004). Beyond the basics: Effects of the Eden Alternative model on quality of life issues. *Journal of Gerontological Nursing, 30*, 27–34.

Biegel, D., Sales, E., & Schulz, R. (1991). *Family caregiving in chronic illness: Heart disease, cancer, stroke, Alzheimer's disease, and chronic mental illness*. Newbury Park, CA: Sage.

Birks, M., Bodak, M., Barlas, J., Harwood, J., & Pether, M. (2016). Robotic seals as therapeutic tools in an aged care facility: A qualitative study. *Journal of Aging Research, 2016*.

Boczko, F. (1994). The Breakfast Club: A multimodal language stimulation program for nursing home residents with Alzheimer's disease. *American Journal of Alzheimer's Care and Related Disorders and Research, 9*, 35–38.

Bourgeois, M. S. (1992). *Conversing with memory-impaired individuals using memory aids*. Gaylord, MI: Northern Speech Services.

Bourgeois, M. S. (2007). *Memory Books and other graphic cuing systems: Practical communication and memory aids for adults with dementia*. Health Professions Press.

Bourgeois, M. S., Dijkstra, K., Burgio, L. D., & Allen, R. S. (2004). Communication skills training for nursing aids of residents with dementia: The impact of measuring performance. *Clinical Gerontologist, 27*(1/2), 119–138.

Bourgeois, M., Dijkstra, K., Burgio, L., & Allen-Burge, R. (2001). Memory aids as an augmentative and alternative communication strategy for nursing home residents with dementia. *Augmentative and Alternative Communication, 17*(3), 196–210.

Brawley, E. (1997). *Designing for Alzheimer's disease*. New York, NY: John Wiley & Sons.

Brislin, R. (1994). *Understanding cultural diversity: A model* [Videotape 1]. University of Arizona National Center for Neurogenic Communication Disorders, Tucson, Arizona.

Broekens, J., Heerink, M., & Rosendal, H. (2009). Assistive social robots in elderly care: A review. *Gerontechnology, 8*(2), 94–103.

Camp, C. J., Judge, K. S., Bye, C. A., Fox, K. M., Bowden, J., Bell, M., . . . Mattern, J. M. (1997). An intergenerational program for persons with dementia using Montessori methods. *The Gerontologist, 37*(5), 688–692.

Camp, C. J., & Mattern, J. M. (1999). Innovations in managing Alzheimer's Disease. In Biegel, D. E. & Blum, A. (Eds.), *Innovations in practice and service delivery across the lifespan* (pp. 276–294). New York: Oxford University Press.

Campbell, S. S., Kripke, D. F., Gillin, J. C., & Hrubovcak, J. C. (1988). Exposure to light in healthy elderly subjects and Alzheimer's patients. *Physiological Behavior, 42,* 141–144.

Cantor, M. H. (1983). Strain among caregivers: A study of experience in the United States. *Gerontologist, 23,* 597–604.

Casado, L. B., Lee, S. E., Hong, M., & Hong, S. (2015). The experience of family caregivers of older Korean Americans with dementia symptoms. *Clinical Gerontologist, 38*(1), 32–48.

Caspar, S., & O'Rourke, N. (2009). The composition and structure of depressive symptomatology among young and older caregivers of persons with dementia. *Ageing International, 34,* 33–41.

Chenoweth, B., & Spencer, B. (1986). Dementia: The experience of family caregivers. *Gerontologist, 26,* 267–272.

Ciorba, A., Bianchini, C., Pelucchi, S., & Pastore, A. (2012). The impact of hearing loss on the quality of life of elderly adults. *Clinical Interventions in Aging, 7,* 159.

Clark, L. (1975). The *ancient art of color therapy.* New York, NY: Pocket Books.

Cohen-Mansfield, J., & Taylor, J. W. (2004). Hearing aid use in nursing homes, part 1: Prevalence rates of hearing impairment and hearing aid use. *Journal of the American Medical Directors Association, 5*(5), 283–288.

Collette, F., Van der Linden, B. M., & Salmon, E. (1999). Phonological loop and central executive functioning in Alzheimer's disease. *Neuropsychologia, 37,* 905–918.

Connors, M. H., Ames, D., Woodward, M., & Brodaty, H. (2017). Predictors of driving cessation in dementia: Baseline characteristics and trajectories of disease progression. *Alzheimer Disease and Associated Disorders.* doi: 10.1097/WAD.0000000000000212.

Cooper, B. (1994). Long-term care design: Current research on the use of color. *Journal of Healthcare Design, 6,* 61–67.

Cruickshanks, K. J., Tweed, T. S., Wiley, T. L., Klein, B. E. K., Klein, R., Chappell, R., . . . Dalton, D. S. (2003). The 5-year incidence and progression of hearing loss: The epidemiology of hearing loss study. *Archives of Otolaryngology-Head and Neck Surgery, 129,* 1041–1046.

Czaja, S. J., Schulz, R., Lee, C.C., & Belle, S. H. (2003). A methodology for describing and decomposing complex psychosocial and behavioral interventions. *Psychology and Aging, 18,* 385–395.

Dawes, P., Emsley, R., Cruickshanks, K. J., Moore, D. R., Fortnum, H., Edmondson-Jones, M., . . . Munro, K. J. (2015). Hearing loss and cognition: The role of hearing aids, social isolation and depression. *PLoS One, 10*(3), e0119616.

Demir, E., Köseoğlu, E., Sokullu, R., & Şeker, B. (2017). Smart home assistant for ambient assisted living of elderly people with dementia. *Procedia Computer Science, 113,* 609–614.

Dijkstra, K., Bourgeois, M., Burgio, L., & Allen, R. (2002). Effects of a communication intervention on the discourse of nursing home residents with dementia and their nursing assistants. *Journal of Medical Speech-Language Pathology, 10,* 143–157.

Doherty, K. A., & Brangman, S. A. (2011). Improving communication for older hospital patients with assistive listening devices. *Update,* Publication of the SUNY Upstate Medical University, pp. 2, 6.

Ducak, K., Denton, M., & Elliot, G. (2018). Implementing Montessori Methods for Dementia™ in Ontario long-term care homes: Recreation staff and multidisciplinary consultants' perceptions of policy and practice issues. *Dementia, 17*(1), 5–33.

Duffy, M. (2016). Normal vision changes. American Foundation for the Blind: Vision Aware. Retrieved from http://www.visionaware.org/info/your-eye-condition/eye-health/normal-vision-changes/125.

El Haj, M., Gallouj, K., & Antoine, P. (2017). Google Calendar enhances prospective memory in Alzheimer's disease: A case report. *Journal of Alzheimer's Disease, 57*(1), 285–291.

Enmarker, I., Olsen, R., & Hellzen, O. (2011). Management of person with dementia with aggressive and violent behaviour: A systematic literature review. *International Journal of Older People Nursing, 6*(2), 153–162.

Farran, C. J., Miller, B. H., Kaufman, J. E., Donner, E., & Fogg, L. (1999). Finding meaning through caregiving: Development of an instrument for family caregivers of persons with Alzheimer's disease. *Journal of Clinical Psychology, 55,* 1107–1125.

Figueiro, M. G., Plitnick, B. A., Lok, A., Jones, G. E., Higgins, P., Hornick, T. R., & Rea, M. S. (2014). Tailored lighting intervention improves measures of sleep, depression, and agitation in persons with Alzheimer's disease and related dementia living in long-term care facilities. *Clinical Interventions in Aging, 9,* 1527.

Fitting, M., Rabins, P., Lucas, M. J., & Eastham, J. (1986). Caregivers for dementia patients: A comparison of husbands and wives. *Gerontologist, 26,* 248–252.

Froehlich, T. E., Bogardus, S. T., Jr., & Inouye, S. K. (2001). Dementia and race: Are there differences between African Americans and Caucasians? *Journal of the American Geriatrics Society, 49,* 477–484.

Gagnon-Roy, M., Bourget, A., Stocco, S., Courchesne, A. C. L., Kuhne, N., & Provencher, V. (2017). Assistive technology addressing safety issues in dementia: A scoping review. *American Journal of Occupational Therapy, 71*(5), 7105190020p1–7105190020p10.

Gallicchio, L., Siddiqi, N., Langenberg, P., & Baumgarten, M. (2002). Gender differences in burden and depression among informal caregivers of demented elders in the community. *International Journal of Geriatric Psychiatry, 17,* 154–163.

García-Betances, R. I., Jiménez-Mixco, V., Arredondo, M. T., & Cabrera-Umpiérrez, M. F. (2015). Using virtual reality for cognitive training of the elderly. *American Journal of Alzheimer's Disease & Other Dementias®, 30*(1), 49–54.

Gates, G. A., Cobb, J. L., Linn, R. T., Rees, T., Wolf, P. A., & D'agostino, R. B. (1996). Central auditory dysfunction, cognitive dysfunction, and dementia in older people. *Archives of Otolaryngology-Head and Neck Surgery, 122,* 161–167.

Geiger, J. R., Wilks, S. E., Lovelace, L. L., Chen, Z., & Spivey, C. A. (2015). Burden among male Alzheimer's caregivers: Effects of distinct coping strategies. *American Journal of Alzheimer's Disease & Other Dementias, 30*(3), 238–246.

George, L. K., & Gwyther, L. P. (1986). Caregiver well-being: A multidimensional examination of family caregivers of demented adults. *Gerontologist, 26,* 253–259.

Gillespie, A., Best, C., & O'Neill, B. (2012). Cognitive function and assistive technology for cognition: A systematic review. *Journal of the International Neuropsychological Society, 18*(1), 1–19.

Gold, M., Lightfoot, L. A., & Hnath-Chisolm, T. (1996). Hearing loss in a memory disorders clinic: A specially vulnerable population. *Archives of Neurology, 53,* 922–928.

Gouin, J. P., Hantsoo, L., & Kiecolt-Glaser, J. K. (2008). Immune dysregulation and chronic stress among older adults: A review. *Neuroimmunomodulation, 15*(4–6), 251–259.

Hanford, N., & Figueiro, M. (2013). Light therapy and Alzheimer's disease and related dementia: Past, present, and future. *Journal of Alzheimer's Disease, 33*(4), 913–922.

Hantsoo L., & Kiecolt-Glaser J. K. (2008). Immune dysregulation and chronic stress among older adults: A review. *Neuroimmunomodulation, 15*(4–6), 251–259.

Hattie, J. A. C., Donoghue, G. M. (2016). Learning strategies: A synthesis and conceptual model. *Science of Learning, 1,* Article number 16013.

Health in Aging. (2015). *Caregiver Self-Assessment Questionnaire.* Retrieved August 30, 2017, from www.healthinaging.org/resources/resource:caregiver-self-assessment/

Hewitt, D. (2017). Age-related hearing loss and cognitive decline: You haven't heard the half of it. *Frontiers in Aging Neuroscience, 9,* 112.

Hoerster, L., Hickey, E. M., & Bourgeois, M. S. (2001). Effects of memory aids on conversations between nursing home residents with dementia and nursing assistants. *Neuropsychological Rehabilitation, 11*(3–4), 399–427.

Hopper, T., Bayles, K. A., & Tomoeda, C. K. (1998). Using toys to stimulate communicative function in individuals with Alzheimer's disease. *Journal of Medical Speech-Language Pathology, 6,* 73–80.

Hull, R. H. (2011). *Hearing in aging.* San Diego, CA: Plural Publishing.

Humes, K. R., Jones, N. A., & Ramirez, R. R. (2015). Overview of race and Hispanic origin, 2010. United States Census 2011.

Hung, S. C., Liao, K. F., Muo, C. H., Lai, S. W., Chang, C. W., & Hung, H. C. (2015). Hearing loss is associated with risk of Alzheimer's disease: A case-control study in older people. *Journal of Epidemiology, 25*(8), 517–521.

Imbeault, H., Gagnon, L., Pigot, H., Giroux, S., Marcotte, N., Cribier-Delande, P., . . . Bier, N. (2016). Impact of AP@

LZ in the daily life of three persons with Alzheimer's disease: Long-term use and further exploration of its effectiveness. *Neuropsychological Rehabilitation,* 1–24.

Irvine, A. B., Ary, D. V., & Bourgeois, M. S. (2003). An interactive multimedia program to train professional caregivers. *Journal of Applied Gerontology, 22,* 269–288.

Judge, K. S., Camp, C. J., & Orsulic-Jeras, S. (2000). Use of Montessori-based activities for clients with dementia in adult day care: Effects on engagement. *American Journal of Alzheimer's Disease and Other Dementias, 15*(1), 42–46.

Kiecolt-Glaser, J. K., Dura, J. R., Speicher, C. E., Trask, O. J., & Glaser, R. (1991). Spousal care givers of dementia victims: Longitudinal changes in immunity and health. *Psychosomatic Medicine, 53,* 345–352.

Kiecolt-Glaser, J. K., Glaser, R., Gravenstein S., Malarkey, W. B., & Sheridan, J. (1996). Chronic stress alters the immune response to influenza virus vaccine in older adults. *Proceedings of the National Academy of Sciences of the USA, 94,* 3043–3047.

Kiecolt-Glaser J. K., Glaser, R., Shuttleworth, E. C., Dyer, C. S., Ogrocki, P., & Speicher, C. E. (1987). Chronic stress and immunity in family caregivers of Alzheimer's disease victims. *Psychosomatic Medicine, 49,* 523–535.

Kiecolt-Glaser, J. K., Marucha P. T., Malarkey W. B., Mercado, A. M., & Glaser, R. (1995). Slowing of wound healing by psychological stress. *Lancet, 346,* 1194–1196.

Kiely, K. M., Gopinath, B., Mitchell, P., Luszcz, M., & Anstey, K. J. (2012). Cognitive, health, and sociodemographic predictors of longitudinal decline in hearing acuity among older adults. *Journals of Gerontology Series A: Biomedical Sciences and Medical Sciences, 67*(9), 997–1003.

King A. C., Oka, R. K., & Young, D. R. (1994). Ambulatory blood pressure and heart rate responses to the stress of work and caregiving in older women. *Journal of Gerontology, 49,* 239–245.

Kleinman, A. (1988). *The illness narratives: Suffering, healing, and the human condition.* New York, NY: Basic Books.

Kleinman, A., Eisenberg, L., & Good, B. (1978). Culture, illness and care: Clinical issues from anthropologic and cross-cultural research. *Annals of Internal Medicine, 88,* 251–258.

Knight, B. G., & Sayegh, P. (2010). Cultural values and caregiving: The updated sociocultural stress and coping model. *Journals of Gerontology: Series B, 65*(1), 5–13.

Kunik, M. E., Snow, A. L., Davila, J. A., Steele, A. B., Balasubramanyam, V., Doody, R. S., . . . Morgan, R. O. (2010). Causes of aggressive behavior in patients with dementia. *Journal of Clinical Psychiatry, 71*(9), 1145–1152.

Lazarou, I., Karakostas, A., Stavropoulos, T. G., Tsompanidis, T., Meditskos, G., . . . Kompatsiaris, I., (2016). A novel and intelligent home monitoring system for care support of elders with cognitive impairment. *Journal of Alzheimer's Disease, 54,* 1561–1591.

Lee, Y., & Bronstein, L. R. (2010). When do Korean-American dementia caregivers find meaning in caregiving?: The role of culture and differences between spouse and child caregivers. *Journal of Ethnic & Cultural Diversity in Social Work, 19*(1), 73–86.

Libin, A. V., & Libin, E. V. (2004). Person-robot interactions from the robopsychologists' point of view: The robotic psychology and robotherapy approach. *Proceedings of the IEEE, 92,* 1789–1803.

Lin, F. R., Metter, E. J., O'Brien, R. J., Resnick, S. M., Zonderman, A. B., & Ferrucci, L. (2011b). Hearing loss and incident dementia. *Archives of Neurology, 68*(2), 214–220.

Lin, F. R., Niparko, J. K., & Ferrucci, L. (2011a). Hearing loss prevalence in the United States. *Archives of Internal Medicine, 171*(20), 1851–1853.

Lin, F. R., Yaffe, K., Xia, J., Xue, Q. L., Harris, T. B., Purchase-Helzner, E., . . . Health ABC Study Group, F. (2013). Hearing loss and cognitive decline in older adults. *JAMA Internal Medicine, 173*(4), 293–299.

Llanque, S. M., & Enriquez, M. (2012). Interventions for Hispanic caregivers of patients with dementia: A review of the literature. *American Journal of Alzheimer's Disease & Other Dementias, 27*(1), 23–32.

LoPresti, E. F., Mihailidis, A., & Kirsch, N. (2004). Assistive technology for cognitive rehabilitation: State of the art. *Neuropsychological Rehabilitation, 14,* 5–39.

Luchsinger, J. A., Tipiani, D., Torres-Patiño, G., Silver, S., Eimicke, J. P., Ramirez, M., . . . Mittelman, M. (2015). Characteristics and mental health of Hispanic dementia caregivers in New York City. *American Journal of Alzheimer's Disease & Other Dementias, 30*(6), 584–590.

Lustig, M. W., & Koester, J. (2013). *Intercultural competence.* Boston, MA: Pearson, Allyn & Bacon.

Mace, N. L., & Rabins, P. V. (2017). *The 36-hour day: A family guide to caring for persons with Alzheimer's disease, related dementing illnesses, and memory loss in later life.* Baltimore, MD: Johns Hopkins University Press.

Mahendra, N., Bayles, K. A., & Harris, F. P. (2005). Effect of presentation modality on immediate and delayed recall in individuals with Alzheimer's disease. *American Journal of Speech-Language Pathology, 14,* 144–155.

Mayo Clinic (2017). Alzheimer's: when to stop driving. Retrieved from: https://www.mayoclinic.org/healthy-lifestyle/caregivers/in-depth/alzheimers/art-20044924.

McCallion, P., Toseland, R. W., & Freeman, K. (1999). An evaluation of a family visit education program. *Journal of the American Geriatrics Society, 47,* 203–214.

McCallion, P., Toseland, R. W., Lacey, D., & Banks, S. (1999). Educating nursing assistants to communicate more effectively with nursing home residents with dementia. *Gerontologist, 39,* 546–558.

McCleary, L., Munro, M., Jackson, L., & Mendelsohn, L. (2005). The impact of SARS visiting restrictions on families of long term care residents. *Journal of Social Work and Long-Term Care, 3,* 3–20.

Meyer, O. L., Nguyen, K. H., Dao, T. N., Vu, P., Arean, P., & Hinton, L. (2015). The sociocultural context of caregiving experiences for Vietnamese dementia family caregivers. *Asian American Journal of Psychology, 6*(3), 263–272.

Mills, P. J., Yu, H., Ziegler, M. G., Patterson, T., & Grant, I. (1999). Vulnerable caregivers of patients with Alzheimer's disease have a deficit in circulating CD62L-T lymphocytes. *Psychosomatic Medicine, 61,* 168–174.

Mordoch, E., Osterreicher, A., Guse, L., Roger, K., & Thompson, G. (2013). Use of social commitment robots in the care of elderly people with dementia: A literature review. *Maturitas, 74*(1), 14–20.

National Center for Health Statistics. (2015). National Health Interview Survey, 2015. Retrieved from https://www.cdc.gov/nchs/nhis/index.htm.

National Center for Health Statistics. (2017). National Health Interview Survey, 2017. Retrieved from https://www.cdc.gov/nchs/nhis/index.htm. For further information, see Schiller, J. S., Lucas, J. W., Ward, B. W., & Peregoy, J. A. (2012). Provisional Report: Summary health statistics for U.S. adults: National health interview survey, 2010. National Center for Health Statistics. *Vital Health Statistics, 10*(252), 7.

National Institute on Aging. (2005). *Aging and your eyes.* AgePages. Bethesda, MD: Author.

Nguyen-Tri, D., Overbury, O., & Faubert, J. (2003). The role of lenticular senescence in age-related color vision changes. *Investigative Ophthalmology and Visual Science, 44,* 3698–3704.

Nirmalasari, O., Mamo, S. K., Nieman, C. L., Simpson, A., Zimmerman, J., Nowrangi, M. A., . . . Oh, E. S. (2017). Age-related hearing loss in older adults with cognitive impairment. *International Psychogeriatrics, 29*(1), 115–121.

Nolan, J. M., Loskutova, E., Howard, A. N., Moran, R., Mulcahy, R., Stack, J., . . . Thurnham, D. I. (2014). Macular pigment, visual function, and macular disease among subjects with Alzheimer's disease: An exploratory study. *Journal of Alzheimer's Disease, 42*(4), 1191–1202.

Ohta, R. J., Carlin, M. R., & Harmon, B. M. (1981). Auditory acuity and performance on the mental status questionnaire in the elderly. *Journal of the American Geriatrics Society, 27,* 476–478.

Orange, J. B., & Colton-Hudson, A. (1998). Enhancing communication in dementia of the Alzheimer's type. *Topics in Geriatric Rehabilitation, 14,* 56–75.

Orengo, C. A., Khan, J., Kunik, M. E., Snow, A. L., Morgan, R., Steele, A., . . . Graham, D. P. (2008). Aggression in individuals newly diagnosed with dementia. *American Journal of Alzheimer's Disease & Other Dementias®, 23*(3), 227–232.

O'Rourke, N., Kupferschmidt, A. L., Claxton, A., Smith, J. Z., Chappell, N., & Beattie, B.L. (2010). Psychological resilience predicts depressive symptoms among spouses of persons with Alzheimer disease over time. *Aging and Mental Health, 14,* 984–993.

Ory, M. G., Hoffman, R. R., Yee, J. L., Tennstedt, S., & Schulz, R. (1999). Prevalence and impact of caregiving:

A detailed comparison between dementia and nondementia caregivers. *Gerontologist, 39,* 177–185.

Palmer, C. V., Adams, S. W., Bourgeois, M., Durrant, J., & Rossi, M. (1999). Reduction in caregiver-identified problem behaviors in patients with Alzheimer disease post-hearing-aid fitting. *Journal of Speech, Language, and Hearing Research, 42,* 312–328.

Parker, J., Young, A., & Rogers, K. (2010). "My Mum's Story" A Deaf daughter discusses her Deaf mother's experience of dementia. *Dementia 9*(1), 5–20.

Paveza, G. J., Cohen, D., Eisdorfer, C., Freels, S., Semla, T., Ashford, J. W., . . . Levy, P. (1992). Severe family violence and Alzheimer's disease: Prevalence and risk factors. *Gerontologist, 32,* 493–497.

Petersen, S., Houston, S., Qin, H., Tague, C., & Studley, J. (2017). The utilization of robotic pets in dementia care. *Journal of Alzheimer's Disease, 55*(2), 569–574.

Pillemer, K., & Suitor, J. J. (1992). Violence and violent feelings: What causes them among family caregivers? *Journal of Gerontology, 47,* S165–S172.

Pinquart, M., & Sörensen, S. (2003). Differences between caregivers and noncaregivers in psychological health and physical health: A metaanalysis. *Psychology and Aging, 18,* 250–267.

Pinquart, M., & Sörensen, S. (2005). Ethnic differences in stressors, resources, and psychological outcomes of family caregiving: A metaanalysis. *The Gerontologist, 45*(1), 90–106.

Pinquart, M., & Sörensen, S. (2006). Gender differences in caregiver stressors, social resources, and health: An updated meta-analysis. *Journal of Gerontology, 61,* P33–P45.

Pinquart, M., & Sörensen, S. (2007). Correlates of physical health of informal caregivers: A meta-analysis. *The Journals of Gerontology Series B: Psychological Sciences and Social Sciences, 62*(2), P126–P137.

Poulshock, S. W., & Deimling, G. T. (1984). Families caring for elders in residence: issues in the measurement of burden. *Journal of Gerontology, 39,* 230–239.

Pruchno, R. A., Kleban, M. H., Michaels, J. E., & Dempsey, N. P. (1990). Mental and physical health of caregiving spouses: Development of a causal model. *Journal of Gerontology, 45,* 192–199.

Quinn, C., Clare, L., & Woods, R. T. (2010). The impact of motivations and meanings on the wellbeing of caregivers of people with dementia: A systematic review. *International Psychogeriatrics, 22*(1), 43–55.

Ramakrishnan, S., & Pollack, M. E. (2000). Intelligent monitoring in a robotic assistant for the elderly. *Proceedings of the 16th National Conference on Artificial Intelligence,* Orlando, FL.

Resnick, O., & Ransom, S. (2001). The search for Eden: An alternative path for nursing homes. *Long-Term Care Interface, 2,* 45–48.

Ripich, D. N. (1994). Functional communication with AD patients: A caregiver training program. *Alzheimer Disease and Associated Disorders, 8,* 95–109.

Ripich, D. N., Wycke, M., & Niles, S. (1995). Alzheimer's disease caregivers: The FOCUSED program. *Geriatric Nursing, 16,* 15–19.

Ripich, D. N., & Ziol, E. (2000). Training Alzheimer's disease caregivers for successful communication. *Clinical Gerontologist, 21,* 37–56.

Rochon, E., Waters, G. S., & Caplan, D. (2000). The relationship between measures of working memory and sentence comprehension in patients with Alzheimer's disease. *Journal of Speech, Language, and Hearing Research, 43*(2), 395–413.

Roff, L. L., Burgio, L. D., Gitlin, L., Nichols, L., Chaplin, W., & Hardin, J. M. (2004). Positive aspects of Alzheimer's caregiving: The role of race. *The Journals of Gerontology Series B: Psychological Sciences and Social Sciences, 59*(4), P185–P190.

Salgado-Delgado, R., Osorio, A. T., Saderi, N., & Escobar, C. (2011) Disruption of circadian rhythms: A crucial factor in the etiology of depression. *Depression Research and Treatment, 2011,* 1–9.

Santo Pietro, M. J., & Boczko, F. (1998). Breakfast Club: Results of a study examining the effectiveness of a multi-modality group communication treatment. *American Journal of Alzheimer's Disease and Other Dementias, 13,* 146–158.

Satlin, A., Volicer, L., Ross, V., Herz, L., & Campbell, S. (1992). Bright light treatment of behavioral and sleep disturbances in patients with Alzheimer's disease. *American Journal of Psychiatry, 149,* 1028–1032.

Schneck, M. E., Haegerstrom-Portnoy, G., Lott, L. A., & Brabyn, J. A. (2014). Comparison of panel D-15 tests in a large older population. *Optometry and vision science: Official publication of the American Academy of Optometry, 91*(3), 284.

Schulz, R. (2000). *Handbook on dementia caregiving: Evidence-based interventions for family caregivers.* New York, NY: Springer.

Schulz, R., & Beach, S. (1999). Caregiving as a risk factor for mortality: The caregiver health effects study. *Journal of the American Medical Association, 282,* 2215–2219.

Schulz, R., & Martire, L. M. (2004). Family caregiving of persons with dementia: Prevalence, health effects, and support strategies. *American Journal of Geriatric Psychiatry, 12,* 240–249.

Schulz, R., Newsom, J., Mittelmark, M., Burton, L., Hirsch, C., & Jackson S. (1997). Health effects of caregiving. The caregiver health effects study: An ancillary study of the cardiovascular Health Study. *Annals of Behavioral Medicine, 19,* 110–116.

Schulz, R., O'Brien, A. T., Bookwala, J., & Fleissner, K. (1995). Psychiatric and physical morbidity effects of dementia caregiving: Prevalence, correlates, and causes. *Gerontologist, 35,* 771–791.

Schumock, G. T. (1998). Economic considerations in the treatment and management of Alzheimer's disease. *American Journal Health-System Pharmacy, 55*(Suppl. 2), 17–21.

Serino, S., Pedroli, E., Tuena, C., De Leo, G., Stramba-Badiale, M., Goulene, K., . . . Riva, G. (2017). A novel virtual reality-based training protocol for the enhancement of the "Mental Frame Syncing" in individuals with Alzheimer's disease: A development-of-concept trial. *Frontiers in Aging Neuroscience, 9,* 240.

Sharma, N., Chakrabarti, S., & Grover, S. (2016). Gender differences in caregiving among family-caregivers of people with mental illnesses. *World Journal of Psychiatry, 6*(1), 7.

Shaw, W. S., Patterson, T. L., Semple, S. J., Ho, S., Irwin, M. R., Hauger, R. L., & Grant, I. (1997). Longitudinal analysis of multiple indicators of health decline among spousal caregivers. *Annals of Behavioral Medicine, 19,* 101–109.

Shulman, M. D., & Mandel, E. (1988). Communication training of relatives and friends of institutionalized elderly persons. *Gerontologist, 28,* 797–799.

Sloane, P. D., Davidson, S., Buckwalter, K., Lindsey, B. A., Ayers, S., Lenker, V., & Burgio, L. D. (1997). Management of the patient with disruptive vocalization. *Gerontologist, 37,* 675–682.

Smale, B., & Dupuis, S. L. (2004). *Caregivers of persons with dementia: Roles, experiences, supports, and coping.* Waterloo: on: Murray Alzheimer Research and Education Program, University of Waterloo. Retrieved from https://uwaterloo.ca/murray-alzheimer-research-and-education-program/sites/ca.murray-alzheimer-research-and-education-program/files/uploads/files/InTheirOwnVoices1-SurveyResults.pdf.

Smith, M., & Filips, J. (2009). *Info-connect. Disruptive vocalizations.* Iowa Geriatric Education Center, University of Iowa.

Smolensky, M. H., Sackett-Lundeen, L. L., & Portaluppi, F. (2015). Nocturnal light pollution and underexposure to daytime sunlight: Complementary mechanisms of circadian disruption and related diseases. *Chronobiology International, 32*(8), 1029–1048.

Sörensen, S., & Pinquart, M. (2005). Racial and ethnic differences in the relationship of caregiving stressors, resources, and sociodemographic variables to caregiver depression and perceived physical health. *Aging & Mental Health, 9*(5), 482–495.

Sparks, M. B., Farran, C. J., Donner, E., & Keanehagerty, E. (1998). Wives, husbands, and daughters of dementia patients: Predictors of caregivers' mental and physical health. *Scholarly Inquiry for Nursing Practice, 12,* 221–234.

Stalder, T., Tietze, A., Steudte, S., Alexander, N., Dettenborn, L., & Kirschbaum, C. (2014). Elevated hair cortisol levels in chronically stressed dementia caregivers. *Psychoneuroendocrinology, 47,* 26–30.

Stuckey, J. C., Neundorfer, M. M., & Smyth, K. A. (1996). Burden and well-being: The same coin or related currency. *Gerontologist, 36,* 686–693.

Sung, H. C., Chang, S. M., Chin, M. Y., & Lee, W. L. (2015). Robot-assisted therapy for improving social interactions and activity participation among institutionalized older adults: A pilot study. *Asia-Pacific Psychiatry, 7*(1), 1–6.

Takechi, H., Kokuryu, A., Kubota, T., & Yamada, H. (2012). Relative preservation of advanced activities in daily living among patients with mild-to-moderate dementia in the community and overview of support provided by family caregivers. *International Journal of Alzheimer's Disease, 2012,* 1–7.

Talamantes, M. A., Trejo, L., Jimenez, D., & Gallagher-Thompson, D. (2006). Working with Mexican-American families. In Yeo G. and Gallagher-Thompson, D (Eds.), *Ethnicity and the Dementias, 2nd ed.* (pp. 327–340). New York, NY: Routledge Taylor & Francis Group.

Tárraga, L., Boada, M., Modinos, G., Espinosa, A, Diego, S., Morera, A., . . . Becker, J. T. (2006). A randomized pilot study to assess the efficacy of an interactive, multimedial tool of cognitive stimulation in Alzheimer's disease. *Neurology, Neurosurgery, and Psychiatry, 77,* 1116–1121.

Teri, L., Logsdon, R. G., Uomoto, J., & McCurry, S.M. (1997). Behavioral treatment of depression in dementia patients: A controlled clinical trial. *Journals of Gerontology Series B-Psychological Sciences and Social Sciences, 52,* 159–166.

Thies, W., & Bleiler, L. (2011). 2011 Alzheimer's disease facts and figures. *Alzheimer's Dementia, 7*(2), 208–244.

Thomas, W. H. (1996). *Life worth living.* Acton, MA: Vander Wyk & Burnham.

Topo, P. (2012). Technology study to meet the needs of people with dementia and their caregivers: A literature review. *Journal of Applied Gerontology, 28,* 5–37.

Uhlmann, R. F., Larson, E. B., Rees, T. S., Koepsell, T. D., & Duckert, L. G. (1989). Relationship of hearing impairment to dementia and cognitive dysfunction in older adults. *Journal of the American Medical Association, 261,* 1916–1919.

Van Ort, S., & Phillips, L. (1992). Feeding nursing home residents with Alzheimer's disease. *Geriatric Nursing, 13,* 249–253.

van Walsem, M. R., Howe, E. I., Frich, J. C., & Andelic, N. (2016). Assistive technology for cognition and health-related quality of life in Huntington's disease. *Journal of Huntington's Disease, 5*(3), 261–270.

Vedhara, K., Cox, N. K., Wilcock, G. K., Perks, P., Hunt, M., Anderson, S., . . . Shanks, N. M. (1999). Chronic stress in elderly carers of dementia patients and antibody response to influenza vaccination. *The Lancet, 353*(9153), 627–631.

Ventry, I. M., & Weinstein, B. E. (1983). Identification of elderly people with hearing problems. *ASHA, 25*(7), 37–42.

Verhoeven, V., Vanpuyenbroeck, K., Lopez-Hartmann, M., Wens, J., & Remmen, R. (2012). Walk on the sunny side of life—epidemiology of hypovitaminosis D and mental health in elderly nursing home residents. *The Journal of Nutrition, Health & Aging, 16*(4), 417–420.

Vitaliano, P. P., Yi, J., Phillips, P. E. M., Escheverria, D., Young, H., & Siegler, I. C. (2005). Psychophysiological mediators of caregiver stress and differential cognitive decline. *Psychology and Aging, 20*(3), 402–411.

Wada, K., Shibata, T., Musha, T., & Kimura, S. (2005, August). Effects of robot therapy for demented patients evaluated by EEG. In *Intelligent Robots and Systems, 2005. (IROS 2005). 2005 IEEE/RSJ International Conference on* (pp. 1552–1557). IEEE.

Weinstein, B. E., & Amsel, L. (1986). Hearing loss and senile dementia in the institutionalized elderly. *Clinical Gerontologist, 4*, 3–15.

Wells, B. A., Glueckauf, R. L., Bernabe Jr, D., Kazmer, M. M., Schettini, G., Springer, J., . . . Graff-Radford, N. (2017). African American dementia caregiver problem inventory: Descriptive analysis and initial psychometric evaluation. *Rehabilitation Psychology, 62*(1), 25.

Wharton, T. C., & Ford, B. K. (2014). What is known about dementia care recipient violence and aggression against caregivers?. *Journal of Gerontological Social Work, 57*(5), 460–477.

Wilkinson, A., Charoenkitkarn, V., O'Neill, J., Kanik, M., & Chignell, M. (2017). Journeys to engagement: Ambient activity technologies for people living with dementia. In *Proceedings of the 26th International Conference on World Wide Web Companion* (pp. 1103–1110). International World Wide Web Conferences Steering Committee.

Williams, S., & Harvey, S. (2013) Culture, Race, and SES: Application to End of Life Decision Making for African American Caregivers. *Perspectives on Gerontology, 18*, 69–76.

Woods, D. L., & Dimond, M. (2002). The effect of therapeutic touch on agitated behavior and cortisol in persons with Alzheimer's disease. *Biological Research for Nursing, 4*(2), 104–114.

Yang, Y. T., & Kels, C. G. (2017). Ethical considerations in electronic monitoring of the cognitively impaired. *The Journal of the American Board of Family Medicine, 30*(2), 258–263.

Yeager, C. A., Hyer, L. A., Hobbs, B., & Coyne, A. C. (2010). Alzheimer's disease and vascular dementia: the complex relationship between diagnosis and caregiver burden. *Issues in Mental Health Nursing, 31*, 376–384.

Zarit, S. (2006). The history of caregiving in dementia. In S. Lobo Prabhu, V. Molinari, & J. Lomax (Eds.), *Supporting the caregiver in dementia: A guide for health care professionals* (pp. 3–22). Baltimore, MD: Johns Hopkins University Press.

Zarit, S. H., Reever, K. E., & Bach-Peterson, J. (1980). Relatives of the impaired elderly: Correlates of feelings of burden. *Gerontologist, 20*, 649–655.

Zarit, S. H., Todd, P. A., & Zarit, J. M. (1986). Subjective burden of husbands and wives as caregivers: A longitudinal study. *Gerontologist, 26*, 260–266.

Zientz, J., Rackley, A., Chapman, S., Hopper, T., Mahendra, N., Kim, E., & Cleary, S. (2007). Evidence-based practice recommendations for dementia: Educating caregivers on Alzheimer's disease and training communication strategies. *Journal of Medical Speech-Language Pathology, 15*(1), liii–lxiv

Section V

American Speech-Language-Hearing Association (ASHA). (2015). Speech-language pathology medical review guidelines. Retrieved from http://www.asha.org/uploadedFiles/SLP-Medical-Review-Guidelines.pdf.

Bayles, K. A., & Tomoeda, C. K. (1993). *Arizona Battery for Communication Disorders of Dementia*. Austin, TX: Pro-Ed.

Bayles, K. A., & Tomoeda, C. K. (1994). *Functional Linguistic Communication Inventory*. Austin, TX: Pro-Ed.

Centers for Medicare and Medicaid Services (2009). 11 part B billing scenarios for PTs and OTs (individual vs group treatment). Retrieved from http://www.cms.gov/Medicare/Billing/TherapyServices/billing_scenarios.html.

Centers for Medicare and Medicaid Services. (2014). Medicare benefit policy manual (CMS Pub. 100-02, Chap. 15). Retrieved from http://www.cms.gov/Regulationsand-Guidance/Guidance/Manuals/downloads/bp102c15.pdf.

de Vreese, L. P., Neri, M., Fioravanti, M., Belloi, L., & Zanetti, O. (2001). Memory rehabilitation in Alzheimer's disease: A review of progress. *International Journal of Geriatric Psychiatry, 16*(8), 794–809.

Havens, L.A., McCarty, J., Sampson, M., & Warren, S. (2017). Cognitive treatment: Is it covered? Reimbursement policies for SLP-provided cognitive assessment and treatment depend on payer, facility, patient's diagnosis and type of treatment. *ASHA Leader, 22*(3), 24–26.

Hopper, T., Bayles, K. A., Harris, F. P., & Holland, A. (2001). The relationship between minimum data set ratings and scores on measures of communication and hearing among nursing home residents with dementia. *American Journal of Speech-Language Pathology, 10*, 370–381.

Hopper, T., Slaughter, S. E., Hodgetts, B., Ostevik, A., & Ickert, C. (2016). Hearing loss and cognitive-communication test performance of long-term care residents with dementia: Effects of amplification. *Journal of Speech, Language, and Hearing Research, 59*(6), 1533–1542. doi:10.1044/2016_JSLHR-H-15-0135.

Kander, M. (2006). Medicare covers cognitive therapy. *ASHA Leader, 11*(3), 14.

Omnibus Budget Reconciliation Act (OBRA) of 1987. (1987). Publication no. 100–203, 483.15.

Salmon, D. P., Heindel, W. C., & Butters, N. (1992). 5 semantic memory, priming, and skill learning in Alzheimer's disease. In *Advances in psychology* (Vol. 89, pp. 99–118). North-Holland.

Saxton, J., Kastango, K. B., Hugonot-Diener, L., Boller, F., Verny, M., Sarels, C. E., . . . Dekosky, S. T. (2005). Development of a short form of the Severe Impairment Battery. *American Journal of Geriatric Psychiatry, 13*, 999–1005.

Saxton, J., & Swihart, A. A. (1989). Neuropsychological assessment of the severely impaired elderly patient. *Clinics in Geriatric Medicine, 5*, 531–543.

Warren, S. (2017). Get ready for IMPACT New Medicare regulations require a more extensive assessment of patients, and SLPs may be called on to help. Here's what you need to know. *The ASHA Leader, 22*, 26–27. doi:10.1044/leader.PA1.22022017.26

Wiener, J. M., Freiman, M. P., & Brown, D. (2007). *Nursing home care quality: Twenty years after the Omnibus Budget Reconciliation Act of 1987*. Report commissioned by the Kaiser Family Foundation, December 2007.

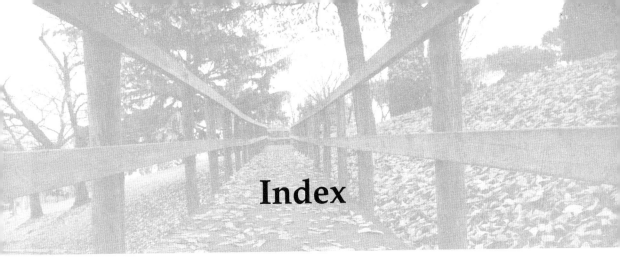

Index

Note: Page numbers in **bold** reference non-text material.